Duke Review of MRI Physics

CASE REVIEW SERIES

Series Editor

David M. Yousem, MD, MBA
Vice-Chairman Radiology, Program Development
Associate Dean, Professional Development
Department of Radiology
Johns Hopkins School of Medicine
Baltimore, Maryland

Volumes in the CASE REVIEW Series

Duke Review of MRI Physics

CASE REVIEW SERIES

Wells I. Mangrum, MD
Partner
Medical X-ray Consultants LLC
Eau Claire, Wisconsin

Timothy J. Amrhein, MD
Assistant Professor
Department of Radiology
Duke University Medical Center
Durham, North Carolina

Scott M. Duncan, MD
Partner
Radiology Associates of Southern Indiana
Prospect, Kentucky

Phil B. Hoang, MD
Staff Radiologist
Department of Radiology
Southeast Louisiana Veterans Health Care
    System
New Orleans, Louisiana

Charles M. Maxfield, MD
Professor
Department of Radiology
Duke University
Durham, North Carolina

Allen W. Song, PhD
Department of Radiology
Duke University
Durham, North Carolina

Elmar M. Merkle, MD
Department of Radiology
University Hospitals
Basel, Switzerland

ELSEVIER

ELSEVIER

1600 John F. Kennedy Blvd.
Ste 1800
Philadelphia, PA 19103-2899

DUKE REVIEW OF MRI PHYSICS: CASE REVIEW SERIES, SECOND EDITION   ISBN: 978-0-323-53038-5

Previous edition copyrighted © 2012 by Mosby, an imprint of Elsevier Inc.

Library of Congress Cataloging-in-Publication Data
Names: Mangrum, Wells I., author.
Title: Duke review of MRI physics / Wells I. Mangrum [and 6 others].
Other titles: Review of MRI physics | Case review series.
Description: Second edition. | Philadelphia, PA : Elsevier, Inc., [2019] |
    Series: Case review series | Preceded by: Duke review of MRI principles /
    Wells I. Mangrum ... [et al.]. c2012. | Includes bibliographical
    references and index.
Identifiers: LCCN 2018000643 | ISBN 9780323530385 (hardcover : alk. paper)
Subjects: | MESH: Magnetic Resonance Imaging | Case Reports | Problems and
    Exercises
Classification: LCC RC386.6.M34 | NLM WN 18.2 | DDC 616.07/548--dc23 LC record available
at https://lccn.loc.gov/2018000643

Executive Content Strategist: Robin Carter
Content Development Specialist: Meghan Andress
Publishing Services Manager: Patricia Tannian
Senior Project Manager: Carrie Stetz
Design Direction: Amy Buxton

Printed in China

Last digit is the print number: 9 8 7 6 5 4 3 2 1

Working together
to grow libraries in
developing countries

www.elsevier.com • www.bookaid.org

For my father. "Our doubts are traitors, and make us lose the good we oft may win, by failing to attempt."

Wells I. Mangrum

To my wife, Jill, and to our two wonderful children, Ty and Kate. Thank you always for your unwavering support and love. The time dedicated to this book was as much your sacrifice as it was mine.

Timothy J. Amrhein

To my wife, Kristen: thank you so much for supporting me through this process and encouraging me to push through.
To my kids, Carter, Tyler, and Chase: you all have grown so much since the first edition came out. I want you to know that you can accomplish anything in life if you work hard and put your mind to it.
To Wells: once again, your persistence, vision, and hard work have made this book possible.
To the Duke Radiology Department: I enjoyed my time at Duke immensely. The training I received was second to none, and there are still several occasions that I refer back to the lessons I learned during residency and fellowship. I am so very proud to be a Duke Radiology alum, and I hope this book will add to the great reputation and tradition of Duke Radiology.

Scott M. Duncan

To my wife, Kim Chi, and our children, Connor, Madeleine, Charles, and Maximus. Y'all are the greatest blessings of my life.

Phil B. Hoang

To Sharon, Charles, and Jack. And to my coauthors, for allowing me to contribute to this tremendous project.

Charles M. Maxfield

To my wife, Christina, the true source of my academic time, and my beloved daughters, Paula and Anna.

Elmar M. Merkle

TIMOTHY J. AMRHEIN, MD
Assistant Professor
Department of Radiology
Duke University Medical Center
Durham, North Carolina

MUSTAFA R. BASHIR, MD
Associate Professor of Radiology
Department of Radiology
Division of Abdominal Imaging
Center for Advanced Magnetic Resonance Development
Duke University Medical Center
Durham, North Carolina

NICHOLAS T. BEFERA, MD
Fellow, Vascular and Interventional Radiology
Department of Radiology
Duke University Medical Center
Durham, North Carolina

SCOTT M. DUNCAN, MD
Partner
Radiology Associates of Southern Indiana
Prospect, Kentucky

PHIL B. HOANG, MD
Staff Radiologist
Department of Radiology
Southeast Louisiana Veterans Health Care System
New Orleans, Louisiana

SPENCER J. HOOD
Department of Neuroscience
Brigham Young University
Salt Lake City, Utah

STEVEN Y. HUANG, MD
Associate Professor
Department of Interventional Radiology
University of Texas MD Anderson Cancer Center
Houston, Texas

ARI KANE, MD
Department of Radiology and Biomedical Engineering
University of California–San Francisco
San Francisco, California

SAMUEL J. KUZMINSKI
Department of Radiological Sciences
University of Oklahoma Health Sciences Center
Oklahoma City, Oklahoma

WELLS I. MANGRUM, MD
Partner
Medical X-ray Consultants LLC
Eau Claire, Wisconsin

CHARLES M. MAXFIELD, MD
Professor
Department of Radiology
Duke University
Durham, North Carolina

ELMAR M. MERKLE, MD
Department of Radiology
University Hospitals
Basel, Switzerland

JEFFREY R. PETRELLA, MD
Professor of Radiology
Division of Neuroradiology
Director, Alzheimer Disease Imaging Research Lab
Duke University Medical Center
Durham, North Carolina

NANCY PHAM, MD
Assistant Professor of Neurosurgery
University of California–Davis
Davis, California

CHRISTOPHER J. ROTH, MD, MMCI
Vice Chair of Radiology for IT & Informatics
Duke University
Director of Imaging IT Strategy, Duke Health
Associate Professor of Neuroradiology
Duke University Medical Center
Durham, North Carolina

FRANCESCO SANTINI, PHD, MRSE
Department of Radiology
Division of Radiological Physics
University Hospital Basel;
Department of Biomedical Engineering
University of Basel
Basel, Switzerland

ALLEN W. SONG, PHD
Department of Radiology
Duke University
Durham, North Carolina

CARLOS TORRES, MD, FRCPC
Associate Professor of Radiology
Department of Radiology
University of Ottawa;
Neuroradiologist
Department of Diagnostic Imaging
The Ottawa Hospital;
Clinical Investigator
Ottawa Hospital Research Institute OHRI
Ottawa, ON, Canada

NEAL K. VIRADIA, MD, MPH
Interventional Radiology Fellow
Department of Radiology
Division of Interventional Radiology
Duke University
Durham, North Carolina

JAMES T. VOYVODIC, PHD
Department of Radiology
Duke University Medical Center
Durham, North Carolina

I am very pleased with the evolution of the second edition of *Duke Review of MRI Physics*. The authors have used a theory of collective wisdom to garner the expertise of many of the great present and future minds in MRI. They think global, but act local, and cover more areas of MR physics than ever before while still keeping the case-based approach that works so well in this forum. This edition adds material on cardiac MRI and safety considerations, is more colorful, and uses "take-home points" to make sure the readers "get it." I got it. You should, too!

Congratulations to Drs. Mangrum, Amrhein, Duncan, Hoang, Maxfield, Song, and Merkle for the incredible teamwork and wisdom they have imparted to this edition. Bravo.

David M. Yousem, MD, MBA

This second edition improves our successful first edition. First, we have added multiple-choice questions to our cases to better fit with the current board exam format. Second, we have improved publication quality by incorporating color images into the main body of the text. Third, we have revised every chapter with up-to-date scientific literature. Fourth, we have added new chapters on cardiac imaging and MRI safety. These changes have required hundreds of hours by many different editors and authors. We hope that you benefit from our work.

CONTENTS

CHAPTER 1

T1 Contrast

Phil B. Hoang, Steven Y. Huang, Allen W. Song, and Elmar M. Merkle

OPENING CASE 1.1

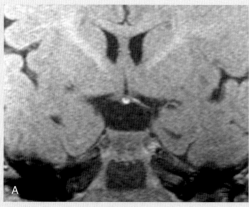 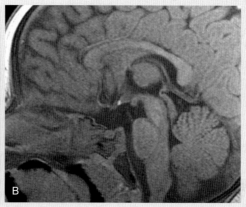

1. In figure A, which of the following MRI parameters produces a T1-weighted sequence?
   A. Short time to repetition (TR), short time to echo (TE)
   B. Long TR, short TE
   C. Short TR, long TE
   D. Long TR, short TE

2. Figure B shows a patient with a clinical history of short stature. What is the most likely diagnosis?
   A. Craniopharyngioma
   B. Saccular aneurysm
   C. Pituitary macroadenoma
   D. Ectopic neurohypophysis

OPENING CASE 1.1

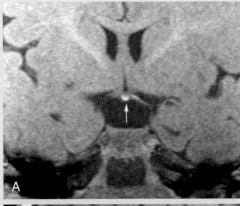

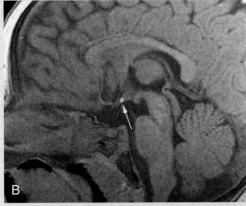

FIG. 1.C1. (A) Coronal and (B) sagittal T1-weighted images of the brain. A small high T1 signal focus at the superior aspect of the infundibulum *(arrows)* is demonstrated. Lack of the expected bright spot of the posterior pituitary gland is noted, and the pituitary stalk is abnormally small.

1. In figure A, which of the following MRI parameters produces a T1-weighted sequence?
   A. Short time to repetition (TR), short time to echo (TE)
2. Figure B shows a patient with a clinical history of short stature. What is the most likely diagnosis?
   D. Ectopic neurohypophysis

Discussion

A short TR and short TE optimize T1 contrast in a MRI image. A long TR and short TE would produce a proton density–weighted image, and a long TR and long TE would produce a T2-weighted image. A short TR and long TE sequence is not used in clinical MRI because this combination produces poor tissue contrast.

The normal T1 bright spot of the neurohypophysis is due to the proteins bound to vasopressin. In this case, the neurohypophysis is not present in the posterior sella, but is instead located in the superior aspect of the pituitary stalk. Note the diminutive appearance of the stalk. These findings are most compatible with ectopic neurohypophysis.

Basic Spin Principles and T1 Relaxation

Because of its abundance in the human body, hydrogen is the most frequently imaged nucleus in clinical MRI. Hydrogen has a considerable angular magnetic moment, with its single, positively charged proton acting as a tiny spinning bar magnet. Protons normally spin in random directions in the absence of an external magnetic field; because of this random movement, the magnetic vector sum of these protons is typically zero.

When placed in a strong external magnetic field (B_0), these protons align parallel (low energy) or antiparallel (high energy) with respect to B_0; more protons tend to align parallel to B_0 because less energy is required to do so. Because they possess magnetic and angular momentum, the protons precess, or wobble, around the axis of B_0 instead of spinning in a tight circle; this precession motion confers both longitudinal (μ_z) and transverse (μ_{xy}) components in the magnetic moments of the protons. Protons tend to precess at a certain frequency while under the influence of B_0, which is called the *Larmor frequency*. The Larmor frequency defines the frequency at which the radiofrequency pulse is broadcast to induce proton resonance, or excitation. The Larmor frequency is defined as $W = \gamma B$, where W is the Larmor frequency, γ is the gyromagnetic ratio in MHz/tesla (T), and B is the strength of the static magnetic field in T. Thus the Larmor frequency is proportional to the strength of the main magnetic field; at 1.5 T, the Larmor frequency of hydrogen protons is 63.8 MHz and approximately 127 MHz at 3.0 T.

The **vector sum** of the magnetic moments of the precessing protons (M_z and M_{xy}) results in a net equilibrium magnetization (M_0). This magnetization vector is primarily in the longitudinal direction (M_z) because more protons align in parallel with B_0. The transverse component (M_{xy}) does not contribute significantly to M_0 because the protons do not spin in phase with each other and effectively cancel each other out. As the energy of B_0 increases, so does the energy differential between protons in the low (parallel) and high (antiparallel) states, with increasing numbers of protons aligning parallel to B_0. This results in a significant directional (vector) component of the net magnetization. However, the receiver coil, which is the component of the MRI machine that detects signals, is sensitive only to variations of the magnetization vector; the original main net magnetization along the z direction, even though it is precessing, is viewed as a stationary vector from the receiver coil perspective. Given this, something must be done to perturb the system (i.e., tip the magnetization away from the z-axis so that the precession motion is visible) and generate detectable signal changes that can be picked up by the receiver coils. This comes in the form of a radiofrequency (RF) excitation pulse.

Application of the RF pulse—a short burst of electromagnetic energy—results in energy absorption by protons. For this energy transfer to occur, the RF pulse and precessing protons must have the same frequency. This results in a change in the protons' energy level, which goes from the low-energy (parallel) state into the high-energy (antiparallel) state. This produces a net *loss* of longitudinal magnetization and a net *gain* in transverse magnetization, respectively. Conceptually speaking, this is better known as the tipping of the net magnetization vector from the longitudinal axis (B_Z) into the transverse plane (B_{XY}), such that the precession motion can be visible and signal changes detectable by the receiver coils. The degree of transverse magnetization generated depends on both the amplitude of the RF pulse and length of time it is administered; *complete rotation of protons into the transverse plane is the result of a 90-degree RF pulse.*

After cessation of the excitation pulse, the resonating protons "relax" back into their equilibrium state, which occurs by two mechanisms—transverse (T2) and longitudinal (T1) relaxation. Although these two mechanisms occur concurrently, they do so at different rates. In brief, transverse relaxation refers to loss of phase coherence due to interactions between spinning protons (spin-spin). This leads to a net decrease in transverse magnetization and is also referred to as T2 decay. This concept is discussed in greater detail in Chapter 2.

In T1 relaxation, the resonating proton returns to its equilibrium state by transferring energy to the other nuclei in its surroundings, or lattice. This energy loss is represented by the transfer of heat into surrounding tissue and is referred to as thermal relaxation or spin lattice relaxation. The end result is a net increase in longitudinal magnetization. *T1 relaxation occurs at an exponential rate; at time T1, longitudinal magnetization has returned to 63% of its final value and, at time 3*T1, longitudinal magnetization has returned to 95% of its final value.* The differences in tissue T1 relaxation are responsible for the contrast on a T1-weighted image and depend on the efficiency of energy transfer from proton to lattice. Tissues with short T1 relaxation times (e.g., fat) generate a high signal, whereas tissues with long T1 relaxation times (e.g., water) generate a low signal.

Differences in T1 relaxation are primarily attributed to the natural movement unique to a molecule. In short, the more similar the molecule's natural motional frequency to that of the Larmor frequency, the more efficient energy transfer to its lattice occurs. This results in a short T1 relaxation time. Small molecules, such as those found in free water (e.g., cerebrospinal fluid), move rapidly; on the other side of the spectrum, macromolecules such as protein move at a slower pace. Although the motional frequencies of these molecules differ immensely, both exhibit long T1 relaxation times because both move at a frequency much different than the Larmor frequency. Intermediate-sized molecules, such as fat, move at frequencies very similar to the Larmor frequency and thus exhibit short T1 relaxation times.

The term *T1 shortening* refers to a decrease in the T1 relaxation time of a tissue, leading to greater signal intensity on a T1-weighted pulse sequence than is expected. This change is usually under the influence of agents that induce T1 relaxivity of nearby free water protons. The mechanisms exhibited by these agents include paramagnetic layer effects (e.g., gadolinium, manganese, methemoglobin) or hydration layer effects (e.g., proteins, ionic calcium). The most commonly known paramagnetic agents are the gadolinium chelates used in contrast-enhanced sequences; these agents, as well as the mechanisms of T1 relaxivity exhibited by these agents, are discussed in greater detail in Chapter 4.

T1 Contrast and Pulse Sequence Considerations

An important point to consider when interpreting any MR image is that image contrast is not exclusively due to differences in T1, T2, or proton density; these contrasts all make some contribution. However, by manipulating certain operator-dependent parameters, we can have *more* of one contrast and *less* of the others. This is why we use the terms T1, T2, and proton density **weighting** when describing the contrast in an image.

Spin Echo

In a conventional spin echo (SE) sequence, the 90-degree RF pulse is followed by a 180-degree refocusing pulse, which is administered at the halfway point of TE and is used to bring the protons back into an in-phase (i.e., synchronized) state. *The parameter with the greatest effect on T1 contrast on a conventional SE sequence is TR, which is the time interval between successive excitation pulses.* The TRs for T1-weighted SE sequences are typically in the range of 400 to 800 ms. As the TR lengthens, most tissues recover their longitudinal magnetization and produce signal; although this will increase overall signal-to-noise ratio in the image, it will diminish T1 contrast (Fig. 1.1).

Although modifying TR can optimize T1 contrast, adjusting the length of the second parameter, the TE, governs T2 contrast. TE is the time interval between the excitation pulse and signal collection; this parameter has the greatest effect on decreasing the contribution from T2 contrast, as illustrated below. To minimize the T2 contrast so that T1 contrast is dominant, the TE should be kept as short as possible (TE = 15–25 ms). A moderate TE would generate significant T2 contrast (Fig. 1.2).

Gradient Recalled Echo

Gradient recalled echo (GRE) pulse sequences use an excitation pulse with a variable flip angle (<90 degrees) and rephase protons with gradients of equal magnitude and duration but *opposite* polarities. This is opposed to conventional SE sequences, which apply a 180-degree refocusing pulse to rephase protons. In GRE acquisitions, the flip angle often plays a role in changing T1 contrast. Small flip angles allow the longitudinal magnetization to recover more rapidly. As such, the TRs used are typically short (<200 ms), as are the TEs (<10 ms to minimize T2 contrast).

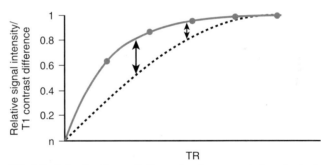

FIG. 1.1. Following the excitation pulse, tissues regain longitudinal magnetization (Mz) at rates determined by its specific T1 relaxation time. A short TR maximizes differences in T1 contrast *(long arrow).* A longer TR minimizes T1 contrast *(short arrow).*

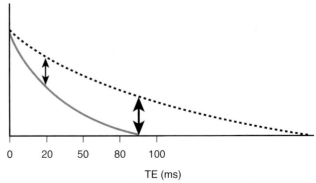

FIG. 1.2. By using a short TE (~20 ms, *short arrow*), differences in T2 contrast in the image are minimized. These differences in T2 contrast would be more significant if a longer TE (~100 ms) were used *(long arrow).*

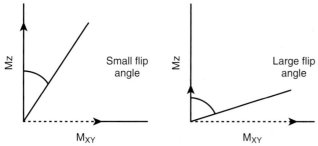

FIG. 1.3. Effect of flip angles for GRE sequences. *Left,* A smaller flip angle tips a smaller number of protons in the transverse plane with a large amount of longitudinal magnetization remaining. *Right,* Conversely, a larger flip angle tips most of the protons into the transverse plane, with a small amount of longitudinal magnetization remaining. Similar to SE sequences, the signal differences between tissues is then dependent on tissue-specific T1 relaxation times.

T1 weighting in GRE sequences is maximized by using an excitation pulse with a large (~50–80 degree) flip angle, a short TR (~100 ms), and a short TE (<10 ms). Both the flip angle and TR have the greatest influence on T1 weighting, with the effect of the flip angle illustrated in Fig. 1.3. Using large flip angles places an emphasis on T1 contrast because the signal intensity produced depends on tissue specific T1 relaxation times. With small flip angles, tissues of different composition retain most of their longitudinal magnetization (Mz, *solid arrows*) and thus appear similar in intensity on a T1-weighted sequence.

Strengths of GRE over conventional SE include faster image acquisition (due to shorter TRs) and decreased RF power deposition (due to the lack of a 180-degree refocusing pulse). In exchange, signal is sacrificed; GRE suffers from irretrievable signal loss due to magnetic field inhomogeneities and susceptibility effects (T2*) because it does not apply a refocusing pulse. Thus GRE sequences are generally lower in signal-to-noise ratio compared with SE sequences.

An important consequence of the short TRs used in GRE is the residual transverse magnetization remaining before the next excitation pulse. If left alone, the transverse magnetization will contribute to the longitudinal component after the next excitation pulse is administered, which eventually alters image contrast. To resolve this issue, a spoiler mechanism is used before the start of the next TR to prevent buildup of a transverse magnetization steady state and makes the magnetization in the longitudinal direction the chief contributor to M_Z at the next alpha pulse.

When extremely short acquisition times are needed, ultrafast GRE sequences are used. These sequences acquire images in 1 second or less by using extremely short TRs (<3 ms) and small flip angles. Because these parameters are generally unfavorable for the T1 weighting needed in contrast-enhanced sequences, an additional step is needed to boost T1 contrast. A preparatory pulse applied prior to the excitation pulse inverts the longitudinal magnetization, which introduces T1 weighting by emphasizing differences in tissue T1 relaxation.

Clinical Applications

The contrast of a T1-weighted sequence provides an important overview of anatomy. The two tissues that produce the most predictable signal intensity on a T1-weighted image are fat and free water. This is a reflection of each tissue's T1 relaxation time, which is short for fat (~250 ms at 1.5 T) and long for water (~2500 ms at 1.5 T). Normal solid organs—brain, muscle, liver, spleen, kidneys—have intermediate relaxation times, ranging from 490 ms (liver) to 970 ms (gray matter) at 1.5 T. The differences in T1 contrast are secondary to the varying ratios of extracellular water and macromolecules. For example, the normal pancreas produces the greatest signal intensity on a T1-weighted image of the solid abdominal organs due to its high protein synthesis and intracellular paramagnetic agents. Bone marrow demonstrates variable signal intensity, depending on its ratio of red to yellow marrow.

CASE 1.2

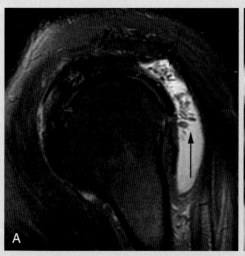
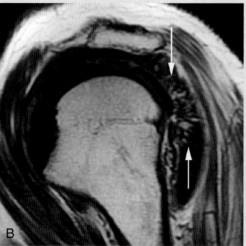

FIG. 1.C2

1. Regarding Fig. 1.C2A, why does fat produce a hyperintense signal on a T1-weighted image?
   A. It has a long T1 relaxation time.
   B. It has a short T1 relaxation time.
   C. It has a long T2 decay time.
   D. Both B and C are correct.

2. The patient in Fig. 1.C2B has subacromial subdeltoid bursitis. Which of the following is the most likely cause for the high signal *(arrows)* within the bursa on the T1-weighted image?
   A. Liposarcoma
   B. Lipoma arborescens
   C. Myelolipoma
   D. Angiomyolipoma

FIG. 1.C2. (A) Sagittal oblique fat-suppressed T2-weighted image of the shoulder demonstrates moderate distention of the subacromial-subdeltoid bursa. A frondlike abnormality within the bursa is present *(arrows)*. (B) Sagittal oblique T1-weighted image of the shoulder. The frondlike abnormallity on the T2-weighted image is hyperintense on the T1-weighted image *(arrows)* and is isointense to subcutaneous fat.

Discussion

Fig. 1.C2A: Due to its short T1 relaxation time, fat characteristically produces hyperintense signal on T1-weighted images (without fat suppression).

Fig. 1.C2B: The frondlike abnormality involving the distended subacromial-subdeltoid bursa represents a villous proliferation of the bursa's synovial lining. The development of benign adipocytes in the subsynovium can occur over time due to a chronic reactive process and appear as fat-containing lesions. This is a typical appearance for lipoma.

CASE 1.2 ANSWERS

1. **B. It has a short T1 relaxation time.**
2. **B. Lipoma arborescens**

CASE 1.3

FIG. 1.C3

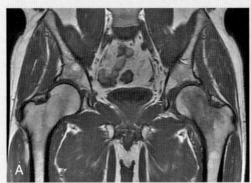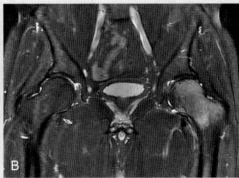

1. What effect does increased extracellular water have on bone marrow on MRI?
   A. Prolongs T1 relaxation
   B. Shortens T1 relaxation
   C. Shortens T2 decay
   D. Both A and C

2. Which of the following diagnoses should be considered in the left hip?
   A. Transient osteoporosis of the hip
   B. Early osteonecrosis
   C. Infection
   D. All of the above

FIG. 1.C3. (A) Coronal T1-weighted image of the pelvis. Homogeneous low T1 signal of the left femoral head and neck is present. The signal abnormality is slightly lower compared with muscle. (B) Coronal T2-weighted image with fat saturation. The left femoral head and neck are high in T2 signal.

Discussion

Fig. 1.C3A: Many pathologic processes are low signal on T1-weighted images, typically because of increased extracellular water content, which prolongs T1 relaxation. Identifying this signal abnormality on a T1-weighted image should alert you to focus on more fluid-sensitive images, such as found on T2-weighted and short tau inversion recovery (STIR) sequences, as well as gadolinium-enhanced T1-weighted sequences, to characterize the pertinent abnormality further.

In Case 1.3, the low signal intensity of the left femoral head and neck is due to bone marrow edema, which results in prolongation of the normal T1 relaxation time of the marrow spaces and produces a low signal abnormality on the T1-weighted sequence. As expected, the extra free water within the marrow produces a hyperintense signal on the corresponding fat-suppressed T2W image.

Fig. 1.C3B: Transient osteoporosis of the hip is a self-limited condition characterized by sudden onset of pain and transitory demineralization of the hip. On MRI, this condition presents as moderate edema involving the femoral head and, to a varying degree, the femoral neck. Other diagnostic considerations for bone marrow edema are early osteonecrosis and infection.

CASE 1.3 ANSWERS

1. **A. Prolongs T1 relaxation**
2. **D. All of the above**

CASE 1.4

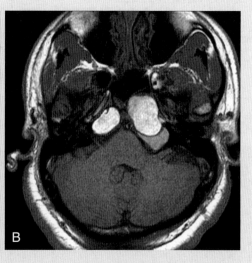

FIG. 1.C4

1. Regarding Fig. 1.C4A, which of the following produces hyperintense signal on a T1-weighted image?
   A. Deoxyhemoglobin
   B. Oxyhemoglobin
   C. Methemoglobin
   D. Hemosiderin

2. Which of the following is the most likely diagnosis?
   A. Petrous apicitis
   B. Cholesteatoma
   C. Cholesterol granuloma
   D. Petrous apex effusion

FIG. 1.C4. (A) Coronal and (B) axial T1-weighted images of the skull base. Bilateral expansile masses involving the petrous apices are identified. The masses are hyperintense, similar to subcutaneous fat.

Discussion

Aside from fat, tissues that contain subacute blood products and/or proteinaceous fluid may exhibit high signal on a T1-weighted image.

Methemoglobin is a breakdown derivative of hemoglobin and is paramagnetic due to its five unpaired electrons. As the oxidation of hemorrhage progresses and methemoglobin accumulates, the integrity of the red blood cell membrane is lost; nearby hydrogen protons from water then freely diffuse across the membrane and interact with the five unpaired electrons of the methemoglobin iron. These protons experience a shortening of their normal T1 relaxation times, which appears as high signal intensity on a T1-weighted image. Of the commonly encountered hemoglobin derivatives in MRI (e.g., oxyhemoglobin, deoxyhemoglobin, methemoglobin, hemosiderin), methemoglobin is the only one that causes significant T1 shortening and a high T1 signal.

The T1 shortening effect of macromolecules (proteins) is different than that exhibited in paramagnetic agents. Proteins bind free water protons onto their surface via hydrophilic side chains, creating a layer of bound water protons; this is referred to as the **hydration layer effect**. Now bound, the water protons' motional frequency is decreased, making energy transfer to the lattice more efficient and leading to T1 shortening.

Outside of methemoglobin and proteins, a variety of agents can promote T1 shortening. Manganese (Mn) is paramagnetic and, until 2004, was previously available in the United States as a T1-shortening chelate (Mn-DPDP, **mangafodipir trisodium** [Teslascan]); Mn is a supplementary addition in total parental nutrition formulations, and its accumulation in the basal ganglia may cause high T1 signal.

Diagnosis

The diagnosis for Figs. 1.C4C–D is manganese deposition secondary to long-term total parenteral nutrition. Although densely calcified tissues are characteristically hypointense on MRI due to a lack of mobile protons, tissues containing microcalcifications may produce hyperintense T1 signal (Fig. 1.C4C–D). The calcium salts form a crystalline lattice in which free water protons settle, which slows the water protons' motional frequency and results in a decrease in the T1 relaxation time. The larger the surface area of the lattice, the higher the number of bound free water protons and the greater the T1 signal intensity.

The diagnosis for Figs. 1.C4E–F is treated glioblastoma multiforme, with mineralizing microangiopathy. Melanoma characteristically is high signal on a T1-weighted sequence due to melanin's ability to bind free radicals and metals (e.g., manganese) as well as the tumor's tendency to hemorrhage (and subsequent production of methemoglobin).

The diagnosis for Fig. 1.C4G is metastatic melanoma.

Discussion

The expansile petrous apices masses that are hyperintense on a T1-weighted sequence are most consistent with cholesterol granulomas. It is the most common lesion of the petrous apex and is due to a chronic foreign body reaction of the

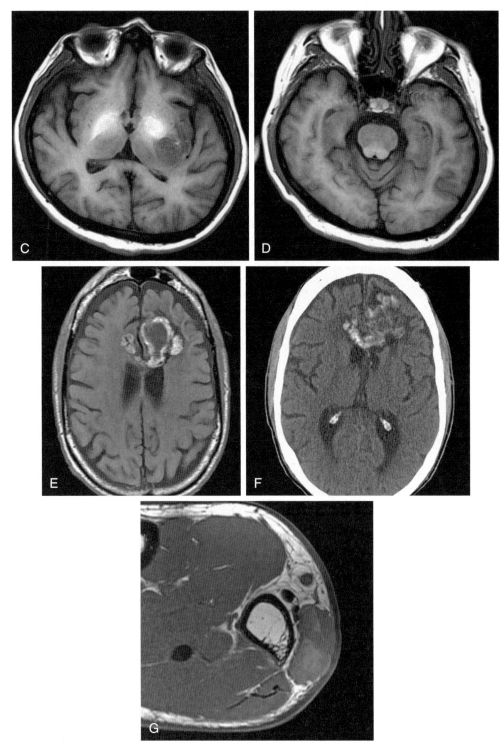

FIG. 1.C4. (C) Axial T1-weighted image of the brain. Symmetric high T1 signals within the globus pallidi are demonstrated. A round low T1 signal focus in the posterior basal ganglia is consistent with acute hemorrhage. (D) Axial T1-weighted image of the pons, same patient as in (C). The high T2 signal intensities of the pontine tegmentum and anterior pituitary gland are noted. (E) T1-weighted image demonstrating an irregular hyperintense lesion that crosses the corpus callosum. (F) Axial noncontrast CT image of the brain. Irregular hyperdensity of the bifrontal mass is consistent with calcifications. (G) Axial T1-weighted image of the right thumb. An oval mass lateral to the cortex of the right thumb's first metacarpal bone demonstrates areas of intrinsic high T1 signal. A well-defined fat plane separates the mass from the metacarpal cortex.

apical air cells to cholesterol crystal deposition. This leads to an accumulation of blood products (methemoglobin) and proteinaceous debris, which produce hyperintense signal on a T1-weighted image.

CASE 1.4 ANSWERS

1. **C. Methemoglobin**
2. **C. Cholesterol granuloma**

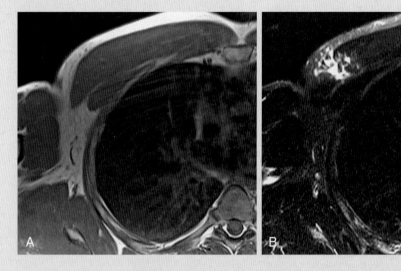

FIG. 1.C5

1. The patient has a ruptured pectoralis major muscle. Which of the following is the most likely explanation for the apparent intact appearance of the muscle on the T1-weighted image?
   A. The hemorrhage and fluid at the site of muscle rupture are hypointense to muscle.
   B. The hemorrhage and fluid at the site of muscle rupture are isointense to muscle.
   C. The hemorrhage and fluid at the site of muscle rupture are hyperintense to muscle.
   D. None of the above; the patient ruptured the muscle between obtaining the T1 and STIR sequences.

FIG. 1.C5. (A) Axial T1-weighted image of the right chest. No focal abnormality is apparent. (B) Axial STIR image of the right chest, same level. Focal increased STIR signal abnormality of the lateral aspect of the right pectoralis major muscle is now evident.

Discussion

Lesions that exhibit similar T1 relaxation times compared to surrounding normal tissues may go virtually undetected on a T1-weighted image. This is illustrated in Case 1.5, in which the fluid and hemorrhage filling the full-thickness pectoralis muscle tear are clearly present on the STIR image (Fig. 1.C5B). However, on the T1-weighted image (Fig. 1.C5A), the fluid-filled tear is isointense to the adjacent musculature, which falsely suggests that the muscle is intact.

CASE 1.5 ANSWER

1. **B. The hemorrhage and fluid at the site of muscle rupture are isointense to muscle.**

TAKE-HOME POINTS

1. T1 represents the efficiency of energy transfer from a resonating proton to its lattice following energy deposition by an RF excitation pulse.
2. Molecules that move at a motional frequency similar to the Larmor frequency quickly transfer energy to the lattice, which results in a short T1 relaxation time and increased signal on a T1-weighted image. An example is a medium-sized molecule such as fat.
3. Small molecules (e.g., bulk water) and large molecules (e.g., proteins) exhibit motional frequencies much different compared with the Larmor frequency, resulting in inefficient energy transfer to the lattice and long T1 relaxation times.
4. MR images have different mix of contrasts (T1, T2, and proton density); operator-adjustable parameters are manipulated to promote a particular weighting, which emphasizes differences of one particular tissue contrast while minimizing the others.
5. In SE sequences, short TR (~600 ms) and shortest possible TE (<10 ms) produce a T1-weighted image. In GRE sequences, an excitation pulse with a large flip angle, a short TR, and the shortest possible TE produces a T1-weighted image.
6. In a T1-weighted image, tissues with short T1 relaxation times produce high signal (e.g., fat, gadolinium-enhanced tissues, proteinaceous fluid), whereas tissues with long T1 times produce low signal (free water, cerebrospinal fluid).
7. T1-weighted sequences provide good anatomic information and are used to evaluate enhancing tissues following intravenous gadolinium chelate administration.
8. Most pathologic tissues are low signal on noncontrast T1-weighted images due to T1 relaxation prolongation from increased extracellular water concentration.
9. T1 shortening refers to the reduction of normal T1 relaxation of tissues due to the effects of external agents, causing them to produce high signal on a T1-weighted sequence.
10. Paramagnetic agents exhibit unpaired electrons, which produce a strong local magnetic field and induce T1 and T2 relaxation of nearby protons. Examples of paramagnetic agents include gadolinium chelates, extracellular methemoglobin, melanin, manganese, and free radicals.
11. The hydration layer effect refers to the binding of water protons to the surface of macromolecules (proteins); this slows down the motional frequency of water protons, making energy transfer to the lattice more efficient and leading to a reduction in its T1 relaxation.

Suggested Readings

Chapman PR, Shah R, Curé JK, Bag AK. Petrous apex lesions: pictorial review. *Am J Roentgenol.* 2011;196(suppl 3):WS26–WS37.

Elster AD. Questions and answers in MRI. MRIQuestions.com.

Ginat DT, Meyers SP. Intracranial lesions with high signal intensity on T1-weighted MR images: differential diagnosis. *Radiographics.* 2012;32(2):499–516.

Pooley RA. Fundamental physics of MR imaging. *Radiographics.* 2005;25(4):1087–1099.

CHAPTER 2

T2 Contrast

Samuel J. Kuzminski, Ari Kane, and Timothy J. Amrhein

OPENING CASE 2.1

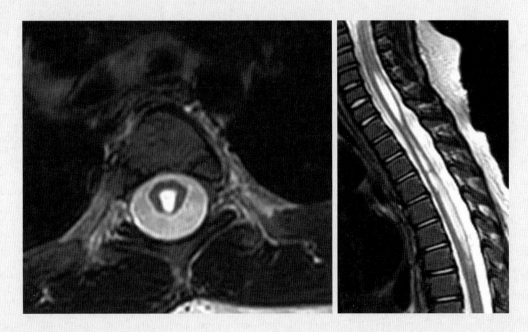

1. Which of the following is true regarding the images in the above and T2-weighted images in general?
   A. The sequence obtained is a T2-weighted spin echo (SE) using a short time to repetition (TR).
   B. Hyperintense (or bright) structures on the images have short T2 relaxation times.
   C. Spoiler gradients were used to maximize contrast.
   D. Time to echo (TE) is longer for SE T2-weighted than SE T1-weighted images.
   E. T2 weighting can only be achieved by SE.
2. T2* is a combination of:
   A. Signal gain in the direction of the main magnetic field and microscopic interactions between adjacent protons
   B. Inhomogeneities in the main magnetic field and microscopic interactions between adjacent protons
   C. Inhomogeneities in the main magnetic field and longitudinal relaxation
   D. Signal loss in the direction of the main magnetic field and microscopic interactions between adjacent protons

3. Compared to SE sequence, gradient recalled echo:
   A. Uses 180-degree refocusing pulses
   B. Is primarily affected by T2 dephasing
   C. Is primarily affected by T2* dephasing
   D. Uses multiple excitation pulses
4. What is the purpose of a 180-degree pulse in SE imaging?
   A. Regains transverse magnetization lost by field inhomogeneities
   B. Increases rate of transverse magnetization loss
   C. Creates T2* weighting factor
   D. Alters microscopic interactions between adjacent protons
5. Steady-state free precession imaging:
   A. Has both T1 and T2 weighting
   B. Applies repeated 180-degree refocusing pulses
   C. Applies spoiler gradients to residual null transverse magnetization
   D. Creates a low signal-to-noise ratio

OPENING CASE 2.1

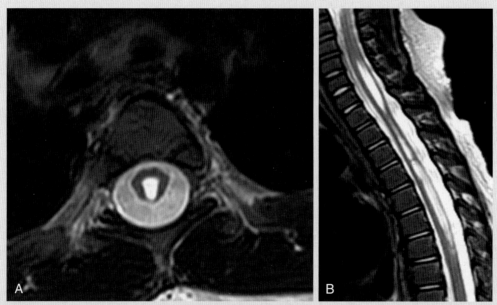

FIG. 2.C1. (A) Axial T2-weighted image of the thoracic spine demonstrates a large T2 hyperintense space in the center of the spinal cord. (B) Sagittal T2-weighted image of the thoracic spine. Vertically oriented central hyperintensity extends throughout the cervical and thoracic cord.

1. Which of the following is true regarding the images in the above and T2-weighted images in general?
   D. Time to echo (TE) is longer for SE T2-weighted than SE T1-weighted images.
2. T2* is a combination of:
   B. Inhomogeneities in the main magnetic field and microscopic interactions between adjacent protons
3. Compared to SE sequence, gradient recalled echo:
   C. Is primarily affected by T2* dephasing
4. What is the purpose of a 180-degree pulse in SE imaging?
   A. Regains transverse magnetization lost by field inhomogeneities
5. Steady-state free precession imaging:
   A. Has both T1 and T2 weighting

Discussion

Figs. 2.C1A–B are *T2-weighted SE images. These are obtained using a long TR and an intermediate to long TE. Tissues with longer T2 relaxation times appear hyperintense on T2-weighted images.* Water, and tissues that contain mostly water, such as cerebrospinal fluid (CSF), have long T2 relaxation times and thus appear hyperintense (bright).

The diagnosis in this case is syringohydromyelia. Syringohydromyelia, often shortened to syrinx, is a pathologic process in which CSF forms a collection in the spinal cord. This term encompasses both syringomyelia (a fluid collection in the spinal cord tissue itself) and hydromyelia (fluid in a dilated central canal of the spinal cord). Because the exact location of the fluid in the spinal cord is difficult to determine on imaging, these terms are lumped together to cover both possibilities (syringohydromyelia).

Syringohydromyelia is often secondary to another process involving the spinal cord, rather than a primary entity. Prior spinal cord trauma, infection, or inflammation can all result in syrinx formation. Degenerative spinal canal stenosis can also cause a syrinx, if severe enough. Congenital causes include tethered spinal cord and Chiari I and II malformations. Spinal cord tumors may have cystic components that can mimic a syrinx or may have an associated adjacent syrinx. As a result, postcontrast images are usually performed during the initial MRI evaluation of a syrinx to exclude the possibility of an underlying neoplasm.

Basic Spin Principles and T2 Relaxation

After a radiofrequency (RF) pulse tips the net (or main) magnetization into the transverse plane, it will gradually lose coherence because individual protons will experience a dephasing process due to spin-spin interactions. This phenomenon is known as *T2, or transverse, relaxation* (or decay). At the same time, the magnetization would also return to its original state via T1 or longitudinal relaxation (or recovery). This chapter focuses on the T2 relaxation.

An RF pulse generates a magnetic field oriented in the transverse (or *xy*) dimension. During its application, the net

magnetization along the longitudinal direction will rotate about the main axis of this magnetic field to the transverse plane. Immediately after this rotation, all protons naturally have the same phase and thus exhibit phase coherence.[1] *Once the RF pulse is turned off, however, there is progressive loss of this phase coherence. This occurs because individual protons begin to precess at slightly different frequencies due to differences in their local microenvironments and secondary interactions between the protons, termed spin-spin interactions. The resultant slight differences in precession frequencies among protons causes phase dispersion, signal cancellation, and loss of transverse magnetization.* It is important to note that transverse relaxation or decay is therefore due to loss of order (i.e., phase dispersion) rather than to loss of magnetization.

Why does this phase dispersion occur if all the hydrogen protons are exposed to the same external magnetic field? This occurs because there are inherent inhomogeneities in the magnetic field that lead to different magnetic microenvironments and, subsequently, slightly different proton precession frequencies. There are two separate causes of magnetic field inhomogeneity:

1. *Inhomogeneities within the external magnetic field (or T2′)*
2. *Microscopic interactions between adjacent protons (or T2)*

The combined loss of signal resulting from both these causes is measured by the T2* decay: T2 + T2′ = T2*.

The dephasing effects from the external magnetic field (T2′) have a much larger contribution to T2* decay than the T2 effects. Unfortunately, T2′ effects are independent of the tissues being imaged and therefore provide little information about the patient. Fortunately, a 180-degree refocusing pulse can be used to reverse the loss of phase coherence from these static inhomogeneities. (This point will become more important in the discussion of SE imaging.) On the contrary, *loss of phase coherence arising from the local microenvironments (T2) is irreversible. However, the resultant differences in extent of T2 signal loss provide information about the microenvironment that the protons are experiencing, allowing for tissue characterization.*

An MR signal can only be detected when the magnetization is in the transverse plane. When an RF pulse is applied, the magnetization vector is "tipped" into the transverse plane while still rotating about the z-axis at the Larmor frequency. The resultant MR signal appears as a sinusoidal wave, peaking when the vector is pointed toward the detector and reaching a trough when the vector is pointed 180 degrees away from the detector. Furthermore, remember that immediately after the RF pulse is turned off, phase dispersion occurs, causing a rapid and continuous fall in signal. The resultant waveform, called *free induction decay* (FID), is a graphic representation of this declining magnetization and the 360-degree rotating signal. As shown in Fig. 2.1, the FID appears as an oscillating waveform that rapidly falls to zero. The FID describes the detected MR signal, which experiences a rapid exponential loss at the rate of T2*.

The component of T2* that provides information about the patient is the T2 relaxation. T2 relaxation occurs at an exponential rate analogous to T2* relaxation, except at the rate of T2. As mentioned previously, the *T2 relaxation time is governed by individual protons' local environments and spin-spin interactions, resulting in phase dispersion.*

In general, all molecules are influenced by their local magnetic microenvironment, which fluctuates over time. Molecular motion is relatively restricted in solid structures and those with larger molecules, resulting in relatively slowly varying magnetic fields. As a result, this more static magnetic field variation results in some areas having persistently stronger local magnetic fields and other areas with weaker local magnetic fields. These relative differences result in different precessing frequencies among the protons, causing significant dephasing. *Smaller molecules (e.g., water), on the other hand, are rapidly moving, leading to an averaging of the magnetic field variability*—that is, the smaller molecules experience a mixture of stronger and weaker magnetic fields that is averaged out over time. This leads to *increased homogeneity of the experienced magnetic field, resulting in less phase dispersion and therefore longer T2 relaxation times.* Unlike T1 relaxation times, T2 relaxation times are less dependent on magnetic field strength. T2 relaxation times for most

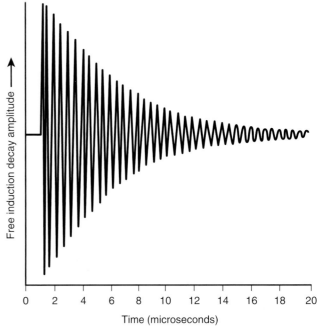

FIG. 2.1. Free induction decay.

tissues within the body range from 30 to 60 ms. The T2 relaxation time for CSF, which is mostly free water, is 1000 ms.

T2-weighted images are well suited for the detection and assessment of most pathologic processes because pathology often results in increased water content, causing T2 hyperintensity relative to the isointense signal of normal soft tissue.

T2 Contrast and Pulse Sequence Considerations

Two general categories of sequences are used to produce images weighted by transverse relaxation times: SE sequences and gradient echo sequences. Pure T2-weighted images can only be obtained with SE sequences. Gradient echo sequences can produce T2*-weighted images but are unable to produce purely T2-weighted images for reasons that are explained later.

Spin Echo

SE imaging involves an initial 90-degree RF pulse that rotates the longitudinal magnetization into the transverse plane and aligns the phase. This is then followed by a 180-degree pulse that realigns the spins. Remember, when the initial 90-degree RF pulse is turned off, the protons immediately begin to dephase. Subsequently, a *180-degree RF pulse (also known as a refocusing pulse) is used to reverse the precession direction of the protons;* that is, instead of rotating clockwise, they begin to rotate counterclockwise about the z-axis or vice versa. This has the intended effect of *reversing the phase dispersion caused by static magnetic field inhomogeneities.*

The reversal occurs because the protons continue to precess at the same rate as when they developed different phases; however, they now do so in the reverse direction. Thus, over the same amount of elapsed time, a faster precessing proton that was able to change phase in relation to its slower precessing counterparts now precesses faster than the slower proton, but in the opposite direction, and effectively catches back up with the slower precessing proton. *By this process, the transverse magnetization that was lost due to magnetic field inhomogeneities will be recovered* (Fig. 2.2). Therefore *any loss of signal in a SE sequence is from*

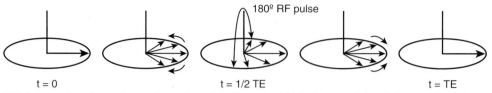

FIG. 2.2. Effect of 180-degree refocusing pulse on phase dispersion. Once the initial 90-degree RF pulse is turned off, the protons begin to dephase. The 180-degree refocusing pulse reverses the phase dispersion and results in rephasing of the protons, which occurs maximally at TE. (From Image Contrast in Biological Imaging. https://users.fmrib.ox.ac.uk/~stuart/thesis/chapter_2/section2_4.html.)

phase dispersion due to microscopic fluctuations in the magnetic field caused by the local molecules—pure T2 relaxation.

In SE sequences, there are two main parameters that affect the weighting of an image (i.e., T1, T2, or proton density weighting)—TR and TE. In generating an image, the protons in a patient are repeatedly exposed to RF pulses to fill each line of k-space. During the first excitation, all the longitudinal magnetization is tipped into the transverse plane. Over time, the longitudinal magnetization returns (or recovers) at a tissue-specific rate, which is based on its T1 relaxation time. If the TR is shorter than the time it takes to recover longitudinal magnetization fully (i.e., another 90-degree RF pulse is introduced prior to complete longitudinal magnetization recovery), there will be less signal available to tip into the transverse plane with the next pulse. Given a short TR, substances with short T1 relaxation times will recover more longitudinal magnetization and will therefore appear hyperintense (bright), whereas substances with long T1 relaxation times will not recover signal prior to the next excitation pulse and will be hypointense (dark). In contradistinction, if the TR is long, then both tissues will recover their longitudinal relaxation, and the T1 relaxation time will not significantly affect the final signal.

TE is defined as the time between the first 90-degree RF pulse and the time of signal acquisition. As previously described, SE sequences use a 180-degree pulse to realign dephased spins and remove signal loss from magnetic field inhomogeneities. To acquire maximal signal in an SE image, *the 180-degree RF pulse is placed at half of the TE. In other words, the spins that dephase during the first half of the TE are subsequently rephased during the second half of the TE, which results in maximal signal at the time of signal acquisition.* All signal loss is therefore secondary to the inherent T2 relaxation of the tissue—fluctuations in the local magnetic field secondary to the structures of the local molecules. *An intermediate to long TE allows enough time for tissues with short T2 relaxation times to lose some signal (and appear hypointense), whereas tissues with long T2 relaxation times still retain most of their signal (and appear hyperintense).* However, if the programmed TE is very short, not enough time will have expired to allow for any significant T2-related signal decay, and no tissue will experience any significant transverse decay.

As can be seen from this description, manipulation of the TR provides separation of tissues based on their T1 relaxation times, and changing the TE results in tissue separation based on inherent T2 relaxation properties. The TE and TR can therefore be adjusted to maximize signal based on the T1 or the T2 relaxation properties of a tissue. This preferential bias toward one relaxation parameter versus another is termed *weighting.* With *T2-weighted images, one minimizes the T1 relaxation effects on signal production by lengthening the TR and maximizes the T2 relaxation effects by choosing an intermediate to long TE.* As a memory aid, one might consider that 1 is a smaller number than 2, and thus has smaller TRs and TEs. For a typical T2-weighted image, the TR is longer than 2000 ms, and the TE is longer than 100 ms.

Recently a new technique allowing for the simultaneous acquisition of multiple sequences has been developed and has received US Food and Drug Administration (FDA) clearance. Known as MAGnetic resonance imaging Compilation (MAGiC), this software allows for the synthetic reconstruction of multiple image series from a single dataset, including T1, T2, and inversion recovery sequences, as well as proton density–weighted images. Purportedly, the result is a time savings up to almost 50%. Although many of the details of this specific technique are proprietary, similar methods have been described in the literature. The basic premise is that an imaging slice—for example, slice *a*—receives a slice-selective saturation pulse followed by a spoiling gradient. This slice is then saturated, meaning that it will not contribute to signal during this excitation. Shortly thereafter, a multiecho SE acquisition is performed on a second slice, slice *b*. In this manner, the transverse (T2) relaxation is measured for slice *b*. On the next acquisition, slice *b* receives the saturation pulse, and slice *a* receives the acquisition pulse. By alternating the slices repeatedly in such a manner, and varying the amount of time between when a slice is exposed to the saturation and acquisition pulses, the longitudinal (T1) relaxation can be determined. The various sequences can then be synthetically created from these data knowing the scan parameters and T1 and T2 relaxation times, thereby circumventing the need to acquire each sequence individually.[2]

Gradient Recalled Echo

Gradient recalled echo (GRE) sequences involve a single excitation RF pulse that transfers some of the longitudinal magnetization into the transverse plane, where it can be used to acquire signal. *A significant difference between GRE sequences and standard SE sequences is the absence of a 180-degree refocusing pulse.* Without this additional pulse, the *phase dispersion caused by inhomogeneities in the main magnetic field are not corrected.* Therefore the loss of signal in a GRE sequence is due to T2* effects. As previously described, these T2* effects are significantly influenced by the inhomogeneity in the external magnetic field and do not provide exclusive information about the relaxation properties of the tissue being imaged. GRE sequences are therefore useful in a select few cases, including the evaluation of magnetic susceptibility artifacts as well as the evaluation of flow.

There are two main types of fast GRE sequences: steady-state GRE sequences and spoiled GRE sequences. In spoiled gradient imaging, any residual transverse magnetization that is available (after the echo has been recorded) is spoiled by the use of a spoiler gradient before the next TR. With *steady-state imaging, however, the residual transverse magnetization is added back to the longitudinal magnetization during the next excitation, resulting in a higher signal-to-noise ratio.* In steady-state imaging, both the longitudinal and transverse magnetizations enter a steady state; that is, their respective magnetizations remain constant from one repetition to the next. Steady-state GRE sequences produce more T2 weighting and negligible T2* weighting. The amount of residual transverse magnetization is based on the T2 time. Substances with long T2 times will have more residual magnetization to add back to the longitudinal magnetization, which can be used in subsequent excitations. In addition, molecules with short T1 times will have recovered more longitudinal magnetization before the next TR, resulting in more magnetization in subsequent excitations. Thus the *steady-state sequences are T2/T1 weighted.* In other words, *substances that have* *long T2 times (water) and short T1 times (fat) will be bright* on these sequences.[1] These sequences are commonly used in cardiac imaging and in the base of the skull, where high-resolution, thin-slice, T2-weighted images are used. Further discussion about steady-state imaging and its role in cardiac imaging is discussed in Chapter 11.

CASE 2.2

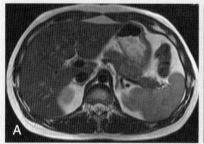
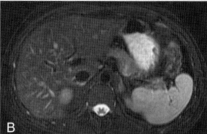
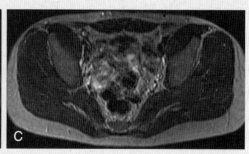

FIG. 2.C2

1. What is true regarding the appearance of the images above?
   A. The patient in Fig. 2.C2A has generalized edema because the fat resembles fluid signal.
   B. The darker appearance of fat on SE, as opposed to FSE, is due to J-coupling.
   C. A lipoma and a cyst would appear the same on the methods used in Fig. 2.C2A and B.
   D. SE is more commonly used for abdominal imaging than FSE.

FIG. 2.C2. (A) Axial T2-weighted fast SE (FSE) image of the abdomen. (B) Axial T2-weighted FSE image with fat saturation of the abdomen. (C) Axial T2-weighted SE image of the pelvis.

Fat on T2-Weighted Imaging

As noted at the beginning of the chapter, T2-weighted images have a relatively long TR to allow the longitudinal magnetization to recover. To shorten the total scan time, *multiple 180-degree refocusing pulses can be applied, and thus multiple echoes collected, during a single TR interval.* The number of refocusing pulses applied during a single TR interval is called the **echo train length** or **turbo factor.** Imaging time reduction is directly proportional to the echo train length; that is, for an echo train length of 9, the imaging time is reduced by a factor of 9. These sequences are known as **turbo** or **FSE.** The number of additional echoes depends on the length of the TR. Sequences with longer TRs, such as T2-weighted images, can fit eight or more TEs into each TR. Because of its significantly more economical imaging times, the fast SE technique has completely replaced conventional SE imaging for T2-weighted imaging. In fact, most residents and young attending physicians have never seen an SE T2-weighted image sequence in clinical practice.

FSE sequences allow T2-weighted images of the abdomen to be obtained in a single breath-hold. This is not possible with the SE technique, which is why the SE image shown in Case 2.2 is of the pelvis rather than the abdomen. Imaging the abdomen with a SE sequence would have resulted in blurring secondary to respiratory motion artifact in the absence of respiratory triggering or a gating method.

One consequence of the FSE technique is a relatively increased signal intensity of fat compared with a conventional SE image. This is one reason why T2-weighted sequences are often fat-saturated or inversion recovery sequences. As you may recall, fat has a relatively short T2 relaxation time secondary to its large molecular size, which results in rapid loss of transverse magnetization. Furthermore, fat molecules are subject to signal loss secondary to a phenomenon called *J-coupling,* which is a complex topic and applies more to nuclear MR spectroscopy than to MR imaging. Macromolecules, such as lipids, share electrons between their nuclei via the electron cloud, causing a slight alteration in the local magnetic fields of different nuclei on the same molecule. This, in turn, results in a change in the precessional frequencies of these different nuclei, leading to a rapid dephasing that occurs in addition to the normal T2 dephasing. This phenomenon is referred to as **J-coupling** *and explains why fat appears as a low to intermediate signal on T2 SE sequences.* Why, then, does fat appear brighter when using FSE techniques? The answer lies in the multiple refocusing pulses used in a FSE sequence, which do not allow sufficient time for J-coupling dephasing to occur. This prolongs the overall T2 relaxation of fat and leads to the relatively higher signal of the fat on the FSE T2-weighted image compared with the conventional SE T2-weighted image.

CASE 2.2 ANSWER

1. **B. The darker appearance of fat on SE, as opposed to FSE, is due to J-coupling.**

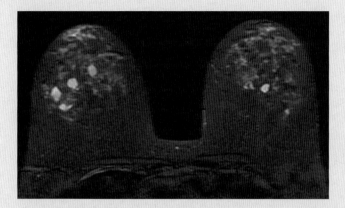

FIG. 2.C3

Multiple Bilateral Simple Breast Cysts

Almost all breast lesions with very high signal on T2-weighted images are benign, with one significant exception: mucinous (or colloid) carcinoma.[3] The criteria for diagnosing a simple cyst within the breast on MRI are similar to those in ultrasound. The cyst is usually homogeneously hyperintense (fluid bright) on a T2-weighted image and should demonstrate a smooth contour. On a T1-weighted image, the cyst is usually uniformly hypointense and should exhibit no internal enhancement after the administration of contrast. A thin rim of peripheral enhancement is acceptable.[4,5]

1. Which is true regarding these lesions in the breasts?
   A. Uniformly fluid signal lesions are always benign.
   B. A thin rim of peripheral enhancement can be seen in a benign cyst.
   C. These lesions require further evaluation with mammography.
   D. The next step for these lesions is biopsy.

FIG. 2.C3. Axial T2-weighted FSE image with fat saturation. There are multiple bilateral T2 hyperintense lesions in the breasts.

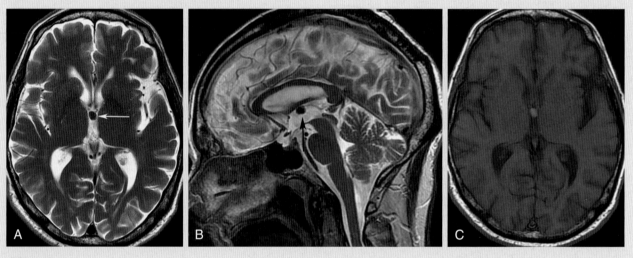

FIG. 2.C4

2. Which of the following is a potential complication of this mass?
   A. Hydrocephalus
   B. Drop metastases
   C. Parinaud syndrome
   D. Gelastic seizures
3. Which of the following is true with regard to the internal signal of a cyst?
   A. Cysts are always T2 hyperintense.
   B. Increasing protein content of a cyst leads to increasing T1 hypointensity.
   C. Increasing protein content of a cyst leads to increasing T2 hyperintensity.
   D. Cysts remain T2 hyperintense until their internal protein concentration exceeds approximately 50%.

Colloid Cysts

Colloid cysts are developmental cysts that occur at a characteristic location, the anterosuperior third ventricle adjacent to the foramina of Monro.[6] Although benign, they can obstruct the foramina of Monro and result in a thunderclap-type headache and acute hydrocephalus. Drop metastases are characteristic of neoplasms, Parinaud syndrome is described with pineal region masses that compress the midbrain tectum, and gelastic seizures are typically described in hamartomas of the tuber cinereum.

Colloid cysts are typically T2 hyperintense. However, in this case, the concentration of internal protein and paramagnetic material is high, which results in T2 hypointensity and T1 hyperintensity. As with other cysts, colloid cysts should be homogeneous and should not exhibit central enhancement.

FIG. 2.C4. (A) Axial T2-weighted image. There is a small homogeneous T2 hypointense mass in the region of the foramen of Monro *(arrow)*. (B) Sagittal T2-weighted image. A T2 hypointense mass was redemonstrated in the region of the foramen of Monro *(arrow)*. (C) Axial T1-weighted image. The mass exhibits T1 hyperintensity.

FIG. 2.C5

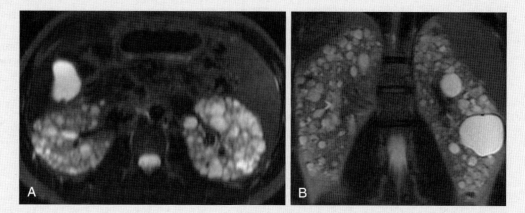

4. What is the most common intracranial complication of this disease?
   A. Ischemic stroke
   B. Glioma
   C. Saccular aneurysm
   D. Incomplete partition defect, type II

5. Which of the following is true regarding T2 relaxation times?
   A. Water has a long relaxation time.
   B. Muscle has a very long relaxation time.
   C. Bone has a very long relaxation time.
   D. Air has a long relaxation time.

FIG. 2.C5. (A) Axial fat-saturated FSE T2-weighted image. (B) Coronal half-Fourier–acquired single-shot turbo SE T2-weighted image. Both images demonstrate innumerable heterogeneous T2 hyperintense foci within the bilateral kidneys.

Autosomal Dominant Polycystic Kidney Disease

Autosomal dominant polycystic kidney disease is an autosomal dominant inherited renal disease characterized by the formation of multiple renal cysts and progressive renal dysfunction. These patients often develop hypertension, flank pain, and hematuria related to the renal cysts. Extrarenal manifestations of the disease include cysts in various other organs (liver, seminal vesicles, pancreas, spleen), cerebral aneurysms, cardiac valve abnormalities, and colonic diverticula.[7]

Variable Appearance of Fluid on T2-Weighted Imaging

Cysts occur throughout the body and typically have a characteristic appearance on MRI scans, regardless of location. *In general, cysts appear fluid bright on T2-weighted images (T2 hyperintense) and dark on T1-weighted images (T1 hypointense).* In addition, simple cysts should be thin walled and contain no internal enhancement on postcontrast T1-weighted images.

However, these classic MR imaging characteristics can be altered by changes in a cyst's internal composition. *The MR appearance of a cyst depends on its protein and free water concentrations,* as well as on the presence or absence of internal paramagnetic material (usually in the form of blood products).[8] Cysts that contain mostly free water and little protein or other material demonstrate the "typical" fluid-bright T2 hyperintense signal and T1 hypointense signal. However, as the concentration of protein and/or paramagnetic material increases in the cyst, it becomes more and more T1 hyperintense. *Cysts typically maintain their T2 hyperintensity until the internal concentration of protein and/or paramagnetic materials increases over 50%. When this occurs, the short T2 relaxation times of the large protein macromolecules (and paramagnetic substances) will dominate, resulting in the cyst appearing dark (hypointense) on T2-weighted images.* This phenomenon is most clearly exemplified in Case 2.4, the colloid cyst. Note also that in Case 2.5, there is variable T2 signal intensity among the many cysts. Although many exhibit fluid-bright T2 hyperintensity, others are intermediate in signal, and a few are T2 hypointense (dark). This heterogeneity reflects variable protein and blood product content in the different renal cysts.

CASES 2.3, 2.4, AND 2.5 ANSWERS

1. **B. A thin rim of peripheral enhancement can be seen in a benign cyst.**
2. **A. Hydrocephalus**
3. **D. Cysts remain T2 hyperintense until their internal protein concentration exceeds approximately 50%.**
4. **C. Saccular aneurysm**
5. **A. Water has a long relaxation time.**

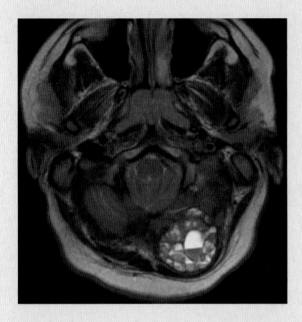

FIG. 2.C6

1. Which of the following is most correct about Fig. 2.C6A?
   A. Internal hemorrhage results in shortening of T2 relaxation times, causing areas of dependent low signal.
   B. Fluid-fluid levels are secondary to internal proteinaceous content, causing T2 prolongation.
   C. Fluid-fluid levels are pathognomonic for aneurysmal bone cysts.
   D. Areas of nondependent T2 hyperintensity in the lesion are secondary to magnetic susceptibility artifact.

Aneurysmal Bone Cysts

Aneurysmal bone cysts (ABCs) are benign osseous lesions, typically in young patients. They usually occur in the metaphysis of long bones, making this case somewhat atypical, and are characteristically expansile, with numerous fluid-fluid levels on MRI scans. Although ABCs usually occur in isolation, in approximately one-third of cases an ABC will occur secondary to another osseous lesion. Precursor lesions that have been described include giant cell tumor, osteoblastoma, chondroblastoma, fibrous dysplasia, eosinophilic granuloma, and osteosarcoma.[9] One tumor of particular note is a telangiectatic osteosarcoma, which can appear identical to an ABC on MRI but is more aggressive appearing on radiographs and CT scans.

FIG. 2.C6. Axial FSE T2-weighted image of the brain. There is a multicystic mass within the left occipital bone containing several fluid-fluid levels.

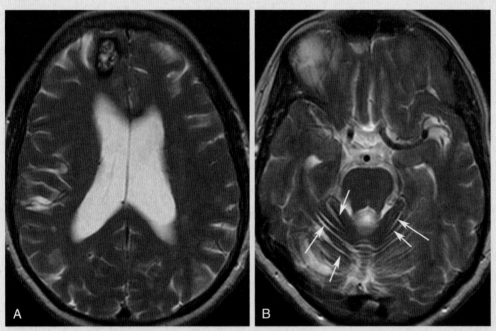

FIG. 2.C7

2. Which of the following intracranial blood products is T2 hyperintense?
   A. Intracellular methemoglobin
   B. Extracellular methemoglobin
   C. Deoxygenated hemoglobin
   D. Hemosiderin

FIG. 2.C7. (A) Axial T2-weighted image FSE of the brain at the level of the lateral ventricles. A heterogeneous mass identified within the right frontal lobe contains a thick rim of black signal. (B) Axial T2-weighted image FSE of the brain at the level of the cerebellum. There is a thin rim of black signal outlining the cerebellar folia (arrows).

Cavernoma With Superficial Siderosis

Cavernous malformations, or cavernomas, are dilated, endothelial cell–lined spaces without interposed normal brain. Cavernomas have a propensity to hemorrhage and often contain blood degradation products of varying stages. This can result in a heterogeneous internal MR signal. However, *cavernomas often demonstrate a characteristic thin rim of dark signal on T2-weighted MR images.* This characteristic finding is well demonstrated in Fig. 2.C7A.

Fig. 2.C7B exhibits findings suggestive of multiple prior hemorrhages within the cavernoma. Note the subtle *lining of T2 hypointensity along the folia of the cerebellum, which is suggestive of diffuse hemosiderin deposition. This finding is termed superficial siderosis* and is the result of multiple repeated hemorrhages within the subarachnoid space. With repeated hemorrhages, and over time, the hemosiderin blood products accumulate dependently within the subarachnoid space, often along the cerebellar folia, as in this example. Superficial siderosis can be the sequelae of any cause of repeated subarachnoid hemorrhage, including cavernomas, arteriovenous malformations, long-term warfarin therapy, and alcoholism.[10]

Appearance of Blood on T2-Weighted Spin Echo Images

Hemorrhage has a complex appearance on MR scans based on its age. It can be hyperintense or hypointense on both T1- and T2-weighted images but is a common cause of T2 hypointensity. This finding occurs because macrophages and microglial cells collect iron from blood breakdown products and transport them to the periphery of the lesion. These iron aggregates are stored as *hemosiderin* and are *extremely paramagnetic.* As described in more detail in Chapter 8, *paramagnetic substances significantly alter the local magnetic field, which results in rapid loss of transverse magnetization and the absence of signal production (i.e., a very short T2 relaxation time).* Hemosiderin deposition is the source of low signal along the periphery of the cavernoma and the cause of the superficial siderosis in Case 2.7.

Hematocrit levels (fluid-fluid levels) occur secondary to stagnant blood products that layer dependently, such as in the ABC found in Case 2.6.[6] The blood products shorten the T2 relaxivity of dependent portions of the lesion, resulting in areas of relative T2 hypointensity.

Intracranial hemorrhage tends to exhibit signal characteristics that fairly reliably reflect the state of the hemoglobin within the hemorrhage. The expected appearance on both T1- and T2-weighted SE sequences for each state of hemoglobin is a common topic found in most neuroradiology texts. On T2-weighted images, oxygenated hemoglobin (hyperacute blood) and extracellular methemoglobin (late subacute blood) result in hyperintense signal due to increased T2 relaxivity.

CASES 2.6 AND 2.7 ANSWERS

1. **A. Internal hemorrhage results in shortening of T2 relaxation times, causing areas of dependent low signal.**
2. **B. Extracellular methemoglobin**

CASE 2.8

FIG. 2.C8

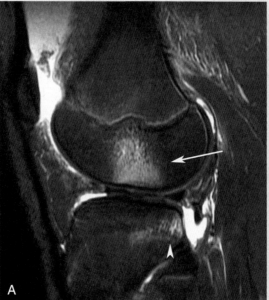 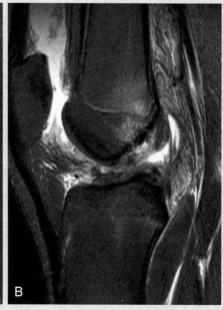

1. What is this pattern of injuries called?
   A. Anterior drawer
   B. Pivot shift
   C. Bucket handle
   D. Contrecoup contusion
2. Which of the following is true?
   A. Water and other small, rapidly moving molecules experience greater magnetic field variability than larger molecules, which results in shorter T2 relaxation times.
   B. A typical T2 relaxation time for free water is approximately 10 ms.
   C. Marrow edema results in increased T2 relaxation times within a voxel, resulting in hyperintense signal.
   D. T2 hyperintensity in marrow edema is secondary to internal hemorrhage.

FIG. 2.C8. (A) Sagittal fat-saturated FSE T2-weighted image along the lateral aspect of the knee. There is increased signal in the bone marrow of the lateral femoral condyle *(arrow)* as well as in the posterolateral aspect of the tibial plateau *(arrowhead)*. (B) Sagittal fat-saturated FSE T2-weighted image centered on the intercondylar notch. There is a conspicuous absence of discernible anterior cruciate ligament (ACL) fibers, which is consistent with an ACL tear.

Pivot Shift Bone Marrow Contusion

Case 2.8 demonstrates T2 hyperintensity within the bone marrow of the lateral femoral condyle and the posterolateral tibial plateau, consistent with edema. This contusion pattern, termed *pivot shift,* occurs with an anterior cruciate ligament (ACL) tear. Absence of the ACL allows the tibia to move anteriorly in relation to the femur, resulting in contact between the posterior aspect of the lateral tibial plateau and the lateral femoral condyle.

Marrow T2 Hyperintensity

T2 hyperintensity within the bone marrow is secondary to extracellular edema. The presence of *increased water content results in a relative increase in the T2 relaxation times within each voxel, leading to increased signal on T2-weighted images.* Edema is a common finding in many pathologic processes throughout the body. There are multiple etiologies for bone marrow edema including trauma (contusions and fractures), neoplasms, and infection.

CASE 2.8 ANSWER

1. **B.** Pivot shift
2. **C.** Marrow edema results in increased T2 relaxation times within a voxel, resulting in hyperintense signal.

CASES 2.9, 2.10, AND 2.11

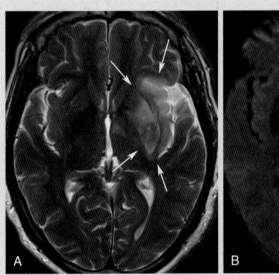
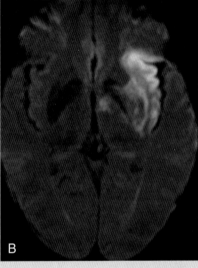

FIG. 2.C9

1. What is the diagnosis?
   A. Glioblastoma
   B. Creutzfeldt-Jakob disease
   C. Cerebral contusion
   D. Ischemic infarct
2. Which of the following is true?
   A. Diffusion-weighted images have intrinsic T1 weighting, requiring correlation with apparent diffusion coefficient maps to confirm the true restriction.
   B. This primarily represents vasogenic edema.
   C. This represents occlusion of the M1 segment of the left middle cerebral artery.
   D. This infarct is at least 2 weeks old.

Acute Ischemic Infarct

This case represents a classic left middle cerebral artery distribution acute ischemic infarct. Given the involvement of the lentiform nucleus, it is due to an M1 segment occlusion because the lenticulostriate vessels must also be involved. Increased T2 signal within the area of infarct arises 6 to 24 hours after the acute occlusion, peaks at 3 to 7 days, and largely represents cytotoxic edema.[11] The edema can persist for 6 to 8 weeks, even after the blood-brain barrier has been restored.

FIG. 2.C9. (A) Axial T2-weighted FSE image. Increased T2 signal is identified within the left insula, internal capsule, and basal ganglia *(arrows).* (B) Axial diffusion-weighted image. A hyperintense signal corresponds to the areas of T2 hyperintensity in part A. This is suggestive of restricted diffusion but should be confirmed by comparison to an apparent diffusion coefficient map (not shown).

FIG. 2.C10

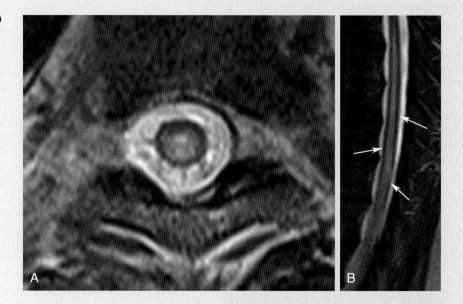

FIG. 2.C11

Spinal Cord Ischemia and Infarct

The involvement of the central gray matter of the cord and the long craniocaudal extent of the abnormality suggest cord ischemia. In ischemia, the gray matter is primarily involved due to its increased energy requirements. However, in severe cases, one may note additional involvement of the white matter. The T2 hyperintensity is a result of cytotoxic edema in a matter analogous to infarctions in the brain.

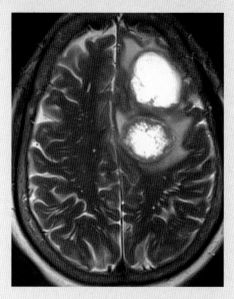

FIG. 2.C10. (A) Axial T2-weighted FSE image of the thoracic spinal cord. There is T2 hyperintensity within the central portion of an expanded cord. (B) Sagittal T2-weighted image of the thoracic spine. T2 hyperintensity and cord expansion *(arrows)* extend from the midthoracic cord inferiorly.

FIG. 2.C11. Axial T2-weighted image at the level of the corona radiata. Two T2 hyperintense masses are identified in the left frontal lobe. T2 hyperintensity consistent with edema is present in the adjacent white matter.

Vasogenic Edema Secondary to Multiple Brain Metastases

In Case 2.11, the two large left frontal lobe masses are surrounded by T2 hyperintensity that is primarily within the white matter, or vasogenic edema. The multiplicity of lesions and surrounding vasogenic edema are findings suggestive of metastatic disease. A known history of a primary malignancy (lung cancer in this case) helps confirm the diagnosis.

Vasogenic Edema and Cytotoxic Edema

Similar to edema in other areas of the body, edema in the central nervous system results in increased water content and resultant relative increases in the T2 relaxation times within each voxel. This causes increased signal on T2-weighted images.

Within the brain, edema is typically divided into cytotoxic and vasogenic subtypes. Although there are often components of both types in a disease process, one usually predominates. It is very important to be able to distinguish between these two patterns of edema because they suggest different causes and therefore different diagnoses. To understand the pattern of edema, it is important to review the pathologic cause of each type of edema.

Cytotoxic edema occurs when there is a breakdown of cellular metabolism, the most common cause of which is infarction. After the initial insult, the sodium potassium pump stops working appropriately, resulting in an influx of water into the intracellular space due to ion imbalances and a resultant osmosis. Thus *cytotoxic edema is secondary to an intracellular accumulation of water. As opposed to vasogenic edema, cytotoxic edema occurs maximally in the gray matter* because of the increased energy demand compared with the white matter.[12] In addition, because it is most often due to infarct, the edema is usually wedge shaped and extends all the way to the cortex.

In contradistinction, *vasogenic edema is due to breakdown of the blood-brain barrier and results in extracellular edema,* as opposed to intracellular edema. The result is that vasogenic edema primarily occurs *within the white matter tracts,* where the extracellular space is less rigid than in the gray matter. The most common causes are tumors, trauma, and ischemic injury.[12]

Both cytotoxic and vasogenic edema can occur in the setting of a cerebral infarct. Initially, due to the lack of oxygen and energy, there is a resultant cytotoxic edema. However, prolonged deprivation leads to cellular death, including death of the cells that establish the blood-brain barrier, which causes a breakdown of the blood-brain barrier tight junctions and a superimposed vasogenic edema.[12] This vasogenic edema is the major component that results in the significant swelling that can occur a few days after a stroke, leading to mass effect and herniation.

CASES 2.9, 2.10, AND 2.11 ANSWERS

1. **D. Ischemic infarct**
2. **C. This represents occlusion of the M1 segment of the middle cerebral artery.**

CASES 2.12, 2.13, AND 2.14

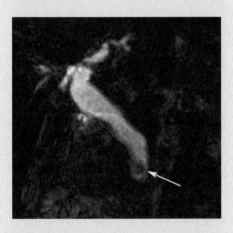

FIG. 2.C12

1. Which of the following decreases the risk of having the finding in Case 2.12?
   A. Pregnancy
   B. Obesity
   C. Coffee consumption
   D. Crohn disease
   E. Weight loss
2. How was this image created?
   A. The TR was considerably shortened.
   B. The flip angle was reduced to less than 20 degrees.
   C. The 180-degree refocusing pulse was removed.
   D. Absence of signal in much of the image was unintended and due to artifact.
   E. The TE was considerably lengthened.

Common Bile Duct Stones and Biliary Ductal Dilation

The MRCP image well delineates a hypointense bile duct stone in the distal common bile duct. There is resultant marked biliary duct dilation. A number of risk factors exist for the development of gallstones, such as high estrogen states (e.g., female gender, oral contraceptives, pregnancy), obesity, weight loss, Crohn disease, and cirrhosis. Coffee has been shown to decrease the risk of gallstones, good news for medical students and residents everywhere.[13]

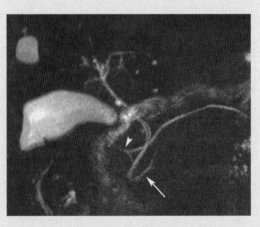

FIG. 2.C13

3. What is true about what is shown in Fig. 2.C13?
   A. It can be associated with recurrent bouts of cholelithiasis.
   B. It is due to a stricture of the major papilla of the pancreatic duct.
   C. It predisposes to malignancy.
   D. It has an association with an annular pancreas.

FIG. 2.C12. Coronal MR cholangiopancreatography (MRCP) image through the common bile duct. There is a rounded focus of hypointensity within the common bile duct (*arrow*), with resultant moderate to severe biliary duct dilation.

FIG. 2.C13. MRCP maximum intensity projection showing nondilated pancreatic and biliary ducts. Note that the ducts of Wirsung (*arrow*) and Santorini (*arrowhead*) empty into the duodenum at different locations.

Pancreas Divisum

During embryologic development, the pancreas begins in two sections, the ventral and dorsal anlages, each with its own drainage pathways. The ventral anlage, which becomes the pancreatic head and uncinate, contains the duct of Wirsung and drains via the major papilla. The body and tail of the pancreas (at this stage called the dorsal anlage) contain the duct of Santorini and drain via the minor papilla. Typically, as a normal part of development, the ducts for these two segments fuse. When the ducts fail to fuse, the result is pancreas divisum. Pancreas divisum is the most common anatomic anomaly of the pancreas and occurs in 5% to 14% of the population.[14] Although the clinical significance of this finding is debatable, many patients with this anatomic variant are reported to have increased rates of abdominal pain and pancreatitis. MRCP well demonstrates a duct crossing the common bile duct to empty into the duodenum. Identification of this anomalous, so-called *crossing duct sign* allows one to make the diagnosis of a pancreas divisum.

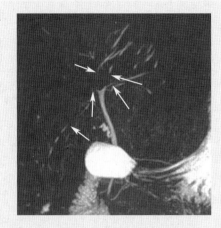

FIG. 2.C14

4. What is the diagnosis?
   A. Primary sclerosing cholangitis
   B. Primary biliary cirrhosis
   C. Caroli disease
   D. Choledocholithiasis

FIG. 2.C14. MRCP maximum intensity projection. Focal areas of narrowing *(arrows)* are noted in the central intrahepatic bile ducts. Note also the prominent intrahepatic biliary ductal dilation in the left hepatic lobe.

Primary Sclerosing Cholangitis

Focal areas of alternating stricture and dilation of the biliary system are characteristic of primary sclerosing cholangitis. Realizing that the central intrahepatic ducts are not visible secondary to severe narrowing and that the peripheral intrahepatic ducts are dilated within the left hepatic lobe is critical to establishing this diagnosis. Remember, the biliary ductal system should always increase in caliber, moving centrally toward the hilum. The reverse is occurring in this case.

MR Cholangiopancreatography

MRCP has become an integral technique for the evaluation of the biliary system. It has several obvious advantages over endoscopic retrograde cholangiopancreatography in that it is noninvasive, less expensive, often provides better and more detailed delineation of the anatomy, and can provide additional information about extraductal pathology. Although MRCP images may appear to be the result of a drastically different type of MR sequence and technique, they are, in actuality, simply a heavily T2-weighted sequence. The resultant images exhibit extreme contrast, with very little in the way of intermediate shades of gray.

How is this type of image produced? Recall that lengthening the TE of a sequence allows the protons more time to lose their transverse magnetization secondary to pure T2 relaxation. Standard T2-weighted sequences use an intermediate to long TE time, which allows for the differences in the T2 relaxation times between different tissues to become more apparent. Care is taken with these sequences to assign a TE that is not too long because this will result in loss of the entirety of the transverse magnetization within the imaged tissues and subsequently lead to absence of signal. *With MRCP images, the TE is drastically lengthened so that the transverse magnetization from short T2 molecules (essentially everything in the body except water) is almost completely lost, resulting in absence of signal. Because water has a very long T2 relaxation time, it is able to retain some of its transverse magnetization and continues to appear hyperintense.* Because bile is mostly composed of water, it too has a long T2 relaxation and produces considerable signal, despite the very long TE. This is the basis for an MRCP image, which essentially eliminates all signal except that within the biliary system.

The previous explanation of the MRCP technique applies to an SE-based sequence. However, MRCP can also be performed using a steady-state GRE sequence, which has both T1 and T2 weighting. Because GRE MRCP is T1 and T2 weighted, not only will water appear bright (because of its T2 properties), but fat and blood can also appear bright (because of their T1 properties).

Gadolinium-based contrast agents with significant biliary excretion (e.g., gadoxetate disodium [Eovist]) allow for an alternative methodology in the MR evaluation of the biliary system. With these agents, contrast is excreted into the biliary system, allowing for the acquisition of an MR cholangiogram on delayed images. This can be conceptualized as analogous to an evaluation of the collecting system via CT urography and renally excreted iodinated contrast. However, it is important to recognize that evaluation of the pancreatic system is not possible with this method because the contrast agent will only be present in the bile. This technique is of considerable utility, particularly for the purposes of problem solving and further evaluation when a traditional T2-weighted MRCP image is nondiagnostic secondary to patient motion. Furthermore, imaging with biliary-excreted contrast agents can provide physiologic information about the biliary system not otherwise available with the use of traditional imaging techniques.[15]

CASES 2.12, 2.13, AND 2.14 ANSWERS

1. C. Coffee consumption
2. E. The TE was considerably lengthened.
3. D. It has an association with an annular pancreas.
4. A. Primary sclerosing cholangitis

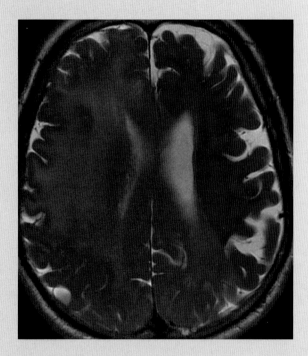

FIG. 2.C15

1. Which of the following is true of T2 weighting?
   A. It is highly dependent on the main magnetic field strength.
   B. T2 weighting is achieved through lengthening the TR and TE.
   C. T2 weighting is achieved through shortening the TR.
   D. T2 weighting is achieved through shortening the TE.

Gliomatosis Cerebri

Gliomatosis cerebri is a diffusely infiltrative glioma that occupies most of one cerebral hemisphere. In this case, there is relative preservation of the underlying neural architecture. Characteristically, MR images demonstrate an area of diffuse T2 hyperintensity involving predominantly the white matter, with some involvement of the gray matter as well. These areas typically do not enhance after the administration of contrast. *Although the pattern and appearance are similar to those of vasogenic edema, the findings actually represent diffuse tumor involvement.* Furthermore, involvement of the gray matter (as in this case) is not typically seen with vasogenic edema.

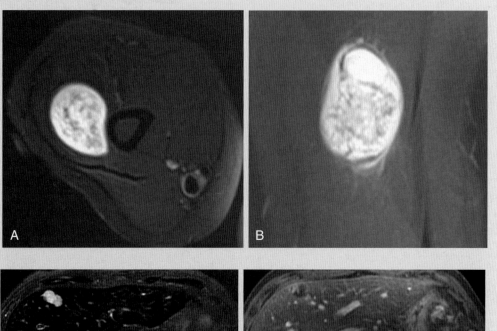

FIG. 2.C16

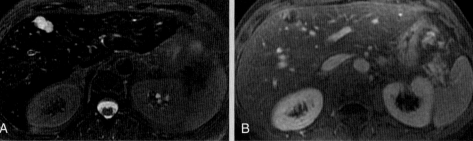

FIG. 2.C17

FIG. 2.C15. Axial T2-weighted image at the level of the corona radiata. There is diffuse T2 hyperintensity throughout the right cerebral hemisphere, with thickening of the gyri.

FIG. 2.C16. Fat-saturated T2-weighted FSE images of the distal humerus in the (A) axial and (B) coronal planes. A T2 hyperintense mass is adjacent to the humerus.

FIG. 2.C17. (A) Axial fat-saturated T2-weighted image of the liver. There is a homogeneously T2 hyperintense lesion within the anterior aspect of the right hepatic lobe. (B) Axial fat-saturated postcontrast T1-weighted image of the liver. Note the peripheral nodular enhancement of the lesion.

Peripheral Nerve Schwannoma

Peripheral nerve tumors exhibit characteristic T2 hyperintensity. Identifying a solid lesion with these signal characteristics in the soft tissues of an extremity can help narrow the differential diagnosis to synovial cell sarcoma and a peripheral nerve tumor. Furthermore, identifying an association between the lesion and an adjacent nerve is essentially diagnostic of a peripheral nerve tumor. Differentiating between a schwannoma and a neurofibroma (types of peripheral nerve tumors) is often not possible. However, schwannomas are considered to be typically located eccentric to the nerve, whereas neurofibromas are often centered on the nerve.[16]

Hepatic Hemangioma

Similar to schwannomas, hemangiomas are benign neoplasms that demonstrate fluid-bright T2 hyperintensity. In addition, hemangiomas often exhibit a characteristic peripheral nodular enhancement on postcontrast T1-weighted images, which establishes their diagnosis (Fig. 2.C17B).

T2 Hyperintense Neoplasms

Cases 2.15, 2.16, and 2.17 all represent T2-hyperintense neoplasms. Neoplasms are often T2 hyperintense for a variety of reasons. Case 2.15 provides an excellent opportunity to elucidate the physics behind T2 hyperintensity further, as well as point out a common misunderstanding in MR neuroradiology. *Anaplastic astrocytomas and glioblastoma multiforme (GBM) exhibit adjacent T2 hyperintensity that is often erroneously described as vasogenic edema.* Although the appearance of this "edema" is very similar to the vasogenic edema identified in the setting of other intracranial pathology (e.g., as in the metastatic lesions in Case 2.11), *pathologic evaluation of these areas demonstrates a combination of both edema and tumor cells.* Thus in the setting of an astrocytoma, *any* adjacent T2 hyperintensity is assumed to represent tumor infiltration. Consider the underlying physics. Any process that results in T2 relaxation prolongation will cause hyperintensity on a T2-weighted image. *Avoid the common pitfall of assuming that all areas of T2 hyperintensity represent edema alone.*

In Case 2.16, a peripheral nerve sheath tumor, the cause of the T2 hyperintensity is multifactorial and includes a combination of cystic changes, the generalized increased vascularity of these tumors, and a high intrinsic water content. This results in T2 prolongation and hyperintense signal.

In Case 2.17, the T2 hyperintensity occurs secondary to slow-flowing blood coursing through dilated vascular spaces within the hemangioma.[17] Flowing oxygenated blood contains intrinsically long T2 relaxation times (with resultant T2 hyperintensity) secondary to its high free water component. The slow velocity of the blood within the hemangioma prevents signal loss from flow voids (discussed further in Chapter 11).

CASES 2.15, 2.16, AND 2.17 ANSWER

1. **B. T2 weighting is achieved through lengthening the TR and TE.**

CASE 2.18

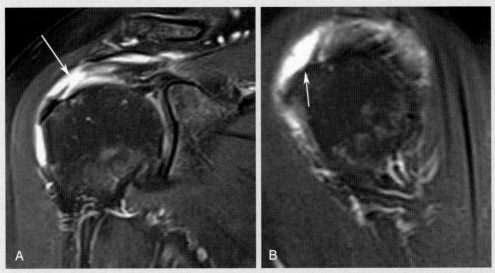

FIG. 2.C18. (A) Coronal oblique T2-weighted image of the shoulder. T2 hyperintensity is completely disrupting the supraspinatus tendon *(arrow)*, with mild retraction of the tendon. (B) Sagittal oblique T2-weighted image of the shoulder. There is fluid-bright T2 hyperintensity in the expected location of the supraspinatus tendon *(arrow)*.

Full-Thickness Tear of the Supraspinatus Tendon

Fluid-bright T2 hyperintense signal replaces the supraspinatus tendon, which is retracted. Findings are diagnostic for a full-thickness tear of the rotator cuff.

CASE 2.19

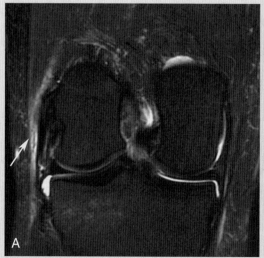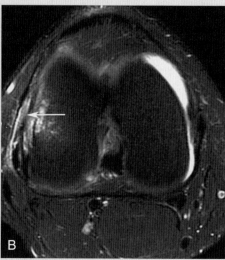

FIG. 2.C19

1. Why are tendons and ligaments typically T2 hypointense?
   A. They consist of small and disorganized collagen fibers.
   B. This is due to the rapid and free motion of internal water molecules.
   C. Magnetic susceptibility from blood products results in signal loss.
   D. There is very little internal water content.
   E. This is due to the linear morphology in the phase-encoding direction.

FIG. 2.C19 (A) Coronal fat-saturated T2-weighted image of the knee. There is T2 hyperintensity in the tissues adjacent to the fibulocollateral ligament *(arrow)*. (B) Axial fat-saturated T2-weighted image of the knee at the level of the femoral condyles. There is T2 hyperintensity adjacent to and within the fibulocollateral ligament *(arrow)*.

Fibulocollateral Ligament Sprain

The T2 hyperintensity within the soft tissues immediately adjacent to the fibulocollateral ligament is representative of edema. In addition, note the increased T2 signal in the substance of the fibulocollateral ligament, which implies internal injury and a more severe sprain.

Physics of Low T2 Signal in Tendons and Ligaments

Tendons and ligaments both consist of large ordered collagen fibers containing very little internal water and therefore very few freely mobile protons. As a result of this relative paucity of mobile protons, *variations in the magnetic field cannot be readily dispersed, and rapid loss of transverse magnetization occurs due to dephasing.*

This produces the dark (almost black) signal identified in these structures on T2-weighted images. Perhaps one of the benefits of this expected background absence of signal is that it facilitates the detection of pathology, which typically manifests as edema and T2 hyperintensity. For this reason, MRI has a very high sensitivity and specificity for ligament and tendon pathology. Fluid-bright T2 hyperintensity in both tendons and ligaments represents fluid intercalation in its substance and implies fiber disruption or a tear. Descriptions of the subtypes of tendon injury and tears are beyond the intended scope of this chapter, but can be found in many excellent clinically oriented musculoskeletal MRI texts.

CASE 2.19 ANSWER

1. **D. There is very little internal water content.**

FIG. 2.C20

1. Which of the following is true about MRI of cartilage?
   A. Cartilage contains few water molecules, resulting in low T2 signal.
   B. Water molecules within cartilage are freely mobile.
   C. The microstructure of cartilage results in rapid dispersion of magnetic field variations, resulting in signal loss.
   D. A rigid molecular structure causes persistence of field inhomogeneities, resulting in dephasing and signal loss.
   E. Cartilage is normally T2 hyperintense.

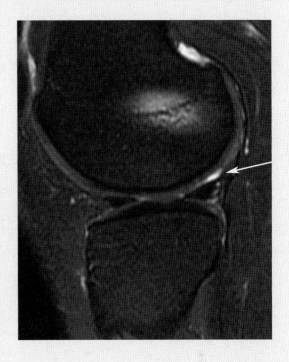

FIG. 2.C20. Sagittal fat-saturated T2-weighted image of the knee through the lateral femoral condyle. There is a focal area of T2 hyperintensity along the posterior aspect of the lateral femoral condyle (arrow).

MR Appearance of Cartilage

Evaluating for cartilage abnormalities is an integral component in the interpretation of musculoskeletal MRI. Although several viable options exist, T2-weighted MR sequences are excellent for detecting cartilage pathology. Cartilage irregularities and defects represent loss of normal cartilage, which is replaced by intraarticular fluid (as with the partial defect in Case 2.20). Therefore these *defects are hyperintense on T2-weighted sequences and are rather conspicuous secondary to their excellent contrast with the adjacent intermediate to low signal cartilage.*[18] *Cartilage actually contains an abundance of water molecules. However, they are bound within the rigid molecular structure of the*

cartilage molecule, precluding their free mobility. This prevents dispersion of the magnetic field variations and results in a persistence of the inhomogeneities that cause dephasing and signal loss. Although this principle results in signal loss, the bound water molecules still exhibit relatively long T2 relaxation times compared with other tissues in the body (just less than those of free water). Therefore the combination of these effects leads to the resultant intermediate to low signal of cartilage on T2-weighted images.

CASE 2.20 ANSWER

1. **D. A rigid molecular structure causes persistence of field inhomogeneities, resulting in dephasing and signal loss.**

CASE 2.21

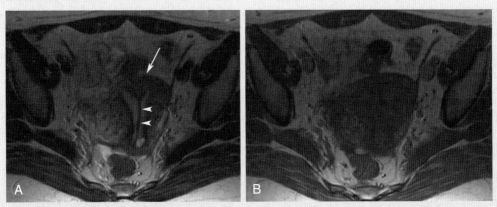

FIG. 2.C21. (A) Axial T2-weighted image of the pelvis. A uterus with two separate cavities is separated by a thin black septum (arrowheads). Note that the uterine fundal contour is convex (arrow). (B) Axial T1-weighted image of the pelvis. The uterus is homogeneously gray, precluding accurate evaluation of uterine anatomy.

Septate Uterus

Differentiating a septate uterus from a bicornuate uterus can be difficult. However, the distinction is important because it changes the treatment options and the prognosis for pregnancy. A septate uterus is the result of failure of resorption of the septum after fusion of the müllerian ducts. A bicornuate uterus is the result of failure of fusion of the müllerian ducts.

A bicornuate uterus will have endometrium and myometrium separating the two cavities, whereas a septate uterus will have only a separating fibrous septum. Patients with a bicornuate uterus have fewer problems with infertility. If one is unable to distinguish distinct endometrial and myometrial tissue separating the two cavities, evaluating the fundal contour may be helpful. The fundal contour is convex in a septate uterus (as in this case) and concave in a bicornuate uterus.[19]

CASE 2.22

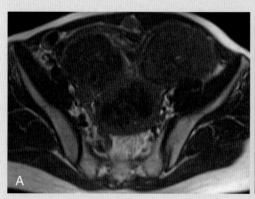 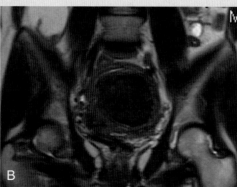

FIG. 2.C22

1. Certain neoplasms such as lymphoma can appear T2 hypointense, in part due to which of the following?
   A. Hypercellularity causing increased extracellular water content
   B. Cell swelling causing increased intracellular water content
   C. Increased water movement in the extracellular space
   D. Hypercellularity causing decreased extracellular water content

FIG. 2.C22. (A) Axial T2-weighted image of the pelvis. There are multiple low signal masses throughout the uterus. (B) Coronal T2-weighted image of the pelvis. A dominant low signal intrauterine mass is redemonstrated.

Uterine Leiomyomas

Uterine leiomyomas, or fibroids, are the most common solid benign uterine neoplasm. They arise from the myometrial layer of the uterus and consist of smooth muscle cells, with variable amounts of intervening connective tissue. Although many are found incidentally on imaging, some become symptomatic, necessitating treatment.

Uterine Anatomy and Tight Cell Packing

T2-weighted images provide an excellent evaluation of the female pelvis because they clearly demarcate the zonal anatomy of the uterus.[20] The central endometrium is T2 hyperintense secondary to the presence of mucinous glands and a highly vascularized stroma. *The junctional zone, or inner myometrium, is dark on T2-weighted images because it contains densely organized smooth muscle fibers and a paucity of free water.* This morphology results in shortening of the T2 relaxation time and a decrease in resultant signal. The outer myometrial layer exhibits a relative T2 hyperintensity secondary to a higher free water content and to the presence of less densely packed smooth muscle fibers.[19] *The zonal anatomy of the uterus is therefore well delineated on T2-weighted images* secondary to the differences in the T2 relaxivity of the zonal layers, a property related to the underlying morphology and content of the tissue.

It is often difficult to identify the type of pulse sequence used to produce a female pelvic MR image, particularly when only a single image is offered (e.g., in a case conference setting). When this situation arises, an evaluation of the uterus may be particularly helpful in determining the sequence type. The uterus is characteristically homogeneously gray in signal on T1-weighted sequences (see Fig. 2.C21B). In contradistinction, if the trizonal anatomy of the uterus is identifiable, then the sequence is T2 weighted.

In a manner analogous to the junctional zone, *leiomyomas contain numerous tightly packed smooth muscle cells and very little free water and intercellular space. This results in an abundance of large molecules and a tissue structure that contains short T2 relaxation times, producing low signal on T2-weighted images.* It should be noted, however, that fibroids may contain some areas of internal T2 hyperintensity if they have undergone degeneration or necrosis.

Densely packed cells are also typically found in several other neoplasms, such as *medulloblastomas, pineoblastomas, and central nervous system lymphoma.* In addition to the *sparse intercellular space, there is also a high nuclear-to-cytoplasm ratio* in these tumors. This results in a relative paucity of free-flowing intracellular water, which decreases the T2 relaxation time of the tissue and manifests on MR images as *uniform low T2 signal* within the mass. This is an important MR concept that can often help narrow a differential diagnosis when confronted with one of these neoplasms.

CASE 2.22 ANSWER

1. **D. Hypercellularity causing decreased extracellular water content**

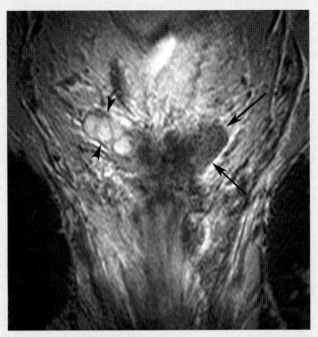

FIG. 2.C23. Coronal T2-weighted image through the seminal vesicles. The expected normal T2 hyperintensity, as visualized in the right seminal vesicle *(arrowheads),* has been replaced by T2 hypointensity in the left seminal vesicle *(arrows).*

Prostate Adenocarcinoma Invasion into the Left Seminal Vesicles

Prostate MRI is not typically used for the diagnosis of prostate cancer, but rather for staging the disease. MRI is used to determine tumor respectability. Findings that preclude surgical intervention include invasion into the periprostatic fat, invasion into the seminal vesicles, the presence of lymph node involvement, and the presence of osseous metastatic disease.

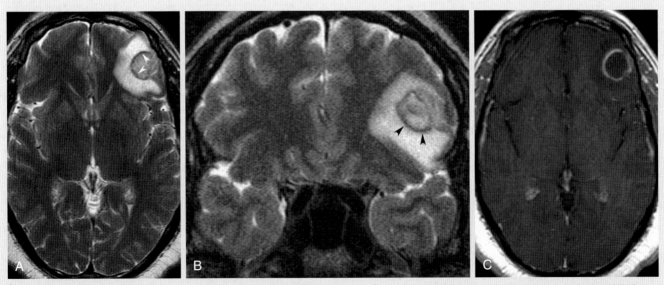

FIG. 2.C24. (A) Axial and (B) coronal T2-weighted FSE images of the brain. There is an intermediate signal mass with a subtle rim of T2 hypointensity *(arrowheads).* (C) Axial postcontrast T1-weighted image of the brain. The mass demonstrates a peripheral rim of enhancement.

Brain Abscess With a Thin T2 Hypointense Rim

The differential diagnosis for an intraaxial rim-enhancing mass is lengthy and nonspecific. There is, however, an MR imaging finding that can narrow the differential diagnosis. Brain abscesses often exhibit a peripheral rim of low signal intensity on T2-weighted images representing their capsule.

Pathology Manifesting as T2 Hypointensity

Although many pathologic processes are T2 hyperintense, some replace an expected area of normal T2 hyperintensity with low T2 signal. This is the situation in Case 2.23. The normal seminal vesicles are T2 hyperintense secondary to the physiologic fluid that they produce and contain. However, invasion with *prostate adenocarcinoma causes a fibrotic reaction that replaces the seminal vesicle and manifests as T2 hypointensity.* The low signal is secondary to the relative paucity of free water and to the presence of macromolecules in the fibrotic tissue, both of which cause shortening of the T2 relaxation time.

Occasionally, identifying T2 hypointensity can help suggest a diagnosis, which is the situation in Case 2.24, a brain abscess with a thin rim of T2 hypointensity. A proposed cause for this rim of hypointensity is the high concentration of oxygen free radicals secondary to macrophages entering the capsule. These free radicals are highly paramagnetic, which causes magnetic susceptibility and considerable effective shortening of the T2 relaxation time, with concomitant low T2 signal. Of note, acute abscesses do not demonstrate this peripheral T2 hypointense rim because they have not yet formed a capsule.

TAKE-HOME POINTS

Physics

1. T2 relaxation reflects the process by which the transverse magnetization loses phase coherence, which is an exponential decay at the rate of T2.
2. Loss of transverse magnetization is primarily due to phase dispersion (loss of phase coherence) among the precessing protons.
3. Loss of phase coherence is due to inhomogeneities in the main magnetic field and the spin-spin interactions of protons in their local microenvironment; together, they create T2* effects.
4. FID is the oscillating waveform that occurs when the RF pulse is turned off and reflects the decaying transverse magnetization. T2* effects determine the rate at which FID occurs.
5. T2 is the loss of magnetization solely due to proton spin-spin interactions in their microscopic environment.
6. Quantitatively, the T2 time for a tissue is the time at which 63% of the original signal is lost during the exponential T2 decay.
7. Because T2 reflects time to loss of signal, tissues with long T2 times will be bright, and tissues with short T2 times will be dark on T2-weighted images.
8. Macromolecules have short T2 times (T2 hypointense). Water has a long T2 time (T2 hyperintense).
9. A T2-weighted sequence has a long TR and an intermediate to long TE.
10. Gradient sequences can produce a T2*-weighted sequence but cannot produce a purely T2-weighted image because they do not use an 180-degree, phase-refocusing pulse.
11. Image acquisition times can be reduced in SE sequences by applying multiple 180-degree RF excitation pulses per each TR. This allows for the collection of multiple lines of k-space during each TR; this is called a turbo or fast SE sequence.
12. The decrease in image acquisition time is proportional to the number of RF pulses that occur during each TR. This is called the turbo factor or echo train length.
13. Fat appears brighter on T2-weighted FSE images than on T2-weighted SE images because the repeated RF pulses disrupt J-coupling.
14. MRCP is a heavily T2-weighted sequence that allows enough time for phase dispersion to occur in just about all tissues, except those containing abundant free water (e.g., bile).
15. Tissues that are highly ordered, have a paucity of water, or have tightly packed cells are T2 hypointense.
16. Paramagnetic substances such as blood degradation products and oxygen free radicals are also hypointense on T2-weighted images secondary to magnetic susceptibility effects.

Clinical Considerations

1. The central canal of the spinal cord is usually not identifiable and is considered pathologic if larger than 3 mm.
2. Cysts are typically bright on T2-weighted images, but can be isointense to hypointense on T2-weighted images with greater concentrations of protein and blood product content.
3. Fluid-fluid levels within a lytic bone lesion were thought to be pathognomonic for an ABC; however, several benign and malignant bone lesions can exhibit this MR finding.
4. Identification of a crossing duct sign on MRCP is diagnostic of a pancreas divisum.
5. The two most common causes of edema in the brain are cytotoxic and vasogenic factors.
6. Cytotoxic edema results from increased intracellular water secondary to dysfunction of the sodium potassium pump. The most common cause for cytotoxic edema is an infarct.
7. Vasogenic edema occurs secondary to breakdown of the blood-brain barrier and is usually secondary to malignancy.
8. The T2 hyperintensity often identified around gliomas does not represent vasogenic edema alone, but may also represent tumor extension.
9. Peripheral nerve sheath tumors are characteristically hyperintense on T2-weighted images.
10. Hepatic hemangiomas are typically T2 hyperintense, with peripheral nodular enhancement.
11. T2-weighted images are excellent for evaluating the zonal anatomy of the uterus. The endometrium is hyperintense, the junctional zone is hypointense, and the outer myometrium is hyperintense.
12. Ligament and tendon injuries are well demonstrated on T2-weighted images secondary to the strong contrast between the hyperintense edema and the hypointense normal ligament or tendon.
13. T2 hypointensity within the seminal vesicle is suggestive of fibrotic prostate tumor invasion.
14. The hypointense peripheral rim exhibited by cerebral abscesses on T2-weighted images can help narrow an otherwise extensive differential diagnosis.

References

1. Lee VS. *Cardiovascular MRI: Physical Principles to Practical Protocols.* Philadelphia: Lippincott Williams & Wilkins; 2005.

2. Warntjes JB, Dahlqvist O, Lundberg P. Novel method for rapid, simultaneous T1, T2*, and proton density quantification. *Magn Reson Med.* 2007;57(3):528–537.

3. Dhillon G, Bell N, Ginat D, et al. Breast MR imaging: what the radiologist needs to know. *J Clin Imaging Sci.* 2011;1(1): 48–48.

4. El Yousef SJ, Duchesneau RH, Alfidi RJ, et al. Magnetic resonance imaging of the breast. Work in progress. *Radiology.* 1984;150(3):761–766.

5. Dash N, Lupetin A, Daffner R, et al. Magnetic resonance imaging in the diagnosis of breast disease. *Am J Roentgenol.* 1986;146(1):119–125.

6. Edelman RR. *Clinical Magnetic Resonance Imaging.* 3rd ed. Philadelphia: Saunders Elsevier; 2006.

7. Martínez V. Autosomal dominant polycystic kidney disease: review and management update. *Eur Med J Nephrol.* 2014;1:61–66.

8. Runge VM. *Clinical MRI.* Philadelphia: Saunders; 2002.

9. Kransdorf MJ, Sweet DE. Aneurysmal bone cyst: concept, controversy, clinical presentation, and imaging. *AJR Am J Roentgenol.* 1995;164(3):573–580.

10. Offenbacher H, Fazekas F, Schmidt R, et al. Superficial siderosis of the central nervous system: MRI findings and clinical significance. *Neuroradiology.* 1996;38:S51–S56.

11. Brant WE, Helms CA. *Fundamentals of Diagnostic Radiology.* Philadelphia: Lippincott, Williams & Wilkins; 2007.

12. Klatzo I. Pathophysiological aspects of brain edema. *Acta Neuropathol.* 1987;72(3):236–239.

13. Zhang YP, Li WQ, Sun YL, et al. Systematic review with meta-analysis: coffee consumption and the risk of gallstone disease. *Aliment Pharmacol Ther.* 2015;42(6):637–648.

14. Kamisawa T, Tu Y, Egawa N, et al. MRCP of congenital pancreaticobiliary malformation. *Abdom Imaging.* 2007;32(1):129–133.

15. Gupta RT, Brady CM, Lotz J, et al. Dynamic MR imaging of the biliary system using hepatocyte-specific contrast agents. *AJR Am J Roentgenol.* 2010;195(2):405–413.

16. Goodwin RW, O'Donnell P, Saifuddin A. MRI appearances of common benign soft-tissue tumours. *Clin. Radiol.* 2007;62(9):843–853.

17. Bartolozzi C, Lencioni R, Donati F, Cioni D. Abdominal MR: liver and pancreas. *Eur Radiol.* 1999;9(8):1496–1512.

18. Bredella MA, Tirman PF, Peterfy CG, et al. Accuracy of T2-weighted fast spin-echo MR imaging with fat saturation in detecting cartilage defects in the knee: comparison with arthroscopy in 130 patients. *AJR Am J Roentgenol.* 1999;172(4):1073–1080.

19. Kennedy AM, Gilfeather MR, Woodward PJ. MRI of the female pelvis. *Semin Ultrasound CT MR.* 1999;20(4):214–230.

20. Proscia N, Jaffe TA, Neville AM, et al. MRI of the pelvis in women: 3D versus 2D T2-weighted technique. *AJR Am J Roentgenol.* 2010;195(1):254–259.

CHAPTER 3

Proton Density

Charles M. Maxfield

OPENING CASE 3.1

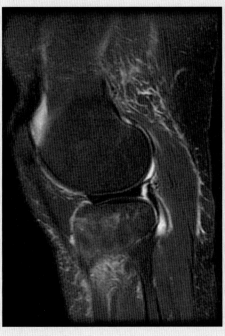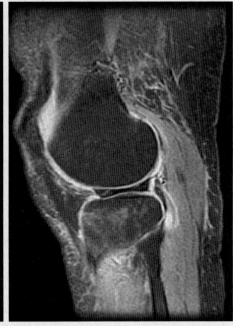

1. Which of the following parameter adjustments are respon-
   sible for the tissue contrast in the proton density–weighted
   (PDW) image?
   A. Adding an additional 180-degree inversion pulse at a set
      time before the 90-degree pulse
   B. Eliminating T2*
   C. Minimizing effects of T1 and T2 contrast
   D. Using flip angles of less than 90 degrees

2. What is the best diagnosis?
   A. Synovitis
   B. Tear of anterior horn of lateral meniscus
   C. Tibial contusion
   D. Normal

OPENING CASE 3.1

FIG. 3.C1. Two corresponding sagittal images of the knee. (A) T2-weighted image. (B) PDW image.

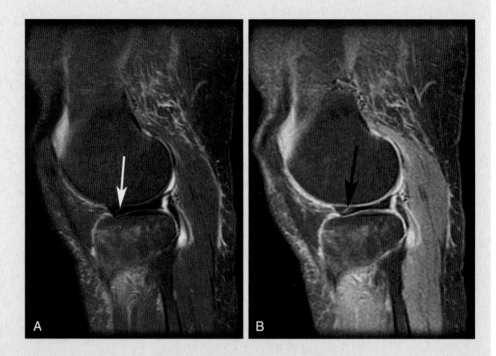

1. Which of the following parameter adjustments are responsible for the tissue contrast in the PDW image?
   C. Minimizing effects of T1 and T2 contrast
2. What is the best diagnosis?
   B. Tear of anterior horn of lateral meniscus

Discussion

By varying time to repetition (TR) and time to echo (TE), MRI can produce images based on three types of contrast: T1 weighted, T2 weighted, and proton density weighted (PDW). PDW is always present to some extent, but when the effects of T1 and T2 weighting are minimized (by using a long TR and a short TE), tissue contrast becomes based, by default, on proton density. PDW provides good overall signal and good anatomic detail, but because tissues do not differ significantly in proton density, contrast resolution is limited.

Fig. 3.C1 demonstrates an oblique tear of the anterior horn of the lateral meniscus. The linear area of high signal is better visualized on the PDW image (see Fig. 3.C1B), where it is clearly seen to extend to the articular surface *(arrow)*. A meniscal tear is defined as abnormal signal in a meniscus that extends to the articular surface. In this case, the tear is seen on both the T2-weighted image (long TE) and PDW image (short TE); however, recognition of the tear and visualization of the tear extent to the articular surface are better seen on the PDW image. The meniscus is best evaluated with short TE sequences (T1 weighted, PDW, and gradient recalled echo). PDW is particularly sensitive because of its superior signal-to-noise ratio (SNR). In recent years, fast spin echo (FSE)-PD sequences have been implemented in evaluating the menisci, with the primary advantage being shorter acquisition times. The disadvantage of using FSE-PD includes increased blurring of the image and brighter appearance of fat on FSE compared with spin echo (SE).

Physics

As discussed in Chapter 2, MR contrast can arise from density (proton) differences or relaxation time (e.g., T1 or T2) differences, which can be typically manipulated by two parameters, TR and TE. Different combinations of TR and TE produce three major types of tissue contrast: T1 weighted, T2 weighted, and PDW contrast. T1-weighted imaging enhances the T1 effect and minimizes T2 weighting by shortening TR and TE. T2-weighted imaging enhances the T2 effect and minimizes T1 weighting by lengthening TE and TR. PDW imaging minimizes both T1 and T2 by *lengthening* TR and *shortening* TE.

The long TR (longer than T1 of fat and water) used in PDW minimizes the T1 relaxation effects by allowing fat and water to fully recover their longitudinal magnetization. The short TE does not allow fat or water time to decay, thereby diminishing T2 weighting. Because T1 and T2 effects are both minimized, signal intensity, by default, becomes proportional to the number of protons per unit of tissue (i.e., proton density). The higher the number of protons in a given unit of tissue, the greater the transverse component of magnetization and the greater the signal. The PD of each voxel forms the image matrix.

The main practical advantage of PDW imaging is that the SNR is higher than any comparable T1-weighted or T2-weighted image. High SNR is achieved because longitudinal recovery is maximized and transverse decay is minimized.

PDW imaging, however, demonstrates little intrinsic contrast because variations in proton density between different tissue elements are often small (<10%). In "true" PDW imaging, pure water will have the most signal because its proton density is higher than that of any tissue. In practice, however, sequence parameters for PDW imaging are modified so that T1 and/or T2 contributions are moderately increased to optimize contrast within the tissue of interest.

In the brain, for example, PDW imaging sequences are designed to depict edema as brighter than cerebrospinal fluid (CSF), even though CSF has a higher PD. TR is shortened to reintroduce more T1 contribution and take advantage of the differences in T1 relaxation between edema and CSF. Although CSF has a higher PD, edema has a shorter T1 recovery. For PDW imaging in the brain, TR is shortened to a time when T1 contrast between CSF and edema is present, and signal intensity related to T1 recovery is still higher for edema.

Historically, PDW images were obtained "free" during conventional SE T2-weighted sequences, using the first echo of a dual-echo, T2-weighted sequence. PD signal was collected at an intermediate TE within the same TR. Therefore PD images were acquired without additional imaging time. Currently, FSE is used to give PD weighting quickly, but it must be run as a stand-alone sequence. A long echo train decreases the time of an FSE-PD sequence but introduces blurring along tissue margins.

Clinical Considerations

Historically, PDW imaging has made its greatest contribution in neuroimaging because it offers good gray-white contrast, especially for the posterior fossa and spine, and in musculoskeletal imaging because of its high SNR as well as the intrinsic PD contrast between musculoskeletal tissue elements. In the past decade, however, PDW has been largely replaced by FSE sequences, especially those with inversion recovery preparatory pulses (e.g., fluid-attenuated inversion recovery [FLAIR], short tau inversion recovery [STIR]), which provide excellent tissue contrast in less time.

Most musculoskeletal protocols still include PDW sequences, especially for the knee, shoulder, foot and ankle, and shoulder. There is controversy in the literature over whether FSE techniques perform as well as SE techniques in evaluating meniscal pathology. PDW images may provide additional information about the tendons, cartilage, and labra. There is debate about the use of fat saturation with PD imaging. Fat saturation narrows the grayscale range, allowing for increased contrast, and some think that this increases the conspicuity of meniscal tears.

CASE 3.2

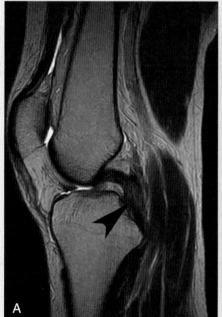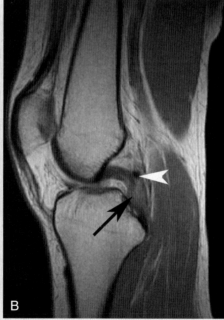

FIG. 3.C2

1. Which of the following statements is true regarding tears of the posterior cruciate ligament?
   A. More common than tears of anterior cruciate ligament (ACL)
   B. Physical examination is usually diagnostic
   C. Associated with tears of the ACL or collateral ligament in almost half of cases
   D. Typically injured in a noncontact deceleration injury

2. Of the following, which best characterizes PDW imaging compared with conventional T1-weighted and/or T2-weighted SE imaging?
   A. High tissue contrast and low SNR
   B. High tissue contrast and high SNR
   C. Low tissue contrast and low SNR
   D. Low signal contrast and high SNR
   E. Low tissue contrast and high SNR

FIG. 3.C2. Two corresponding sagittal images of the knee. (A) T2-weighted image. (B) PDW image.

Discussion

The sagittal T2-weighted image (Fig. 3.C2A) and sagittal PDW image (see Fig. 3.C2B) demonstrate thickening (*black arrowhead* in Fig. 3.C2A) and increased signal (*arrow* in Fig. 3.C2B) in the posterior cruciate ligament (PCL). The PCL should be uniformly dark in signal. The bright signal seen best on the PDW image is indicative of a tear. Note that the signal intensity is more conspicuous on the PDW image. The *white arrowhead* denotes the posterior meniscofemoral ligament (ligament of Wrisberg), just posterior to the PCL. The stark contrast between the very low signal posterior meniscofemoral ligament and the bright signal PCL is more conspicuous on the PDW image than on the T2-weighted image.

Tears of the PCL account for about 10% of all knee injuries as depicted on MRI. They are less common than ACL tears but are associated with ACL tears, as well as tears of the medial and lateral collateral ligaments and menisci, and bone contusions. Isolated PCL tears, which typically occur from posterior tibial displacement on a flexed knee, hyperextension of the knee, or rotation with an abduction or adduction force, may be relatively asymptomatic and produce few findings on physical examination.

PDW imaging results in an SNR higher than comparable T1-weighted or T2-weighted images. A high SNR is achieved with PDW imaging because longitudinal recovery is maximized and transverse decay is minimized. However, intrinsic tissue contrast is poor with PDW imaging because variations in proton density between different tissue elements are often small (<10%). PDW imaging continues to contribute to imaging in settings in which SNR is at a premium, and the advantages of a high SNR outweigh the disadvantages related to lower intrinsic tissue contrast.

CASE 3.3

FIG. 3.C3

1. Of the following, which would best result in PDW?
   A. TR 3000 ms and TE 100 ms
   B. TR 2000 ms and TE 20 ms
   C. TR 500 ms and TE 20 ms
   D. TR 500 ms and TE 100 ms
2. What is the most likely diagnosis in this patient?
   A. Acute disseminated encephalomyelitis
   B. AIDS-related myelitis
   C. Leukemia
   D. Neuromyelitis optica

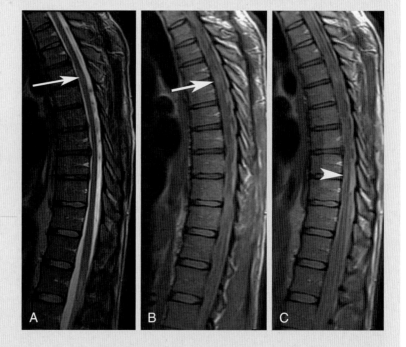

FIG. 3.C3. (A) Sagittal T2-weighted image. (B–C) Sagittal PDW images of the thoracic spine in a patient with new-onset blindness.

Discussion

Fig 3.C3A (T2-weighted image) and Fig. 3.C3B (PDW image) both demonstrate high T2 signal within the spinal cord (denoted by *white arrows*) at the T5–T6 level. Fig. 3.C3C (PDW image) demonstrates an additional T2 bright lesion at T9–T10 that is not seen on the T2-weighted image.

The PDW images (see Fig. 3.C2B–C) were obtained with a TR of 2000 ms and a TE of 20 ms. A long TR (longer than the T1 of both fat and water) allows both fat and water to fully recover their longitudinal magnetization, which minimizes T1 effects. The short TE of 20 ms receives signal before fat and water have had time to lose transverse magnetization, which minimizes T2 weighting. Because both T1 and T2 effects are diminished, tissue contrast, by default, is proportional to the number of protons per unit tissue (proton density.) The superior SNR of PDW allows visualization of the additional spinal cord lesion not seen on the T2-weighted image.

T2 bright lesions in the thoracic spinal cord can be seen with myelitis (inflammation of the spinal cord), tumors, spinal cord infarction and trauma. Myelitis can be due to multiple sclerosis (MS), acute disseminated encephalomyelitis, or neuromyelitis optica (NMO). The new-onset blindness in this patient with thoracic cord lesions makes NMO the most likely diagnosis.

NMO, also known as Devic disease, is a demyelinating disease caused by an autoantibody to the aquaporin-4 water channel. NMO is characterized by bilateral optic neuritis and myelitis. Patients typically present with blindness and paraplegia. NMO shares several features with MS, including a relapsing and remitting course, but is thought to be a distinct entity. The spinal lesions of NMO are characteristically long, extending for at least three vertebral body segments, and involve the central cord, unlike MS, which tends to involve the peripheral white matter tracts.

CASE 3.3 ANSWERS

1. **B. TR 2000 ms and TE 20 ms**
2. **D. Neuromyelitis optica**

TAKE-HOME POINTS

1. T1-weighted images are produced with a short TR and short TE. T2-weighted images are obtained with a long TR and long TE. A third combination—long TR and short TE—produces PDW images. The fourth (theoretical) combination of a short TR and long TE is not at all useful in clinical practice.
2. To produce a truly PDW image, the longitudinal magnetization of all tissues is allowed to recover completely between excitations (infinitely long TR) while allowing no transverse magnetization (zero TE). In reality, some T1 and T2 contrast is always present in all MR images.

3. PDW images have a higher SNR than comparable T1-weighted and T2-weighted images because recovery is maximized and transverse decay is minimized.
4. PDW imaging is most helpful in settings in which SNR is limited and inherent differences in PD between tissue elements are high, providing images that have both excellent contrast and high SNR.
5. Specific clinical applications of PDW imaging include evaluation of the meniscus in musculoskeletal imaging and evaluation of the cervical spine in neurologic imaging.

Suggested Readings

Blackmon GB, Major NM, Helms CA. Comparison of fast spin-echo versus conventional spin-echo MRI for evaluating meniscal tears. *AJR Am J Roentgenol.* 2005;184:1740–1743.

Edelman RR, Hesselink J, Zlatkin M. *Clinical Magnetic Resonance Imaging.* 2nd ed. Philadelphia: Saunders; 1996.

Filippi M, Yousry T, Baratti C, et al. Quantitative assessment of MRI lesion load in multiple sclerosis. *Brain.* 1996;119:1349–1355.

Gawne-Cain ML, O'Riordan JI, Thompson AJ, et al. Multiple sclerosis lesion detection in the brain: a comparison of fast fluid-attenuated inversion recovery and conventional T2-weighted dual spin echo. *Neurology.* 1997;49:364–370.

Kaplan PA, Dussault R, Helms CA, Anderson MW. *Musculoskeletal MRI.* Philadelphia: Saunders; 2001.

Miller DH, Grossman RI, Reingold SC, et al. The role of magnetic resonance techniques in understanding and managing multiple sclerosis. *Brain.* 1998;121:3–24.

Mitchell DG, Cohen M. *MRI Principles.* 2nd ed. Philadelphia: Elsevier; 2004.

Rubin D, Kneeland JB, Listerud J, et al. MR diagnosis of meniscal tears of the knee: value of fast spin-echo vs conventional spin-echo pulse sequences. *AJR Am J Roentgenol.* 1994;162:1131–1135.

Wolff AB, Pesce LL, Wu JS, et al. Comparison of spin echo T1-weighted sequences versus fast spin-echo proton density-weighted sequences for evaluation of meniscal tears at 1.5 T. *Skeletal Radiol.* 2009;38:21–29.

CHAPTER 4

Gadolinium-Based Contrast Agents

Charles M. Maxfield

OPENING CASE 4.1

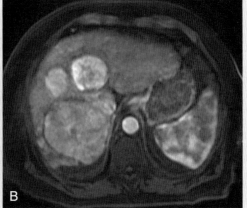

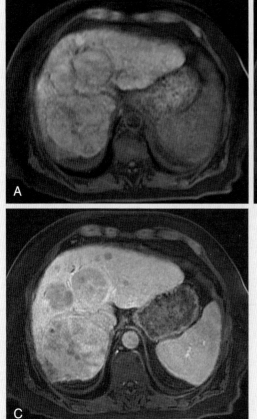

FIG. 4.C1. Fat-suppressed three-dimensional gradient recalled echo (GRE) T1-weighted (A) precontrast, (B) postcontrast arterial phase, and (C) portal venous phase images in a 58-year-old man with hepatitis C cirrhosis.

1. How do gadolinium-based contrast agents create contrast in clinical MRI?
   A. Gadolinium has a short inherent T1 relaxation time.
   B. Gadolinium has a long T2 relaxation time.
   C. Gadolinium manipulates the relaxation time of adjacent molecules.
   D. Gadolinium accentuates MRI sensitivity to flow.
2. Which of the following is a term used to reflect the effectiveness of an MRI contrast agent in shortening relaxation times?
   A. B_0
   B. Relaxivity
   C. Paramagnetism
   D. Coherence
3. Given the images provided in Figs. 4.C1, which of the following is the most likely diagnosis to explain the multiple liver masses?
   A. Multiple hemangiomas
   B. Regenerating nodules
   C. Hepatocellular carcinoma
   D. Fungal infection

OPENING CASE 4.1

FIG. 4.C1. Fat-suppressed three-dimensional, GRE, T1-weighted (D) precontrast and (E–F) postcontrast images demonstrate hyperenhancement of multiple large liver masses in the arterial phase (E), with rapid washout of contrast in the portal venous phase (F).

1. How do gadolinium-based contrast agents create contrast in clinical MRI?
   C. Gadolinium manipulates the relaxation time of adjacent molecules.
2. Which of the following is a measure of the effectiveness of an MR contrast agent in shortening relaxation times?
   B. Relaxivity
3. Given the images provided in Figs. 4.C1D–F, which of the following is the most likely diagnosis to explain the multiple liver masses in a 58-year-old man with hepatitis C cirrhosis?
   C. Hepatocellular carcinoma

Discussion

Question 1: Unlike iodinated contrast used in CT imaging, gadolinium is not directly seen on an MRI scan. Rather, this paramagnetic ion shortens the T1 relaxation time of molecules in the tissue in which it accumulates, so the tissue appears bright on T1-weighted images. It does this through an interaction between the protons of the tissues being imaged and the unpaired electrons of the paramagnetic gadolinium ion.

Question 2: The effectiveness of MRI contrast agents can be measured by their relaxivity, which can be thought of as the ability of the agent to decrease the relaxation rate of adjacent protons. The relaxivity of gadolinium-based contrast agents decreases as the magnetic field strength increases.

Question 3: Dynamic serial imaging with gadolinium-based contrast agents can characterize hepatic lesions. The multifocal hepatocellular carcinoma (HCC) shown in Figs. 4.C1D–F demonstrates the characteristic enhancement pattern, which can provide a definitive diagnosis in the appropriate clinical setting.

Because the typical HCC lacks a portal venous blood supply, it is supplied entirely by abnormal hepatic arteries. For this reason, HCC characteristically enhances during the arterial phase of imaging (Fig. 4.C1D), at which time it appears hyperenhanced relative to the surrounding liver parenchyma, which receives most of its blood supply from the portal veins. During the portal venous phase (Fig. 4.C1D), gadolinium reaches the liver parenchyma, which appears hyperintense relative to the mass and appears relatively hypointense due to its lack of portal venous supply. This so-called washout effect is characteristic of HCC and distinguishes it from other hepatic lesions. Occasionally, a fourth delayed phase of imaging is necessary to demonstrate the washout.

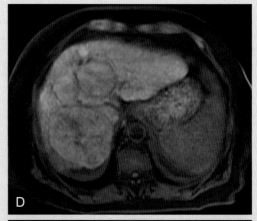

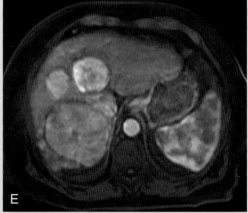

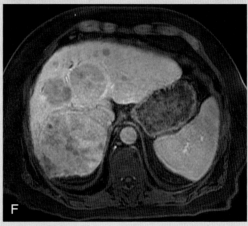

Physics

Gadolinium is an effective MRI contrast agent due to its paramagnetic properties, which enhance MRI contrast by shortening the T1 relaxation time of adjacent molecules. Paramagnetism is an intrinsic property of certain metals that have unpaired electrons. Because gadolinium has seven unpaired electrons, it is strongly paramagnetic. In the presence of an external magnetic field, these unpaired electrons create an oscillating magnetic field. If this magnetic field oscillates at or near the Larmor frequency, dipolar interactions occur with hydrogen protons in adjacent water molecules, resulting in spin lattice relaxation, which shortens the T1 relaxation time for these protons.

These interactions require that the water molecules be in very close proximity and bind transiently to the gadolinium complex. They are released in a microsecond, a process that is repeated, so the gadolinium ion can relax more than 1 million water molecules per second.

FIG. 4.C2

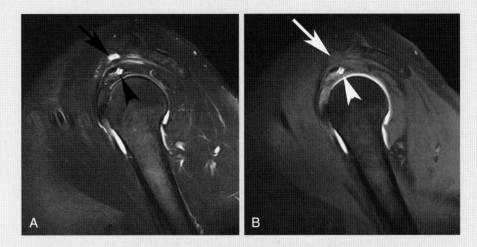

1. Given the images provided, which of the following is the most likely diagnosis?
   A. Partial-thickness supraspinatus tendon tear
   B. Full-thickness supraspinatus tendon tear
   C. Ganglion cyst
   D. Solid mass
2. Which administrative routes have been approved by the US Food and Drug Administration (FDA) for gadolinium administration? (Select all that apply.)
   A. Intravascular
   B. Intrathecal
   C. Oral
   D. Intraarticular

3. Of the following, which is the appropriate dilution of gadolinium for intraarticular administration?
   A. 2 mmol/L
   B. 100 mmol/L
   C. 500 mmol/L
   D. 1 mol/L

FIG. 4.C2. Sagittal oblique (A) T2-weighted and (B) T1-weighted MR arthrogram with fat saturation.

Discussion

Fig. 4.C2 demonstrates high signal in the supraspinatus tendon *(black and white arrowheads)*, consistent with a tear. The signal is bright on both T1- and T2-weighted imaging, suggesting that there is gadolinium within the tear. There is also high T2 signal within the subacromial-subdeltoid bursa *(black arrow* in A), which is low in signal on the T1-weighted image *(white arrow* in B), consistent with fluid without gadolinium, suggesting that this may be a partial-thickness tear.

Gadolinium-based contrast agents (GBCAs) have been approved by the FDA only for intravascular administration. This does not preclude their oral, intraarticular, or intrathecal administration. In fact, GBCAs are routinely administered by these routes. The FDA, like regulatory government agencies in many countries, permits the discretionary use of approved drugs for nonapproved purposes (off-label use). This policy allows physicians to administer an FDA-approved drug by an alternative route or dose when it may benefit a patient.

Gadolinium-enhanced MR arthrography has proven valuable in demonstrating small tears in cartilage or ligaments that are not visible on routine MRI. Gadolinium has been used orally as an enteric contrast agent and intrathecally when evaluating for suspect cerebrospinal fluid leaks.

Gadolinium is typically prepared at a concentration of 500 mmol/L for intravascular administration but must be highly diluted with saline solution for intraarticular administration, normally to a concentration of 2 mmol/L. The exact dilution and volume injected can vary according to which joint is being studied. This dilute gadolinium results in T1 shortening and increased signal. In combination with joint expansion and fat suppression, sensitivity is increased for lesions of the labrum and other capsular ligamentous structures. If gadolinium were injected into the joint without first being diluted, the joint space would display low signal because of the significant T2-shortening effects.

CASE 4.2 ANSWERS

1. **A. Partial-thickness supraspinatus tendon tear**
2. **A. Intravascular**
3. **A. 2 mmol/L**

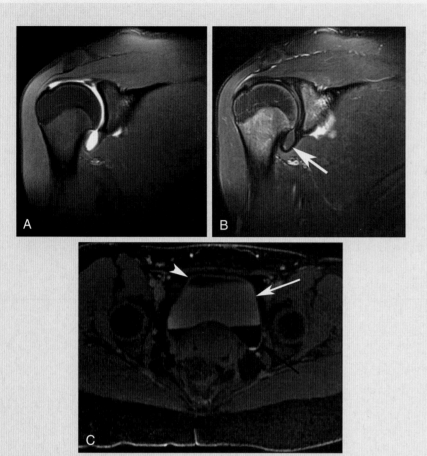

FIG. 4.C3

1. The intraarticular fluid on the T2-weighted image (Fig. 4.C3B) is unexpectedly dark. Which of the following is the best explanation for this finding?
   A. Joint hemorrhage
   B. Iodinated contrast agent injected along with gadolinium to confirm intraarticular position of needle
   C. Insufficiently diluted gadolinium
   D. Overly dilute gadolinium

FIG. 4.C3. Coronal oblique fat-saturated (A) T1-weighted image and (B) coronal oblique T2-weighted image from an MR arthrogram. (C) Axial GRE delayed, postcontrast, T1-weighted image demonstrates layering of fluid of different signal intensities in the bladder (parfait effect).

Discussion

Note that on the T1-weighted image (Fig. 4.C3A), there is a small tear of the superior glenoid labrum. Also note on the T2-weighted image (Fig. 4.C3B) that the intraarticular fluid *(white arrow)* is unexpectedly low in signal. This is the result of the administration of a gadolinium solution that was 10 times more concentrated than what is normally used, resulting in T2- shortening effects of fluid on the T2-weighted image.

Low-dose gadolinium has mild T2-shortening effects, but these are overwhelmed by the more dominant T1-shortening effects that increase signal intensity. At high concentrations, however, gadolinium's T2-shortening effects can predominate over its T1-shortening properties, resulting in a decrease in signal (on both T1-weighted and T2-weighted) sequences, as seen in Fig. 4.C3B.

A similar phenomenon is demonstrated in Fig. 4.C3C. The so-called parfait effect can be seen in the bladder or renal pelvis on supine patients on delayed, postcontrast, T1-weighted excretory phase images. A middle layer *(white arrow)*, in which the gadolinium concentration is diluted with urine, is hyperintense on T1 because the T1-shortening effects of gadolinium predominate at lower gadolinium concentrations—the gadolinium is diluted by urine. The top layer *(white arrowhead)* is hypointense because it contains only urine, without gadolinium. The bottom layer *(black arrow)* is low in signal because of the higher concentration of gadolinium, in which case the T2-shortening effects predominate over the T1-shortening effects.

CASE 4.3 ANSWERS

1. **C. Insufficiently diluted gadolinium**

FIG. 4.C4

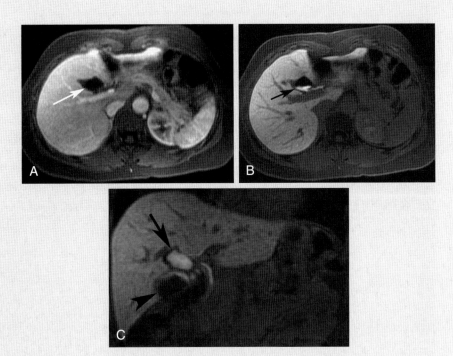

1. Of the following gadolinium-based contrast agents, which is most likely to have been used in this case?
   A. A blood pool agent
   B. An extracellular contrast agent
   C. A hepatocyte (hepatobiliary) agent
   D. A manganese agent

2. Based on the images provided, which of the following is the most likely diagnosis in an 8-year-old with jaundice and abdominal pain?
   A. Acute cholecystitis
   B. Acalculous cholecystitis
   C. Cholangiocarcinoma
   D. Choledochal cyst

FIG. 4.C4. (A) Portal venous phase. This three-dimensional GRE volumetric interpolated breath-hold examination sequence demonstrates a low-signal region in the anterior segment of the right hepatic lobe *(arrow)*. (B) Axial image acquired 20 minutes after contrast administration demonstrates biliary excretion of contrast into this low-signal area *(arrow)*. (C) Coronal image shows that this structure *(arrow)* is separate from the gallbladder *(arrowhead)* but that they both contain contrast.

Discussion

Gadolinium-based contrast agents can be classified by their biodistribution into extracellular, blood pool, and hepatobiliary agents. The **extracellular agents** are the most commonly used and are the least expensive MRI contrast agents. Common trade names include MultiHance (gadobenate), Omniscan (gadodiamide), Dotarem (gadoterate), ProHance (gadoteridol), Optimark (gadoversetamide), and Magnevist (gadopentetate). These extracellular agents can be further categorized by their chemical structure as macrocyclic or linear. Gadolinium ions are more tightly bound and less likely to disassociate from macrocyclic agents, which are therefore considered more stable and potentially safer than the linear (or open-chain) agents. The pharmacokinetics of these agents is similar to those of iodine—their excretion is almost entirely though passive glomerular filtration in the kidneys. Following the arterial first pass, these agents diffuse out of the blood pool fairly rapidly and are distributed into the extracellular interstitium.

Gadolinium-based **blood pool agents** are characterized by prolonged intravascular circulation, allowing for steady-state vascular imaging for up to 60 minutes postinjection. These agents bind reversibly to albumin, resulting in large macromolecules that limit diffusion across the endothelial membrane. There are no commercially available blood pool agents currently on the US market, although Ablavar (gadofosveset) has FDA approval as an agent for contrast-enhanced MR angiography.

Because approximately 50% of the **hepatobiliary MR contrast agents** is excreted into the biliary system (50% is excreted through the kidneys), they can be used to assess function and integrity of the biliary system. Because these contrast agents accumulate in hepatocytes, they are also valuable for the detection and characterization of focal hepatic lesions, particularly in cases of suspected focal nodular hyperplasia (FNH). As a rule, images following the administration of these hepatocyte-specific contrast agents are acquired after a longer delay compared with the extracellular agents, particularly for the evaluation of the biliary system. Eovist (gadoxetate) is the most commonly used hepatobiliary MR contrast agent.

The images provided demonstrate a cystic mass in the porta hepatitis, which is separate from the gallbladder. Excretion of the hepatobiliary MR contrast agent (Eovist) into the cyst confirms its communication with the biliary system and establishes the diagnosis of choledochal cyst.

CASE 4.4 ANSWERS

1. **C. A hepatocyte (hepatobiliary) agent**
2. **D. Choledochal cyst**

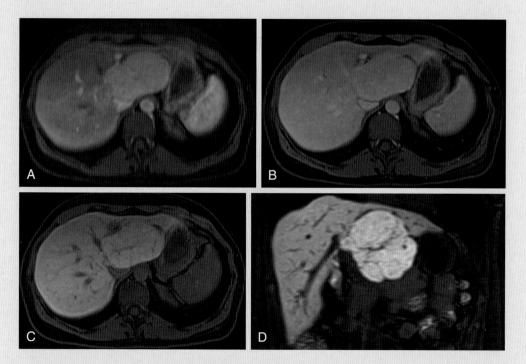

FIG. 4.C5

1. Which of the following gadolinium-based contrast agents would be the agent of choice to characterize a hepatic mass detected on another imaging study further?
   A. A blood pool agent
   B. An extracellular contrast agent
   C. A hepatocyte (hepatobiliary) agent
   D. A manganese agent

2. Based on the images provided, which of the following is the most likely diagnosis?
   A. Hemangioma
   B. Hepatic adenoma
   C. Focal nodular hyperplasia
   D. Hepatocellular carcinoma

FIG. 4.C5. (A) Three-dimensional GRE, volumetric interpolated breath-hold examination. This postcontrast (Eovist) arterial phase image demonstrates a large hyperenhancing mass in the left hepatic lobe. (B) The mass is isointense to the liver parenchyma on the portal venous phase image. Hepatocyte phase images in the axial (C) and coronal (D) planes demonstrate hyperenhancement of the mass relative to the liver parenchyma.

Discussion

Any of the gadolinium-based MR contrast agents can help characterize liver lesions. The enhancement characteristics during the arterial and portal venous phases of imaging assist in narrowing diagnostic considerations for liver lesions. Hepatobiliary agents can add further specificity to the diagnostic workup of a liver mass, particular in the case of FNH. Because these agents are actively transported into the hepatocytes before being excreted in the bile ducts, they can reliably differentiate FNH, which contain hepatocytes and bile ducts, from tumors that do not—hemangiomas, metastases, adenomas, and poorly differentiated hepatocellular carcinomas.

There is a broad differential for a hyperenhancing mass with rapid fade-in of contrast enhancement during the arterial phase of imaging. The delayed phase images distinguish this mass. Notice the persistent enhancement of the mass on the delayed phase images (Fig. 4.C5C–D). This

is characteristic of focal nodular hyperplasia (FNH). FNH contains hepatocytes that take up hepatobiliary contrast agents. Because the bile ducts are malformed in FNH, they excrete the contrast agent inefficiently. This explains why they retain contrast on delayed imaging long after other liver lesions have washed out.

Note that in this case the mass demonstrates greater hyperintensity on the coronal image (Fig. 4.C5D) than on the axial image (Fig. 4.C5C), although both are delayed. This is explained by the fact that the flip angle on the axial image is 10 degrees, and it is 30 degrees for the coronal image. The higher flip angle increases the T1 weighting.

CASE 4.5 ANSWERS

1. **C. A hepatocyte (hepatobiliary) agent**
2. **C. Hepatocellular carcinoma**

FIG. 4.C6

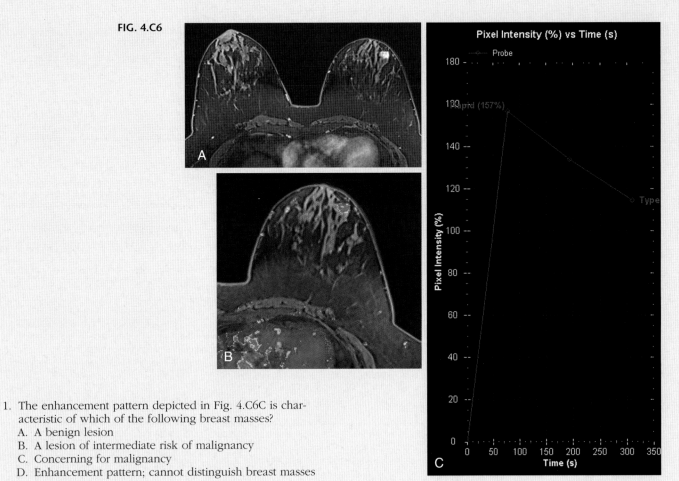

1. The enhancement pattern depicted in Fig. 4.C6C is characteristic of which of the following breast masses?
   A. A benign lesion
   B. A lesion of intermediate risk of malignancy
   C. Concerning for malignancy
   D. Enhancement pattern; cannot distinguish breast masses

FIG. 4.C6. (A) Axial first-pass postcontrast T1-weighted image with fat suppression. (B) Postcontrast image of breast mass with color overlay. (C) Graph demonstrating the enhancement curve of the mass.

Discussion

Enhancement kinetics are used in MRI of the breast to help characterize breast lesions better. Three enhancement patterns plotted on a signal intensity–time curve have been described (Fig. 4.1).

- Type I is a pattern of steadily increasing or persistent enhancement. This type of enhancement pattern typically represents a more benign pattern of enhancement.
- Type II is a pattern of initial rapid enhancement that then plateaus. This enhancement pattern is associated with an intermediate risk of malignancy.
- Type III is a pattern of early initial enhancement with rapid washout. This pattern of enhancement is the most concerning for malignancy.

Fig. 4.C6C demonstrates a rapid washout of contrast after an initial early enhancement, which is characteristic of malignancy. Biopsy confirmed an invasive ductal carcinoma.

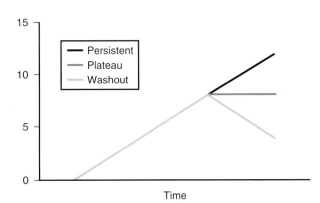

FIG. 4.1. Graph demonstrating various potential enhancement curves of a breast lesion.

CASE 4.6 ANSWERS

1. **C. Concerning for malignancy**

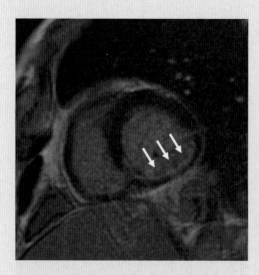

FIG. 4.C7

1. Based on the image, which of the following is the most likely diagnosis?
   A. Right coronary artery (RCA) distribution infarction
   B. RCA distribution ischemia
   C. Myocarditis
   D. Sarcoidosis
2. Which of the following is the greatest risk factor for nephrogenic systemic fibrosis (NSF)?
   A. Chronic kidney disease
   B. Immunosuppression
   C. Liver dysfunction
   D. Acute kidney disease
3. Which of the following is a finding of the FDA's 2017 review of safety ramifications of gadolinium accumulation in the brain?
   A. There is no retention of gadolinium in the brain.
   B. Gadolinium is retained in the brain only in patients with renal or liver failure.
   C. Retention of gadolinium in the brain is dose dependent.
   D. Retention of gadolinium in the brain is associated with adverse health effects.

FIG. 4.C7. This short-axis, delayed-enhancement MR image of the heart of a 51-year-old man with chest pain (segmented inversion recovery prepared fast GRE sequence) demonstrates subendocardial delayed enhancement in the inferior wall of the left ventricle (*arrows*).

Discussion

Myocardial delayed enhancement images are produced by a 180-degree inversion recovery preparatory pulse, followed by a GRE sequence. The inversion recovery pulse time to inversion is set to null the myocardium and enhance T1 relaxation, which increases the contrast between the myocardium and region of enhancement. Delayed enhancement imaging is helpful in demonstrating infarcted myocardium and in establishing whether there is viable myocardium that would benefit from reperfusion. It has been postulated that delayed enhancement occurs in regions of acute myocardial infarction secondary to cell membrane breakdown, which allows gadolinium chelate to enter the cell. The gadolinium chelate remains within the ischemic tissue while it washes out of the nonaffected myocardium, which leads to T1 shortening and increased signal. Delayed enhancement is also seen within areas of chronic myocardial infarction. It is currently believed that fibrous tissue (infarct) has a greater area of interstitial space in which the gadolinium chelate can disperse when compared with the interstitial space surrounding normal packed cells. Viability is defined as myocardium in the region of ischemia that could survive if coronary revascularization is performed. If the hyperenhancement involves less than 50% of the myocardial wall, then remaining viable myocardium would benefit from coronary revascularization.

NSF is a progressive debilitating disease characterized by widespread fibrosis in the skin and subcutaneous tissues. In severe cases, the lungs, esophagus, heart, and skeletal muscles may be involved. NSF develops in patients with moderate to end-stage renal impairment who have had exposure to GBCAs. It typically presents weeks to months after the administration of gadolinium for MR scanning.

Although the exact mechanism remains unclear, it has been postulated that free gadolinium ions are disassociated from the chelate in patients with poor renal function due to the prolonged clearance time of GBCA. This leads to activation of circulating fibroblasts, which results in inflammation and fibrosis.

Less stable GBCAs (e.g., gadodiamide, gadoversetamide, gadopentetic acid), in which the gadolinium more easily dissociates from its chelate, have the strongest association with NSF. The ionic macrocyclic gadolinium chelates are the most stable GBCAs and are thought to have the best safety profile in patients with renal failure.

The American College of Radiology (ACR) has recommended that a screening glomerular filtration rate (GFR) be determined in any patient with suspected renal disease. GBCA should not be used in patients with a GFR below 30 mL/min per 1.73 m^2 or those requiring dialysis.

A 2013 report noted that gadolinium is retained in the brain of patients who had received multiple doses of gadolinium. The deposition of gadolinium was found to be most concentrated in the dentate nucleus and globi pallidi. The retention correlates with the number of gadolinium administrations and may also depend on the chemical structure of the administered gadolinium complex. Macrocyclic agents appear to present less risk than linear agents.

The FDA has reviewed the safety ramification of this discovery and, in early 2017, released a drug safety communication confirming that small amounts of gadolinium can be retained in the brain (and other tissues) in patients with normal renal function, but found no adverse health effects. Gadolinium use was not restricted, although the safety of gadolinium will continue to be assessed.

CASE 4.7 ANSWERS

1. **B. RCA distribution infarction**
2. **A. Chronic kidney disease**
3. **C. Retention of gadolinium in the brain is dose dependent.**

TAKE-HOME POINTS

1. Gadolinium is a paramagnetic element that results in T1 shortening (increased signal on T1-weighted images).
2. Relaxivity is a measure of the efficiency of a contrast agent to decrease T1 and T2 relaxation times.
3. At low contrast medium concentrations, the T1 relaxation effect predominates as a result of the fast inherent transverse relaxation in tissue. The result is increased signal on T1-weighted images. However, at high concentrations of contrast medium, the T2 relaxation time is so short that low signal results.
4. The relaxivity of contrast agents decreases as the magnetic field strength increases.
5. Unlike CT, in which the iodine molecule itself generates the contrast, gadolinium changes signal through its effects on the surrounding protons during MRI.
6. Extracellular contrast agents are the most commonly used.
7. Eovist (and, to a lesser extent, MultiHance) is unique in that it is excreted in part by the hepatobiliary system. Eovist has a higher relaxivity because it exhibits low-level binding to plasma proteins and can stay in the blood pool longer; thus it has a shorter half-life because of its dual excretion.
8. Eovist can aid in differentiating tumors that contain bile ducts from tumors that do not.
9. Ablavar is an FDA-approved agent for contrast-enhanced MRA. It has a very long plasma half-life and very high relaxivity, which allows for a much lower administered dose and increased flexibility in imaging the vasculature.
10. Ionic, macrocyclic gadolinium chelates are the most stable and therefore thought to have the best safety profile in patients with renal failure.

Suggested Readings

American College of Radiology. ACR Committee on Drugs and Contrast Media: ACR Manual on Contrast Media, Version 10.3. https://www.acr.org/Quality-Safety/Resources/Contrast-Manual/.

Beomonte Zobel B, Quattrocchi CC, Errante Y, Grasso RF. Gadolinium-based contrast agents: did we miss something in the last 25 years? *Radiol Med*. 2016;131:478–481.

Edelman RR, Hesselink JR, Zlatkin MB, Crues JV III. *Clinical Magnetic Resonance Imaging*. Philadelphia: Elsevier; 2006.

Gandhi SN, Brown MA, Wong JG, et al. MR contrast agents for liver imaging: what, when, how. *Radiographics*. 2006;26:1621–1636.

Hadizadeh DR, Gieseke J, Lohmaier SH, et al. Peripheral MR angiography with blood pool contrast agent: prospective intraindividual comparative study of high-spatial-resolution steady-state MR angiography versus standard-resolution first-pass MR angiography and DSA. *Radiology*. 2008;249:701–711.

Juluru KM, Vogel-Claussen J, Macura K, et al. MR imaging in patients at risk for developing nephrogenic systemic fibrosis: protocols, practices, and imaging techniques to maximize patient safety. *Radiographics*. 2009;29:9–22.

Kanda T, Ishii H, Kawaguchi K, et al. High signal intensity in the dentate nucleus and globus pallidus on unenhanced T1-weighted MR images: relationship with increasing cumulative dose of a gadolinium-based contrast material. *Radiology*. 2014;270:834–841.

Macura KJ, Ouwerkerk R, Jacobs MA, Bluemke DA. Patterns of enhancement on breast MR images: interpretation and imaging pitfalls. *Radiographics*. 2006;26:1719–1734.

Morcos SK, Thomsen HS. Nephrogenic systemic fibrosis: more questions and some answers. *Nephron Clin Pract*. 2008;110:c24–c31.

Penfield J, Riley R. Nephrogenic systemic fibrosis risk: is there a difference between gadolinium-based contrast agents? *Semin Dialysis*. 2008;21:129–134.

Rohrer M, Bauer H, Mintorovitch J, et al. Comparison of magnetic properties of MRI contrast media solutions at different magnetic field strengths. *Invest Radiol*. 2005;40:715–724.

US Food and Drug Administration (FDA). Gadolinium-based contrast agents for magnetic resonance imaging (MRI): drug safety communication—no harmful effects identified with brain retention. https://www.fda.gov/safety/medwatch/safetyinformation/safety-alertsforhumanmedicalproducts/ucm559709.htm.

CHAPTER 5

Frequency and Spatial Saturation Pulses

Phil B. Hoang, Allen W. Song, and Elmar M. Merkle

OPENING CASE 5.1

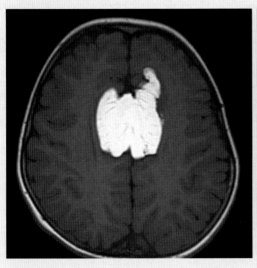 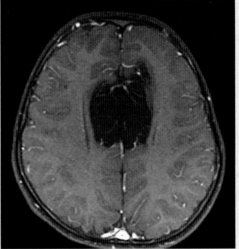

1. In an MRI sequence, when are the radiofrequency (RF) pulse and spoiler gradients used to suppress fat applied?
   A. Before the excitation pulse
   B. Simultaneously with the excitation pulse
   C. Immediately after the excitation pulse
   D. Performed after the entire examination is completed (postprocessing feature)

OPENING CASE 5.1

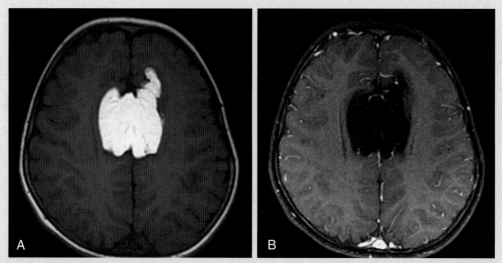

FIG. 5.C1. (A) Axial T1-weighted image demonstrates the mass's interhemispheric position; thin, linear hypointense septa are noted. (B) Axial postcontrast T1-weighted image with fat saturation. The mass exhibits homogeneous signal loss.

1. In an MRI sequence, when are the RF pulse and spoiler gradients used to suppress fat applied?
   A. Before the excitation pulse

Diagnosis

This is a lipoma of the corpus callosum.

Discussion

Fat suppression techniques use a narrow-bandwidth RF pulse tuned to the resonant frequency of hydrogen protons in fat, selectively exciting those protons. This is followed by a spoiler gradient that dephases the magnetized lipid protons, rendering them unable to produce signal. Thereafter the excitation pulse to begin the MR imaging sequence is applied.

Saturation Pulses

The common link between inversion recovery, spatial presaturation, frequency selective, and magnetization transfer techniques is the use of an RF pulse administered before the excitation pulse, which is referred to as the **preparatory pulse**. This chapter covers frequency-selective and spatial saturation pulses; Chapter 6 reviews inversion recovery.

Frequency-selective saturation is a widely used and versatile technique. It is based on the assumption that a hydrogen proton resonates at a certain frequency according to its unique molecular environment. Protons in water and lipid resonate at different frequencies when under the same external magnetic field due to the micromolecular environments unique to each tissue. These differences increase with increases in magnetic field strength. For example, protons in fat precess 74 Hz *slower* than protons in free water at 0.5 T, 220 Hz slower at 1.5 T, and 448 Hz slower at 3 T. Frequency-selective saturation takes advantage of these differences in precessional frequencies, which allows signal suppression of fat or water (Fig. 5.1).

Once the target protons are saturated (Fig. 5.2), they are dephased when a spoiler gradient is applied (Fig. 5.3). This spoiling of the protons' transverse magnetization suppresses their ability to produce signal. The excitation pulse is administered soon after to begin the imaging sequence. As noted, water or fat signal may be suppressed if the appropriate RF saturation pulse is used.

The most common clinical use of frequency-selective saturation is suppression of the normally high signal intensity arising from fat, particularly in T2-weighted and postcontrast T1-weighted images. Benefits of frequency-selective saturation

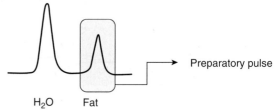

FIG. 5.1. Frequency-selective saturation uses a narrow-range RF preparatory pulse *(box)* that matches the resonant frequency of the target protons, saturating them.

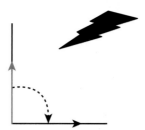

FIG. 5.2. First, a frequency-selective preparatory pulse *(black bolt)* with a narrow range of frequencies matching the resonant frequency of the target proton is administered *(black arrow)*. The remaining protons *(gray arrow)* are unaffected and stay in net longitudinal magnetization.

include its use to confirm or exclude the presence of fat within a high T1 signal intensity mass and to suppress fat on postcontrast T1-weighted sequences, which functions to increase tissue-lesion contrast and margin characterization.

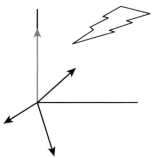

FIG. 5.3. A spoiler gradient (*white bolt*) is subsequently applied, which dephases the protons magnetized by the preparatory pulse and eliminates their ability to produce signal. The excitation RF pulse is sent soon after and excites only the unspoiled protons.

Because the frequency-selective saturation pulse is broadcast at a narrow-range RF to affect the target protons specifically, the quality of signal suppression depends on a uniform magnetic field. The presence of magnetic field inhomogeneities typically results in poor signal suppression and, at times, inadvertent signal suppression of nontarget tissues.

Also, because fat has a short T1 relaxation time, it recovers a measure of its net longitudinal magnetization during the time between the preparatory and excitation pulses. This may require multiple fat saturation pulses to obtain the preferred signal loss, which contributes to energy deposition in the patient.

Frequency-selective techniques are typically not used at lower magnetic field strengths (<1.0 T) because of an excessive overlap of resonant frequencies between water and lipid protons. This leads not only to incomplete saturation of the desired protons but also to saturation of nontarget protons.

Another setting in which a preparatory pulse is administered to affect tissue contrast is **magnetization transfer** (MT). MT refers to the transfer of longitudinal magnetization from restricted water protons to free water protons. This technique is based on the concept that restricted water protons bound to macromolecules (e.g., proteins, lipids) are subject to greater local field inhomogeneities. Free water protons, on the other hand, exist in a comparatively uniform magnetic field environment. The different environments lead to different ranges of resonance frequencies of the water protons; free water will have a narrow resonance frequency range, near 63 MHz (1.5 T), whereas the range of resonance frequencies in bound water protons will be much broader owing to the inherent field inhomogeneities in their environment. Therefore an off-resonance preparatory pulse will preferentially saturate bound water protons. What allows for variable soft tissue contrast, however, is the phenomenon whereby magnetization is then transferred from bound water protons to available adjacent free water protons, leading to a saturation effect. The result is reduced signal from the free water protons in tissues in which the MT phenomenon is prevalent. Because the extent of signal decay depends on the exchange rate between free and bound water protons, MT can be used to provide an alternative contrast method to complement T1,T2, and proton density methods. The most accepted application is in magnetic resonance angiography (MRA), where MT markedly suppresses background tissue signal while leaving flowing blood unaffected. MT is also believed to be a nonspecific indicator of the structural integrity of the tissues and has found promising applicability in highlighting specific tissue abnormalities in the brain (e.g., demyelination in multiple sclerosis).

Spatial selective presaturation is a technique used to suppress signal arising from regions of the body *outside* the imaging area of interest but *inside* the field of view. It is frequently used in spinal imaging, in which reduction of phase-related motion artifact arising from the peristalsing bowel and the tongue during swallowing is achieved with application of a saturation band placed over the abdomen and mouth, respectively.

CASE 5.2

FIG. 5.C2

1. Which of the following is preferred for fat suppression on gadolinium-enhanced, T1-weighted images?
   A. Frequency-selective fat saturation
   B. Short tau inversion recovery (STIR)
   C. Dual-echo opposed-phase imaging
   D. A and B

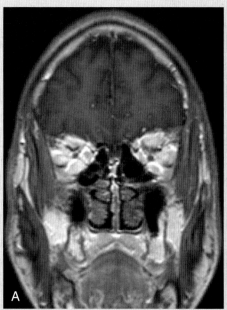
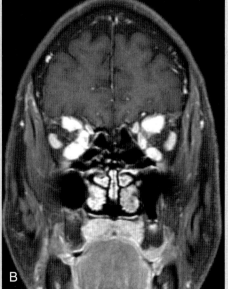

FIG. 5.C2. (A) Coronal postcontrast T1-weighted image demonstrates diffusely hyperintense signal within the bilateral orbits. (B) Coronal postcontrast T1-weighted image with fat saturation demonstrates marked enhancement and enlargement of the bilateral intraocular muscles.

Discussion

Gadolinium-perfused tissues on postcontrast T1-weighted sequences may demonstrate T1 relaxation times similar to those of fat, which can make the distinction between enhancing lesions in a background of fat challenging. There is diffuse high signal intensity present within the bilateral orbits on the postcontrast T1-weighted sequence (Fig. 5.C2A). Using fat saturation (Fig. 5.C2B) to suppress signal from the orbital fat reveals avid enhancement and diffuse enlargement of the intraocular muscles in this patient with Graves disease.

CASE 5.3

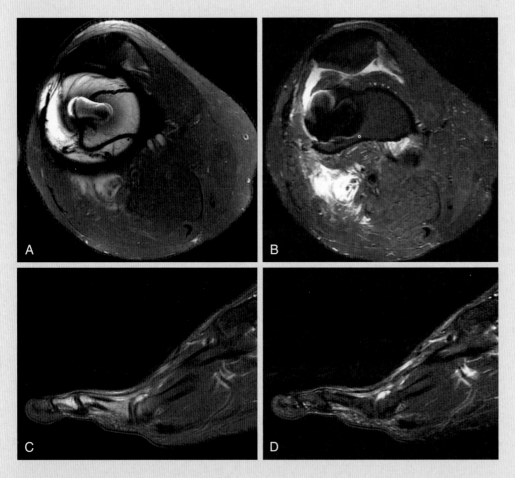

FIG. 5.C3

1. Which of the following is not an ideal setting in which to use frequency-selective saturation?
   A. Air-bone interfaces
   B. Orthopedic hardware
   C. Sharp anatomic contour variations
   D. All of the above

FIG. 5.C3. (A) Axial T2-weighted image with fat saturation of the knee demonstrates an interference screw in the distal femur, which causes geometric distortion, signal loss, signal pile-up, and failed fat suppression in the surrounding tissues. (B) Axial STIR image of the knee at the same level demonstrates near-homogeneous fat suppression in the tissues surrounding the interference screw. Geometric distortion, signal loss, and signal pile-up related to the screw, however, remain. (C) Sagittal T2-weighted image with fat saturation demonstrates increased signal involving the phalanges and soft tissues of the toe. (D) Sagittal STIR image of the same toe demonstrates a homogeneous hypointense signal in the phalanges and soft tissues.

Discussion

Frequency-selective saturation assumes that all protons are precessing at the same resonant frequency, with more uniform signal suppression achieved with greater magnetic field homogeneity. Unfortunately, field inhomogeneities are invariably present, particularly in areas of the body where there are significant differences in magnetic susceptibility. This includes air-tissue interfaces (answer A), orthopedic hardware (answer B), and variations in anatomic contours (answer C).

The significant artifact on the fat-saturated, T2-weighted image of the knee (Fig. 5.C3A) is due to the presence of a titanium interference screw (used for an anterior cruciate ligament reconstruction in this case), which induces large variations in the precession rate of protons and dephasing. This results in signal loss, geometric distortion, failed frequency-selective fat suppression, and signal pile-up—which, in short, represent an accumulation of signals from multiple different positions misregistered into one position and manifest as areas of hyperintense signal.

STIR is less susceptible to magnetic field inhomogeneities and is more effective for fat suppression when metallic hardware is in place, as illustrated in Fig. 5.C3B. STIR provides effective fat suppression in the setting of anatomic contour variations (Fig. 5.C3D), which can cause ineffective fat saturation and present as bone marrow edema on the fat-saturated T2-weighted image (Fig. 5.C3C).

CASE 5.3 ANSWERS

1. **D. All of the above**

CASE 5.4

FIG. 5.C4

1. Which of the following does the left renal mass definitively *not* contain?
   A. Methemoglobin
   B. Protein
   C. Fat
   D. A and B

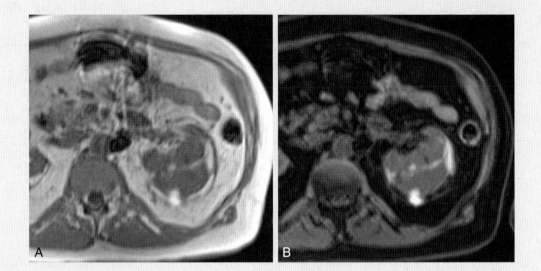

FIG. 5.C4. (A) Axial T1-weighted, dual-echo, in-phase image of the left hemiabdomen. A mixed signal intensity posterior left renal mass demonstrates a peripheral margin of increased T1 signal volumetric interpolated breath-hold examination (VIBE) intensity, which is isointense to fat. (B) Axial T1-weighted VIBE fat-saturated image without intravenous contrast. Subcutaneous and intraabdominal fat signal is hypointense; the high T1 signal arising from the left renal mass persists.

Discussion

Two important uses of fat saturation are as follows: (1) suppression of high signal intensity fat to promote additional contrast; and (2) confirmation of the presence or absence of fat. The left renal mass demonstrates high T1 signal peripherally, which is isointense compared with subcutaneous and intraabdominal fat on the axial in-phase, T1-weighted image (Fig. 5.C4A). This raises the possibility of a fat-containing mass, such as an angiomyolipoma. However, given the lack of signal loss following the administration of fat saturation (Fig. 5.C4B), a fat-containing mass is excluded. As previously discussed in Chapter 1, methemoglobin is a hemoglobin derivative that has T1-shortening properties and can produce a hyperintense T1 signal, as in this case of a subcapsular renal hematoma.

CASE 5.4 ANSWERS

1. **C. Fat**

CASE 5.5

FIG. 5.C5

1. Fig. 5.C5A was obtained before Fig. 5.C5B. What was done to decrease the motion artifact from peristalsis in the bowel loops in Fig. 5.C5B?
   A. Longer breath-hold by the patient
   B. Decreasing the width of the saturation band
   C. Increasing the width of the saturation band
   D. Increasing the time to repetition

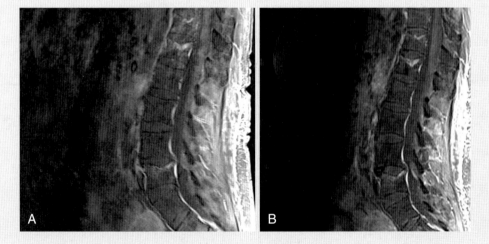

FIG. 5.C5. (A) Sagittal postcontrast T1-weighted image with fat saturation of the lumbar spine. Heterogeneity and poor resolution of the lumbar vertebral bodies and spinal canal are evident. Note a thin hypointense band, which projects over the central abdomen. (B) Sagittal postcontrast T1-weighted image. There is marked improvement in the resolution of the lumbar spine compared with Fig. 5.C5A. A wider hypointense band is evident in the abdomen.

Discussion

Spatial presaturation is used to suppress unwanted signal arising from tissues within the imaging slice, but not in the area of clinical concern. Similar to fat and water saturation, spatial presaturation uses a frequency-selective RF pulse, followed by a spoiler gradient. Localizer images are used to place a saturation band over regions of the body that are potential sources of motion artifact.

Motion arising from peristalsis in the bowel loops in the abdomen produces a phase-related artifact that propagates posteriorly in the lumbar spine. The initial attempt at using a narrow saturation band (Fig. 5.C5A) placed over the abdomen was insufficient in reducing the signals arising from the bowel loops. A wider saturation band covering virtually the entire width of bowel was used, resulting in a reduction in the artifact and improved resolution of the lumbar spine (Fig. 5.C5B).

CASE 5.5 ANSWER

1. **C. Increasing the width of the saturation band**

TAKE-HOME POINTS

1. Preparatory pulses are techniques that use an RF pulse administered before the excitation pulse.
2. Frequency-selective saturation, spatial selective presaturation, MT, and inversion recovery use variations of preparatory pulses to affect tissue contrast.
3. Frequency-selective saturation is a common technique used to suppress signal from fat or water protons. A preparatory pulse selectively excites the targeted region; a spoiler gradient is subsequently applied to dephase the magnetized protons, rendering them unable to produce signal after the excitation pulse is applied.
4. The quality of frequency-selective saturation depends on the magnetic field strength and presence of magnetic field inhomogeneities—the greater the field strength, the more specific the proton saturation.
5. Magnetic field inhomogeneities cause variations of the target proton resonant frequency, resulting in incomplete signal suppression. Scenarios in which fat saturation fails include air-bone interfaces, orthopedic hardware, and asymmetric body parts (e.g., feet, axilla).
6. Preparatory pulses can be used with virtually any imaging sequence. The consequences of this include an increase in imaging time, increased RF energy deposition, and a decrease in the signal-to-noise ratio.
7. Spatial presaturation pulses are administered outside the area of interest in the body. These are primarily used to reduce signal from protons responsible for motion-related artifacts (e.g., peristalsis in the bowel).
8. MT techniques use an off-peak RF pulse to magnetize bound water protons in macromolecules. These protons then transfer their magnetization to free water protons, leading to a saturation effect. The result is decreased signal in areas where this MT phenomenon has occurred.

Suggested Readings

Bogaert J, Dymarkoqwski S, Taylor AM, Muthurangu V, eds. *Clinical Cardiac MRI*. New York: Springer; 2005.

Delfaut EM, Beltran J, Johnson G, et al. Fat suppression in MR imaging: techniques and pitfalls. *Radiographics*. 1999;19:373–382.

Henkelman RM, Stanisz GJ, Graham SJ. Magnetization transfer in MRI: a review. *NMR Biomed*. 2001;14(2):57–64.

Lee MJ, Kim S, Lee SA, et al. Overcoming artifacts from metallic orthopedic implants at high-field-strength MR imaging and multi-detector CT. *Radiographics*. 2007;27:791–803.

Merkle EM, Nelson RC. Dual gradient-echo in-phase and opposed-phase hepatic MR imaging: a useful tool for evaluating more than fatty infiltration or fatty sparing. *Radiographics*. 2006;26(5):1409–1418.

Mitchell DG, Cohen MS. *MRI Principles*. 2nd ed. Philadelphia: Elsevier; 2004.

CHAPTER 6

Inversion Recovery

Phil B. Hoang, Allen W. Song, and Elmar M. Merkle

OPENING CASE 6.1

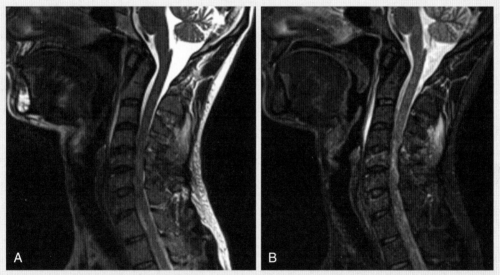

FIG. 6.C1. (A) Sagittal T2 fast spin echo (FSE) of the cervical spine demonstrates mild height loss of the C5 vertebral body and high T2 signal in the prevertebral soft tissues. Cervical spinal canal stenosis is noted at this level, with possible mild high T2 signal within the cord. (B) Sagittal short tau inversion recovery (STIR) at the same level. Prevertebral edema is more evident, with edema now evident in the C5, C6, and C7 vertebral bodies. Persistent, abnormal high signal intensity of the posterior soft tissues is consistent with ligamentous injury. Possible mild high T2 signal in the spinal cord at this level is confirmed on the STIR image.

1. Inversion recovery techniques are based on which of the following tissue-specific properties?
   A. T1 relaxation time
   B. T2 relaxation time
   C. Proton density
   D. Resonance frequency

OPENING CASE 6.1

1. Inversion recovery techniques are based on which of the following tissue-specific properties?
   A. T1 relaxation time

Discussion

Inversion recovery techniques rely on tissue-specific T1 relaxation times to produce the desired tissue contrasts. In the case of the STIR sequence used in Fig. 6.C1B, this results in suppression of signal arising from fat.

Inversion Recovery

Inversion recovery belongs to the family of preparatory pulse sequences. Chapter 5 reviewed both frequency-selective and spatial presaturation pulses; this chapter reviews inversion recovery. Although the use of a preparatory pulse in inversion recovery is similar to frequency-selective techniques, the principle behind the desired signal nulling is different. *Inversion recovery deploys a preparatory pulse that affects all protons in the imaging field and relies on the specific longitudinal recovery rates of the targeted tissue to reach the desired signal-nulling effect.*

The preparatory pulse is often a 180-degree inversion pulse. All protons are flipped in polarity, going from positive ($+M_Z$) to negative ($-M_Z$) magnetization. Protons will begin to recover their net $+M_Z$ longitudinal magnetization as determined by their specific T1 relaxation time (Fig. 6.1).

Tissue-specific T1 recovery times form the foundation for inversion recovery and enable signal suppression, depending on the parameter selected; the most common tissues targeted with this technique are fat, cerebrospinal fluid (CSF), and myocardium. The null point is the position in time following the inversion preparatory pulse, when the targeted protons produce minimal signal; this occurs when the tissue has recovered its equilibrium magnetization to the zero value.

The interval between the administration of the inversion pulse and the excitation pulse is known as the inversion time (TI). The TI to null a particular proton pool can be calculated with the following formula: 0.693 × T1, with T1 being the longitudinal relaxation time of that particular proton pool. At 1.5 T, the radiofrequency (RF) pulse is administered at 175 ms to suppress fat; for CSF, the RF pulse is sent in the range of 2000 to 2500 ms. Because T1 relaxation times are prolonged with increasing magnetic field strengths, TIs will also be prolonged. For example, the TI to nullify fat signal at 3 T is from 200 to 225 ms.

Two inversion recovery techniques are in common clinical use and are primarily discussed in this chapter. The first is short T1 (or tau) inversion time (STIR), and the second is fluid attenuation inversion recovery (FLAIR).

STIR is used both to suppress the signal from fat and to increase contrast in tissues exhibiting long T1 relaxation and T2 decay times. *Contrast in STIR has been described as the inverse of T1 because tissues hypointense on T1-weighted sequences are correspondingly hyperintense on STIR.* In the setting of magnetic field inhomogeneities and low field strengths, STIR is preferred over frequency-selective saturation for fat suppression. *Although STIR provides homogeneous fat suppression, it does so in a nonspecific fashion. As an unintended consequence, any tissue that exhibits a similar T1 relaxation time to fat will also suppress.*

FLAIR is a staple in neuroimaging. The TI is set to eliminate signal from free water and simple fluids (e.g., CSF). Because of the long T1 relaxation time of free water, the TI is longer than what is used in STIR, typically in the range of 2000 to 2500 ms at 1.5 T. *Nulling CSF signal improves lesion-parenchyma contrast, most notably lesions within the CSF itself and lesions at the CSF-brain border.* FLAIR is particularly important for depicting lesions that do not enhance following gadolinium administration. FLAIR techniques can also be applied on T1-weighted imaging, which has been used to accentuate faintly enhancing CNS lesions and to improve gray-white differentiation (Fig. 6.2).

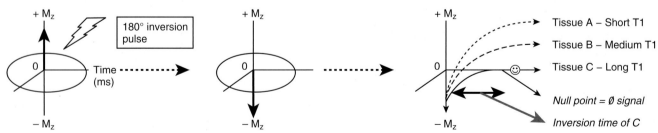

FIG. 6.1. Following administration of the 180-degree inversion preparatory pulse, protons are flipped from positive ($+M_Z$) to negative ($-M_Z$) magnetization. Tissues begin recovering net longitudinal ($+M_Z$) magnetization as determined by individual T1 relaxation times. The null point of a tissue *(smiley face)* is defined as the position in time following the inversion preparatory pulse when the tissue's net longitudinal magnetization is zero.

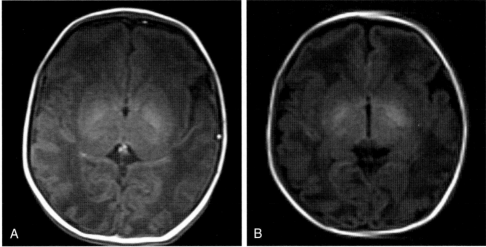

FIG. 6.2. (A) Axial T1 spin echo image of the neonatal brain. The contrast between hypointense CSF and the diencephalon and brain stem, as well as gray-white matter differentiation, are suboptimal. (B) Axial T1-FLAIR image at the same level. The robust suppression of CSF signal and improved gray-white differentiation are now evident. The symmetric high T1 signal in the bilateral pallidi is consistent with newborn myelination.

CASE 6.2

FIG. 6.C2

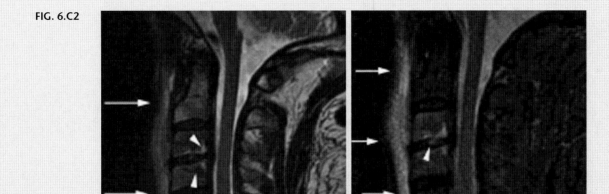

1. Tissues that exhibit long T1 relaxation times produce what type of signal on a STIR sequence?
   A. Hypointense compared with fat
   B. Isointense compared with fat
   C. Hyperintense compared with fat
   D. No signal (signal void)

FIG. 6.C2. (A) Sagittal T2-FSE image of the upper cervical canal demonstrates areas of abnormal hyperintense signal involving the endplates adjacent to the C3–C4 disc *(arrowheads)*. There is also adjacent prevertebral soft tissue swelling and high-intensity signal *(arrows)*. (B) Sagittal STIR image at the same level demonstrates increased conspicuity of the endplate and disc signal abnormalities *(arrowhead)*. A more diffuse high signal involving the C3 and C4 vertebral bodies is now evident. Compare the signal intensity of the prevertebral soft tissue swelling *(arrows)* with that in part A.

Diagnosis

The diagnosis is discitis (osteomyelitis).

Discussion

The abnormal high signal edema of the C3 and C4 vertebral bodies is more conspicuous on a STIR image because the normal high signal from (fatty) bone marrow is suppressed. Note the low signal within the normal C2 and C5 vertebral bodies on the STIR image due to suppression of fat within the bone marrow. The prevertebral soft tissue swelling is also more striking on the STIR image.

This case illustrates an important point about STIR—tissues with long T1 relaxation times, such as the prevertebral soft tissue edema in Case 6.2, will produce hyperintense signal, and tissues exhibiting short T1 (fat) will be low in signal. This pattern is the opposite of that seen in conventional T1-weighted images, which is why the contrast in STIR is referred to as the *inverse* of T1.

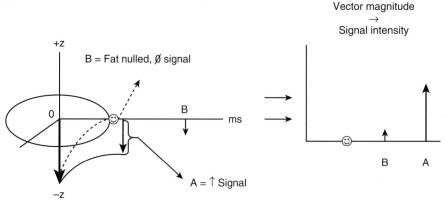

FIG. 6.3. With a short TI *(solid lines)*, the protons with the longest T1 *(A)* (and thus farthest from its respective null point) will create the greatest amount of signal.

Following the 180-degree inversion pulse, fat recovers its equilibrium longitudinal magnetization faster than tissues with longer T1 times. Once fat recovers to its null point, the excitation pulse is sent, rendering the fat unable to produce signal. Most protons in tissues with longer T1 times remain inverted yet maintain a large vector with respect to their null point. In STIR, signal intensity depends on the magnitude (and not polarity) of the protons' longitudinal vector; in other words, it does not matter if the protons are pointing north (+M_Z) or south (−M_Z); how far and how many of those protons are pointing north or south in relation to their respective null points determine the signal intensity. In other words, the size of the protons' longitudinal vector influences signal intensity, not the direction of the protons (Fig. 6.3).

CASE 6.2 ANSWERS

1. **C. Hyperintense compared with fat**

CASE 6.3

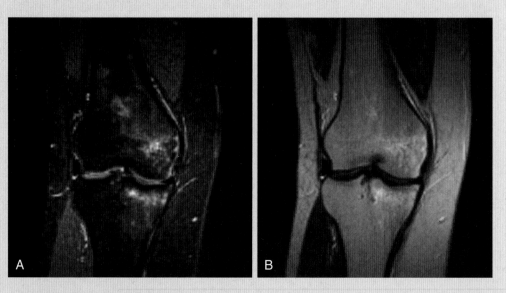

FIG. 6.C3

1. Which of the following provides the most effective fat suppression at low (<1.0 T) magnetic field strengths?
   A. STIR
   B. Frequency-selective fat saturation
   C. FLAIR
   D. Opposed-phase imaging

FIG. 6.C3. (A) Coronal STIR image of the knee. High signal marrow edema is identified in the medial tibial plateau and medial femoral condyle. Fraying of the lateral meniscus free edge represents a degenerative radial tear. (B) Coronal FSE T2-weighted image at the same position. The edema is largely obscured by the high signal intensity marrow.

Diagnosis

This patient was diagnosed as having bone marrow edema.

Discussion

As previously mentioned in Chapter 2, fat is high in signal intensity on an FSE T2-weighted image. This is because of the use of multiple 180-degree refocusing pulses, which disturbs the J-coupling effects normally seen in conventional T2-weighted spin echo sequences. As may be recalled, J-coupling refers to the spin-spin coupling of atomic nuclei in lipid molecules that results in shortening of T2 relaxation. This interruption of J-coupling affects the spin-spin interaction in fat, resulting in T2 prolongation and high signal intensity on a T2-weighted sequence.

This can become problematic when evaluating bone marrow, in which high T2 signal intensity edema may be masked by the similarly high signal intensity fat. In this setting, the use of fat suppression becomes a necessity. The benefit of fat suppression was previously illustrated in Cases 6.1 and 6.2; Case 6.3 demonstrates how high marrow signal on the FSE T2-weighted image (Fig. 6.C3B) virtually obscures the edema in the medial knee, which was clearly depicted on the corresponding STIR image (Fig. 6.C3A).

Fat suppression using a frequency-selective saturation technique would have been just as effective in depicting the edema if only this study had been done at a higher main magnetic field strength; it was performed on a 0.6-T magnet. Recall that the

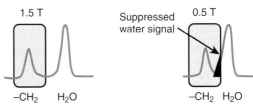

FIG. 6.4. At higher field strengths, there is a greater chemical shift (or separation) between water and methylene (–CH₂) protons, which allows more precise fat suppression with frequency-selective fat saturation. At lower field strengths, there is less chemical shift between water and methylene protons, with some overlap between protons at the ends of the frequency peaks *(black triangle)*; the narrow-frequency RF preparatory pulse would now suppress some water protons.

resonant frequencies of water and lipid protons are very similar at lower magnetic field strengths, resulting in a small chemical shift (approximately 74 Hz at 0.5 T, 224 Hz at 1.5 T, and 448 Hz at 3.0 T). Had the narrow-bandwidth saturation pulse used to suppress fat been applied, the water protons precessing within the frequency range of the saturation preparatory pulse would have also been inadvertently suppressed (Fig. 6.4).

CASE 6.3 ANSWER

1. **A. STIR**

CASE 6.4

FIG. 6.C4

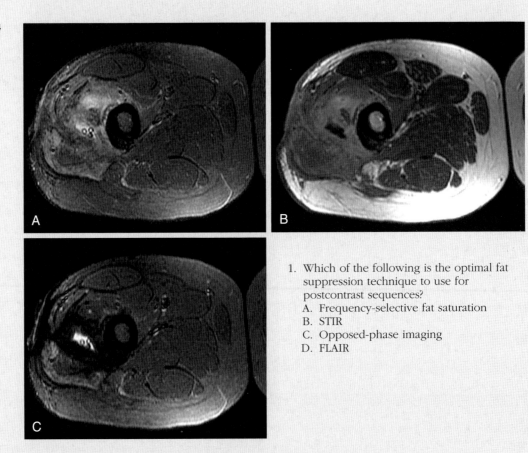

1. Which of the following is the optimal fat suppression technique to use for postcontrast sequences?
   A. Frequency-selective fat saturation
   B. STIR
   C. Opposed-phase imaging
   D. FLAIR

FIG. 6.C4. (A) Axial STIR image of the thigh. High signal tissue in the deep lateral thigh adjacent to the femur extending to the subcutaneous soft tissues is demonstrated. Thickening of the posterior periosteum of the femur compatible with posttraumatic change is present. The three small round foci centrally in the soft tissue abnormality are surgical drains. (B) Axial postcontrast T1-weighted image. The abnormal tissue enhances while the fluid collection centrally does not. (C) Axial STIR image at the same level as A following gadolinium administration. There is a complete dropout in signal intensity in the abnormal tissue; high signal intensity centrally is consistent with simple fluid.

Diagnosis

This was diagnosed as postoperative changes.

Discussion

Gadolinium is a paramagnetic agent that shortens both the T1 and T2 relaxation times of affected tissues. At the concentrations used in diagnostic imaging, the degree of T2 shortening is minimal and should not cause noticeable signal decreases in T1-weighted or T2-weighted sequences.

The abnormal high signal intensity tissue in the lateral thigh seen in the first STIR image (Fig. 6.C4A) became suppressed when a STIR sequence was repeated following gadolinium administration (Fig. 6.C4C). The postcontrast T1-weighted image showed avid enhancement of the tissue (Fig. 6.C4B), meaning that it was perfused with gadolinium.

The drop in signal in the abnormal tissue on the postcontrast STIR image was due to inadvertent signal suppression. Gadolinium caused shortening of T1 relaxation of the tissue, which in turn led to a decrease in its TI. Because the TI of the abnormal tissue now closely approximates that of fat, the addition of the STIR preparatory pulse resulted in inadvertent signal suppression. Because of this, frequency-selective fat saturation is used for fat suppression purposes on postcontrast images.

CASE 6.4 ANSWER

1. **A. Frequency-selective fat saturation**

CASE 6.5

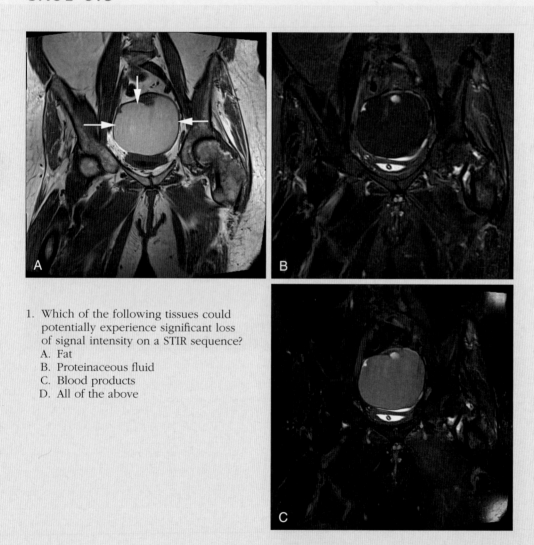

FIG. 6.C5

1. Which of the following tissues could potentially experience significant loss of signal intensity on a STIR sequence?
   A. Fat
   B. Proteinaceous fluid
   C. Blood products
   D. All of the above

FIG. 6.C5. (A) Coronal T1-weighted image of the pelvis. A round, high-signal pelvic mass superior to the bladder is demonstrated (*arrows*). (B) Coronal STIR at the same level as part A. Diffuse hypointense signal is demonstrated within the pelvic mass. High signal nodular tissue is noted along the superior aspect of the mass. (C) Coronal T2-weighted image with fat saturation. The mass is intermediate high in signal intensity and is slightly hypointense to urine.

Diagnosis

This patient was diagnosed as having hemorrhagic melanoma metastasis.

Discussion

The teaching points for this case are as follows: (1) not everything that is high in signal intensity on both T1-weighted and T2-weighted images is fat; and (2) although STIR is primarily used to suppress fat, not everything that is low signal intensity on STIR is fat.

A high T1 signal pelvic mass (Fig. 6.C5A) was low in signal intensity on the STIR image (Fig. 6.C6B), but remained high in signal intensity on the fat-saturated T2-weighted image (Fig. 6.C5C). If STIR were chosen as the sole fat suppression technique in this examination, the imaging pattern might have raised the possibility of a fat-containing mass. However, the lack of marked signal loss on the fat saturation image alerts you that this mass is definitely not fat containing—remember,

fat saturation is lipid specific—and should trigger a search for an alternative diagnosis. This mass was a hemorrhagic metastatic lesion in a patient with melanoma.

The interesting aspect of this case is the appearance of the hemorrhagic pelvic mass, which appears low in signal on the STIR image but high in signal on the fat saturation T2-weighted sequence. This, along with the increased T1 signal of the mass, confirms that the T1 relaxation time of this lesion was shortened by the effects of methemoglobin, a paramagnetic blood breakdown product seen in subacute hemorrhage. The methemoglobin caused a decrease in the TI of the mass, making it susceptible to inadvertent signal nulling by STIR. Proteins can also cause a similar effect on fluid.

CASE 6.5 ANSWER

1. **D. All of the above**

CASE 6.6

FIG. 6.C6

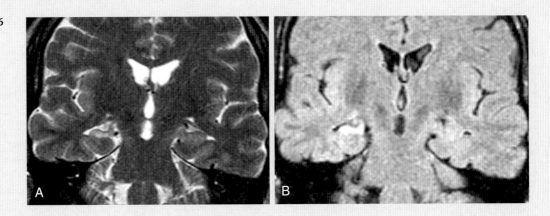

1. Signal from which of the following is intentionally suppressed on a FLAIR sequence?
   A. Fat
   B. Blood
   C. Brain
   D. CSF

2. What is the most likely diagnosis in this patient with a history of seizures?
   A. Multiple sclerosis
   B. Mesial temporal sclerosis
   C. Herpes encephalitis
   D. Chronic traumatic encephalopathy

FIG. 6.C6. (A) Coronal T2-weighted image. A loss of right-sided hippocampal volume is identified. (B) Coronal FLAIR image, same level. Right-sided hippocampal volume loss is again noted, with an abnormal hyperintense signal now evident.

Discussion

Signal suppression of CSF on a FLAIR sequence provides dramatically improved contrast at the CSF-brain border. Although the right-sided hippocampal loss of volume was evident on the coronal T2-weighted image, the hyperintense signal abnormality of the right hippocampus on the FLAIR image further supports a diagnosis of mesial temporal sclerosis.

CASE 6.6 ANSWERS

1. **D. CSF**
2. **B. Mesial temporal sclerosis**

FIG. 6.C7

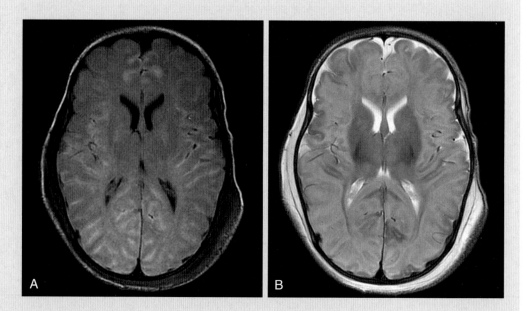

1. Which of the following explains the altered CSF signal
   intensity on the FLAIR image?
   A. CSF flow-related artifacts
   B. Hemorrhage causing an alteration in the T1 relaxation
      time of CSF
   C. TI erroneously set to null fat by the MRI technologist
   D. Nothing; this is a normal appearance of the CSF on a
      FLAIR sequence

FIG. 6.C7. (A) Axial FLAIR image through the level of the basal ganglia. Note the diffuse hyperintense signal within the sulci, as well as high signal dependently layering in the subdural spaces, compatible with both subarachnoid and subdural hematomas. (B) Axial T2-weighted image at the same level. The abnormal CSF signal evident on the FLAIR image is obscured by the hyperintense CSF signal.

Diagnosis

This was patient was diagnosed as having a subarachnoid hemorrhage.

Discussion

Similar to STIR, FLAIR emphasizes differences in T1 contrast by using a nonselective inversion pulse and is frequently incorporated with long echo time sequences to produce heavily T2-weighted images. Unlike STIR, the TI in FLAIR is set to null the usually high-signal CSF; because of CSF's long T1 relaxation time, the time to inversion is typically 2000 to 2500 ms. With this long TI, most tissues regain equilibrium longitudinal magnetization when the excitation pulse is administered; the signal from CSF is normally suppressed.

When a high FLAIR signal in the CSF spaces is present, it frequently means that something is present that is altering *both* the T1 and T2 relaxation times of CSF. The high FLAIR signal within the sulci and posterior convexities is due primarily to the presence of blood, which alters the T1 relaxation time of CSF, resulting in a lack of desired signal suppression. FLAIR is highly sensitive for detecting acute subarachnoid hemorrhage. Other considerations in the setting of high FLAIR signal in the CSF and subarachnoid spaces include meningitis and leptomeningeal spread of disease (Fig. 6.5).

CASE 6.7 ANSWER

1. **B. Hemorrhage causing an alteration in the T1 relaxation
   time of CSF**

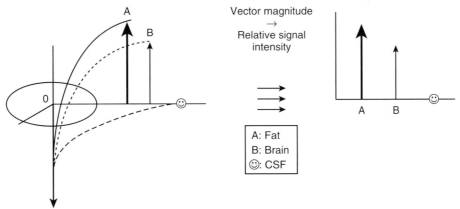

A: Fat
B: Brain
☺: CSF

FIG. 6.5. After the administration of a nonselective 180-degree pulse, the long TI used to suppress CSF *(smiley face)* allows significant longitudinal relaxation of other tissues.

FIG. 6.C8

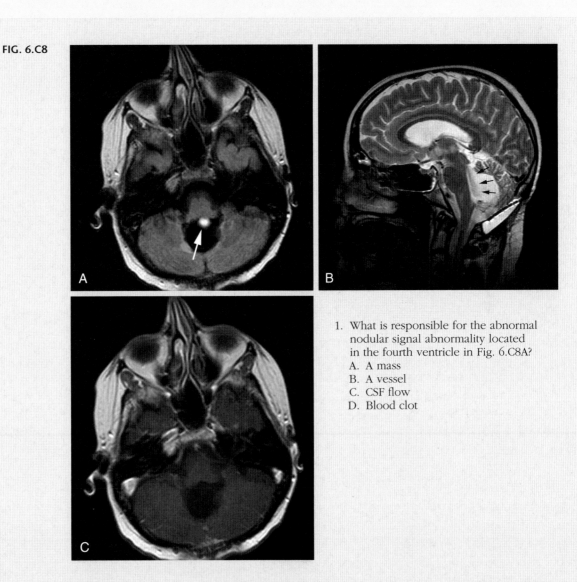

1. What is responsible for the abnormal nodular signal abnormality located in the fourth ventricle in Fig. 6.C8A?
   A. A mass
   B. A vessel
   C. CSF flow
   D. Blood clot

FIG. 6.C8. (A) Axial FLAIR image at the level of the clivus. A round hyperintense focus just posterior to the medulla is present *(arrow)*. A patulous fourth ventricle is in keeping with postresection changes in this patient with a history of medulloblastoma. (B) Sagittal T2-weighted image. The bandlike low signal *(arrows)* within the fourth ventricle is due to the flow of CSF protons through the aqueduct of Sylvius. (C) Postcontrast T1-weighted image at the same level as the FLAIR image. No lesion is detected in the same region as the FLAIR abnormality.

Diagnosis

This was diagnosed as a pseudomass from a CSF flow artifact on FLAIR.

Discussion

In Case 6.8, the CSF flow through the cerebral aqueduct has introduced protons that were not subjected to the inverting 180-degree preparatory pulse and thus were not suppressed at the CSF null point. The high signal "nodule" on the FLAIR sequence might have raised the possibility of disease recurrence; fortunately, the sagittal T2-weighted sequence provided an explanation for the false FLAIR signal because the jet of hypointense T2 signal is readily evident. Absence of the nodule on the postcontrast T1-weighted image excludes a mass (answer A), a vessel (answer B), and a blood clot (answer D) in this region.

CSF flow artifacts can also give the false impression of subarachnoid disease. These artifacts often occur within areas of relative increased CSF flow, including the ventricular foramina and the basilar cisterns. The artifacts are less conspicuous and seen less frequently in regions of reduced CSF flow, such as the cerebral convexities.

Other potential causes of spurious FLAIR signal include delayed excretion of gadolinium into the subarachnoid spaces, which is mainly seen in the setting of renal failure (not much of an issue now given the concern for nephrogenic systemic fibrosis) and sedated patients receiving both propofol and supplemental oxygen.

CASE 6.8 ANSWER

1. **C. CSF flow**

TAKE-HOME POINTS

1. Inversion recovery belongs to the family of preparatory pulse sequences—that is, an RF pulse is delivered before the excitation pulse. The trade-off for using this extra pulse is an increased acquisition time because the TI increases the repetition time.
2. STIR is a popular technique that relies on the T1 recovery time of a lipid to achieve fat suppression.
3. Advantages of STIR over its frequency-selective saturation counterpart include effectiveness at low magnetic field strengths, insensitivity to magnetic field nonuniformities, and increased edema and tumor contrast due to the additive effects of T1 and T2 weighting.
4. Disadvantages include nonspecific suppression of signal from tissues with similar T1 recovery times as lipids, decreased signal-to-noise ratio, decreased spatial resolution due to prolonged acquisition times, and alteration in image contrast.
5. FLAIR is used primarily in neuroimaging to suppress signal from CSF and increase conspicuity of lesions with T2 prolongation. Because of the long T1 relaxation time of CSF, the TI in FLAIR is much longer compared with STIR.
6. FLAIR is most useful to detect abnormalities within the CSF (e.g., blood, proteins), as well as parenchymal lesions in close proximity to CSF.
7. Beware of FLAIR artifacts that mimic CSF abnormalities. Because of CSF flow dynamics, not all CSF protons will be suppressed, resulting in a false high signal in cisterns and foramina.

Suggested Readings

Del Grande F, Santini F, Herzka DA, et al. Fat-suppression techniques for 3-T MR imaging of the musculoskeletal system. *RadioGraphics.* 2014;34(1):217–233.

Delfaut EM, Beltran J, Johnson G, et al. Fat suppression in MR imaging: techniques and pitfalls. *RadioGraphics.* 1999;19(2): 373–382.

Stuckey SL, Goh TD, Heffernan T, Rowan D. Hyperintensity in the subarachnoid space on FLAIR MRI. *AJR Am J Roentgenol.* 2007; 189(4):913–921.

CHAPTER 7

Type 2 Chemical Shift Artifact

Nicholas T. Befera, Mustafa R. Bashir, and Timothy J. Amrhein

OPENING CASE 7.1

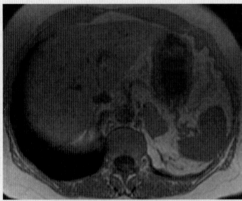
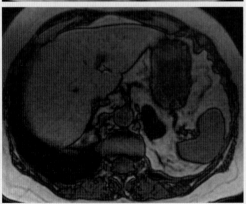

1. What is the most likely diagnosis?
   A. Pheochromocytoma
   B. Adrenal adenoma
   C. Adrenal cortical carcinoma
   D. Metastatic lesion to adrenal gland
2. Which of the following will have the most signal dropout on an out-of-phase T1 gradient recalled echo sequence?
   A. Subcutaneous fat
   B. Hepatic lesion with 40% signal contribution from protons surrounded by fat and 60% signal contribution from protons surrounded by water
   C. Hepatic lesion with 90% signal contribution from protons surrounded by fat and 10% signal contribution from protons surrounded by water
   D. Mesenteric fat
   E. Cerebrospinal fluid
3. Out-of-phase images should always be acquired before in-phase images. Why?
   A. Because in-phase images are derived from out-of-phase images
   B. To minimize the effect of T2* decay on out-of-phase images
   C. Because out-of-phase time to echo (TE) is shorter than in-phase TE
   D. To reduce overall acquisition time

OPENING CASE 7.1

FIG. 7.C1. (A) Axial T1-weighted, out-of-phase image. The large left adrenal nodule *(arrow)* exhibits significant signal loss *(black)*. (B) Axial T1-weighted, in-phase image. The large left adrenal nodule *(arrow)* exhibits signal intensity that is isointense to muscle *(gray)*.

1. What is the most likely diagnosis?
   B. Adrenal adenoma
2. Which of the following will have the most signal drop-out on an out-of-phase T1 gradient recalled echo (GRE) sequence?
   B. Hepatic lesion with 40% signal contribution from protons surrounded by fat and 60% signal contribution from protons surrounded by water
3. Out-of-phase images should always be acquired before in-phase images. Why?
   B. To minimize the effect of T2* decay on out-of-phase images

Discussion

Adrenal adenomas are common benign neoplasms of the adrenal gland. The signal loss on the out-of-phase image is indicative of a combination of water protons and fat protons within the lesion, a finding most consistent with an adrenal adenoma. Rarely, adrenal cortical carcinomas, pheochromocytomas, and metastases from clear cell renal cell carcinoma or hepatocellular carcinoma can also exhibit these MR characteristics.[1] Atypical adrenal nodules (those that are growing rapidly, are inhomogeneous, or have clinical features suggestive of malignancy) warrant further evaluation with positron emission tomography/computed tomography (PET/CT), a dedicated adrenal protocol CT to assess for contrast washout, or a biopsy to confirm the diagnosis.

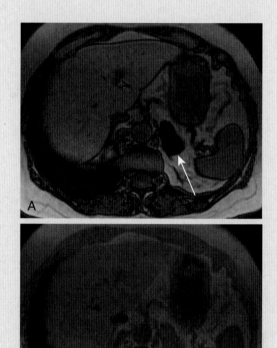

Type 2 Chemical Shift

A type 2 chemical shift artifact forms the basis for in- and out-of-phase MR sequences. These sequences are particularly useful in abdominal imaging, where they are invaluable for assessment of the liver, adrenal glands, and kidneys. In- and out-of-phase sequences take advantage of an artifact termed *chemical shift* to evaluate for the presence of both fat and water protons in the same imaging voxel. There are two types of chemical shift artifacts, type 1 and type 2. Type 1, or chemical shift misregistration artifact, is present on all sequences but is often imperceptible (discussed in Chapter 9). Type 2 artifact, or chemical shift cancellation, is only present on out-of-phase sequences and is the focus of this chapter.

Protons (or hydrogen nuclei) within different types of molecules experience slightly different magnetic field strengths. This occurs due to the various conformations of surrounding electron clouds resulting in unique local electromagnetic microenvironments.[2,3] For this reason, the protons within fat and water molecules precess at slightly different Larmor frequencies. Due to this precession at slightly different frequencies, there are regular intervals when their orientations in the transverse plane are either in phase or out of phase with each other. Setting the TE to these specific time points, when the nuclei are either in or out of phase with each other,

produces the in- and out-of-phases images.[2] The rate of precession for all protons depends on the overall magnetic field strength (see Chapter 1). For this reason, *the time points at which the protons in fat and water molecules are either in or out of phase are different, depending on the main magnet strength.* On a 1.5-T system, there is an approximately 220-Hz frequency difference between the two molecules. This means that approximately every 4.4 ms (1 sec/220 Hz) water protons will have completed exactly one extra rotation and be back in phase with the fat protons. The signals are in directly opposed phases (water will have an extra 180-degree rotation) in between the in-phase TEs, so they will be, for example. at about 2.2 ms and 6.6 ms. The frequency difference for fat and water is doubled on 3.0-T systems, so the above increments are halved (1 sec/440 Hz), as are the TEs (e.g., in phase at ~2.2 ms, ~4.4 ms; opposed phase at ~1.1 ms, 3.3 ms).[4]

In- and out-of-phase images are acquired using a single T1-weighted, GRE sequence. *The out-of-phase images should be acquired before the in-phase image because of the confounding variable of T2* decay.* Remember, T1-weighted GRE sequences use a single-excitation radiofrequency (RF) pulse, after which magnetic field inhomogeneities result in progressive signal loss due to a T2* effect. By

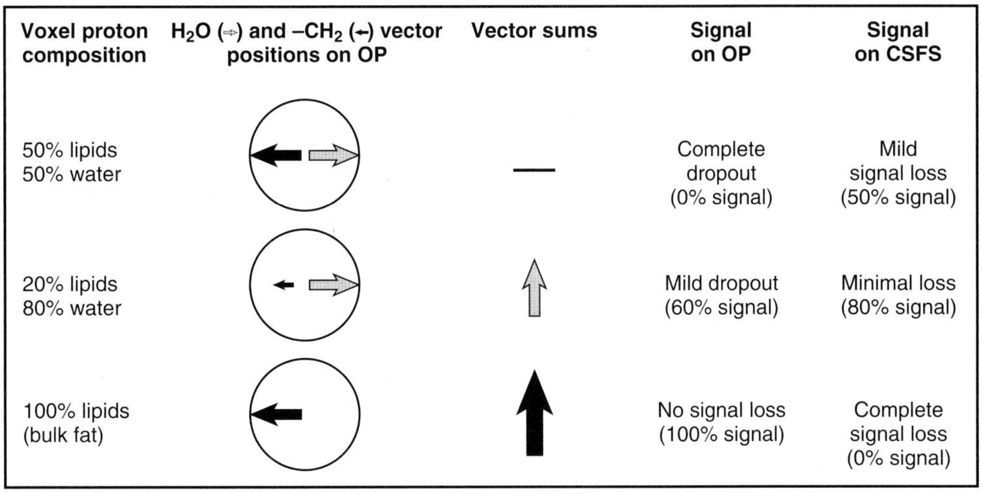

Voxel proton composition	H$_2$O ($\rightarrow$) and –CH$_2$ ($\leftarrow$) vector positions on OP	Vector sums	Signal on OP	Signal on CSFS
50% lipids 50% water		—	Complete dropout (0% signal)	Mild signal loss (50% signal)
20% lipids 80% water			Mild dropout (60% signal)	Minimal loss (80% signal)
100% lipids (bulk fat)			No signal loss (100% signal)	Complete signal loss (0% signal)

FIG. 7.1. The effect of fat on pixel signal intensity in out-of-phase (OP) and chemical-selective fat saturation (CSFS). This illustrates the greater sensitivity of OP imaging for small amounts of fat in water-based tissues compared with CSFS.

acquiring out-of-phase images before in-phase images, we can be sure that any signal loss noted is due to chemical shift artifact—signal dropout due to fat-water cancellation—because there the effect of T2* decay will actually be more pronounced on the in-phase images, which have a longer TE. If the out-of-phase images were acquired after the in-phase images, it would be difficult or impossible to determine whether signal loss on the out-of-phase images was from a chemical shift artifact or T2* decay.[5]

In- and out-of-phase imaging is particularly useful due to its sensitivity to small amounts of fat within a lesion or organ. Although CT and other MR fat suppression techniques (e.g., chemical-selective fat suppression [CSFS] or inversion recovery) can also help detect fat within a lesion, they are less sensitive for small amounts of fat.[6] In certain clinical scenarios, including the example in Opening Case 7.1, confirming the presence of fat within a lesion can help establish a diagnosis or determine if a lesion is benign or malignant. *Lesions with small amounts of fat lose signal on out-of-phase images because there is a proportion of both fat and water within an individual voxel. When these two signals of opposing phases are summed, a portion of the signals will cancel, resulting in loss of signal within the pixel—the pixel appears darker.*

For a better understanding of why out-of-phase images are more sensitive to fat than a T1-weighted, fat-saturated sequence, consider the theoretical example of a lesion in which fat contributes 15% of the signal intensity and water the remaining 85%. In the T1-weighted, fat saturation sequence, 85% of the signal will remain in the lesion after the fat saturation prepulse (i.e., the 15% from fat will be removed). However, in the out-of-phase sequence, the 15% fat signal *cancels* out a portion of the 85% water signal, resulting in only 70% of the original signal. This increased reduction in signal intensity makes the difference much easier to detect. In summary,

out-of-phase sequences magnify the signal loss from fat by a factor of 2 compared with fat-saturated sequences, resulting in increased conspicuity of lesions with minimal fat (Fig. 7.1).

If a pixel's signal contribution is 50% from water and 50% from fat, then the two signal contributions will completely cancel each other out and the resultant pixel will have no signal (i.e., be black). The most common location for this to occur is at an interface of fat and water, such as between abdominal organs (containing nearly 100% water signal) and the surrounding mesenteric or retroperitoneal fat. This is the basis for the characteristic *so-called India ink artifact identified on out-of-phase images, a thin black line that outlines all the organs in the abdomen* (see Fig. 7.C1A). The India ink artifact is identified around the entirety of an organ (on all sides), differentiating it from a type 1 chemical shift artifact, which only occurs in the frequency-encoding direction.[2]

However, unlike with fat suppression techniques, *areas that are composed solely of fat do not lose signal intensity on out-of-phase images* (see Fig 7.C1A; note that the mesenteric fat retains its high signal intensity). This may seem counterintuitive; the mesenteric fat and the adrenal nodule both contain fat, so shouldn't both lose signal? To understand this, one must remember that signal loss on out-of-phase images is due to signal cancellation between protons in fat and water. In tissues such as mesenteric fat, there are very few water protons to cancel the signal from fat protons and, given that there is little resultant cancellation, these voxels remain bright; therefore options A and D for question 2 are incorrect. Thus *the closer a voxel is to having 50% of its signal derived from fat, the more signal loss will be observed on out-of-phase images.* However, if the fat signal content is approximately 0% or 100%, little to no signal loss will occur.

FIG. 7.C2

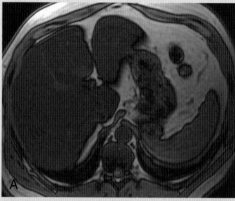

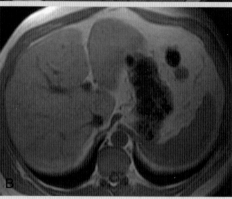

FIG. 7.C3

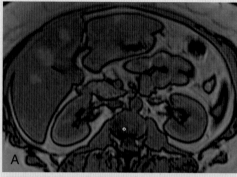

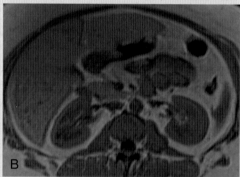

1. What is the diagnosis?
   A. Hemochromatosis
   B. Hepatic cirrhosis
   C. Hepatic steatosis
   D. Glycogen storage disease
2. If the order of acquisition was switched, and the in-phase image (Fig. 7.C2B) was acquired first, how would the relative signal intensity of the liver parenchyma in the two images change?
   A. Difference in liver signal intensity between the two images would be greater (in-phase signal would be increased, out-of-phase signal would be decreased)

B. Difference in liver signal intensity between the two images would be less (in-phase signal would be decreased, out-of-phase signal would be increased)
C. Liver signal would be reversed (out-of-phase signal would be greater than in-phase signal)
D. No change, because order of in-phase/out-of-phase acquisition only matters in the setting of iron deposition

3. What is the diagnosis?
   A. Multifocal hepatocellular carcinoma
   B. Focal nodular hyperplasia
   C. Normal liver with multiple hemangiomas
   D. Hepatic steatosis with areas of focal fatty sparing

FIG. 7.C2. (A) Axial T1-weighted, out-of-phase image showing diffuse signal loss throughout the liver. (B) Axial T1-weighted, in-phase image. This is a normal-appearing liver without lesion.

FIG. 7.C3. (A) Axial T1-weighted, out-of-phase image. There is diffuse loss of signal throughout most of the liver. Note the presence of several well-defined, non–masslike hyperintense areas in segments III, IVB, V, and VI. (B) Axial T1-weighted, in-phase image of a normal-appearing liver.

Hepatic Steatosis and Focal Fat Sparing

Hepatic steatosis occurs when abnormal amounts of triglycerides are deposited in the liver.[6] The result is diffuse fat deposition throughout the liver, which causes signal loss on the out-of-phase images compared with the in-phase images (Fig. 7.C2A).

In Case 7.3, we again see loss of signal throughout the liver, signifying hepatic steatosis. However, in this case we also see several hyperintense lesions. These are not true lesions but are areas of normal liver that appear hyperintense in comparison with the signal loss in the surrounding liver. This occurs because these areas of focal fat sparing lack the internal fat content that leads to the signal cancellation on the opposed-phase images. Focal fat sparing can often

be distinguished from liver masses by its geographic shape, angular margins, and relatively normal contrast enhancement compared with the background liver.[6] A diagnosis of either focal fat infiltration or focal fat sparing can be suggested in part due to its occurrence in characteristic locations, including the gallbladder fossa, adjacent to the teres ligament, anterior to the right portal vein, and in the subcapsular parenchyma.[5]

CASES 7.2 AND 7.3 ANSWERS

1. **C. Hepatic steatosis**
2. **A. Difference in signal intensity would be greater**
3. **D. Hepatic steatosis with areas of focal fatty sparing**

FIG. 7.C4

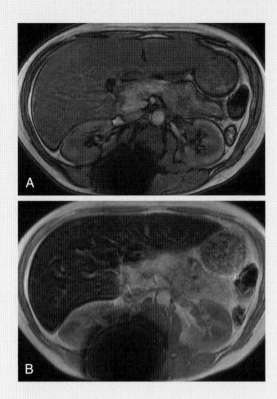

FIG. 7.C5

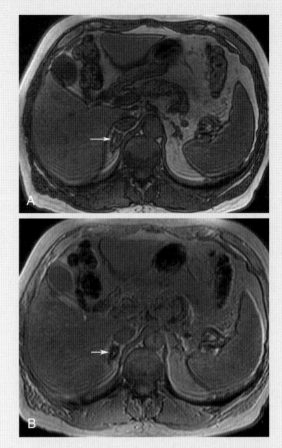

1. What is the diagnosis?
   A. Hemosiderosis
   B. Hepatic steatosis
   C. Normal liver; out-of-phase images mistakenly acquired after in-phase images
   D. Diffuse hepatic fibrosis
2. What is the cause of the diffuse signal loss throughout the liver seen on the in-phase image?
   A. Signal contributions from hemosiderin and water within each voxel cancel each other out.
   B. The magnetic susceptibility artifact is related to presence of hemosiderin, resulting in signal loss.
   C. Hepatic steatosis results in signal loss.
   D. The type 2 chemical shift artifact is related to the presence of hemosiderin, resulting in signal loss.

3. What is the diagnosis?
   A. Lipid-rich adrenal adenoma
   B. Adrenal hyperplasia
   C. Prior adrenal hemorrhage
   D. Adrenal myelolipoma

FIG. 7.C4. (A) Axial T1-weighted, out-of-phase image. There is normal signal intensity of the liver without lesion. The India ink artifact indicates that this is the out-of-phase image. (B) Axial T1-weighted, in-phase image. There is a markedly decreased signal intensity of the liver compared with the out-of-phase image. Note the more prominent susceptibility artifact due to the spinal hardware compared with the out-of-phase image, referred to as *blooming* (T2* effect).

FIG. 7.C5. (A) Axial T1-weighted, out-of-phase image. A heterogeneous adrenal nodule is seen within the right adrenal gland *(arrow)*. The India ink artifact around the organs indicates that this is the out-of-phase image. (B) Axial T1-weighted, in-phase image. There is considerably decreased signal intensity of the adrenal nodule *(arrow)* compared with the out-of-phase image. Note also that the type 1 chemical shift artifact is nicely demonstrated around the spleen.

Hemosiderin Deposition

Iron, a ferromagnetic substance, results in an increase in the rate of T2*-related decay of transverse magnetism (dephasing), causing signal loss. Hemosiderin contains inhomogeneously distributed iron, leading to this signal loss on the in-phase images. The signal loss is more pronounced on the in-phase images because they are acquired after the out-of-phase images, which allows more time for dephasing.

In Case 7.4, the diagnosis is hepatic hemosiderosis. Hepatic hemosiderosis refers to a state of excess hemosiderin deposition within the liver. This can occur as a result of multiple blood transfusions or hemochromatosis or conditions with high red blood cell turnover, such as hemolytic anemia.

Case 7.5 is an example of prior hemorrhage into the right adrenal gland. Adrenal hemorrhage may result from traumatic or nontraumatic causes, including physiologic stress, coagulopathy, or underlying adrenal tumor.[7] If unilateral, patients are often asymptomatic, and the adrenal hemorrhage may be incidentally discovered at the time of imaging performed for other causes. Appropriate diagnosis of this benign condition can prevent unnecessary additional imaging and may even avoid biopsy or resection.

Signal Loss from T2* Decay

Hemosiderin is a ferromagnetic substance that alters the local magnetic field inhomogeneously. As a result, protons in slightly different locations, but still within a single voxel, experience slightly different main magnetic fields, and therefore precess at slightly different frequencies. As a result, the transverse magnetization of the individual protons rapidly becomes misaligned, leading to a rapid reduction in the net transverse magnetization for the entire group of protons. This so-called field inhomogeneity results in a susceptibility artifact, characterized by accelerated proton dephasing and rapid signal loss on GRE sequences, also called the $T2^*$ effect. The more time that passes after the initial excitation pulse, the more time available for dephasing and the greater the resultant susceptibility-induced signal loss. Recall that *in-phase images are acquired after out-of-phase images, allowing the protons more time to dephase and resulting in more signal loss* (compared with out-of-phase images). Thus hemosiderosis appears as diffuse decreased signal throughout the liver on in-phase images, whereas the out-of-phase images appear relatively normal.

It is important to understand the difference between this type of signal loss ($T2^*$ effect) and a type 2 chemical shift (cancellation) artifact. *In- and out-of-phase images are acquired using TEs specific to fat and water. Therefore we would expect to see cancellation of signal within a voxel on out-of-phase images only if both fat and water molecules are present.* Cancellation would not occur in a voxel in which only hemosiderin and water are present. Furthermore, recall that cancellation of the fat-water signal is seen *only* on out-of-phase images, whereas in this case the signal loss was observed on the in-phase images. In cases of severe iron deposition, abnormally low signal in the liver

(when compared with muscle) will be present on the out-of-phase images (because some signal decay will occur), but signal loss will still be more pronounced on the in-phase images (because more signal loss will have occurred).

Note that in Case 7.5 the hemorrhage in the right adrenal gland has higher signal intensity on the out-of-phase images, with relative loss of signal on the in-phase images. The iron-containing hemosiderin within the adrenal hemorrhage results in rapid $T2^*$ decay and progressive signal loss on GRE sequences (longer TE = more signal loss). This is similar to the situation in Case 7.4, in which hemosiderosis of the liver resulted in signal loss on the in-phase images. Again, it is important to understand that this is not due to a chemical shift cancellation artifact. Type 2 chemical shift (cancellation) artifact occurs only when water and fat are present in the same voxel. Also note the increased susceptibility artifact from the spinal hardware in Case 7.4, which is more apparent and appears larger on the in-phase image due to the longer TE. The same holds true for gas-related susceptibility artifacts. The transverse colon in Case 7.5 contains stool mixed with gas bubbles. Theses gas bubbles also lead to susceptibility artifacts (signal loss) on the image with the longer TE (i.e., the in-phase image).

CASES 7.4 AND 7.5 ANSWERS

1. **A. Hemosiderosis**
2. **B. The magnetic susceptibility artifact is related to the presence of hemosiderin, resulting in signal loss**
3. **C. Prior adrenal hemorrhage**

CASES 7.6 AND 7.7

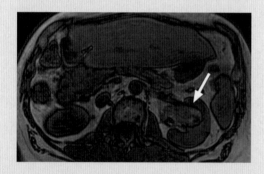

FIG. 7.C6

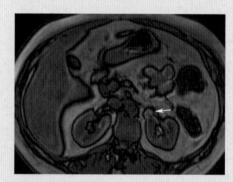

FIG. 7.C7

1. What is the dominant tissue type within the T1 hyperintense lesion?
   A. Blood products
   B. Fat
   C. Proteinaceous fluid
   D. Simple fluid
2. What is the most likely diagnosis of the lesion noted by the arrow?
   A. Hemorrhagic cyst
   B. Angiomyolipoma (AML)
   C. Renal metastasis
   D. Proteinaceous cyst
3. Why is there no signal loss (type 2 chemical shift cancellation artifact) between the lesion and the retroperitoneal fat on out-of-phase images?
   A. Voxels contain predominantly fat molecules.

   B. Voxels contain predominantly water molecules.
   C. Lesions contain only a small amount of fat.
   D. Lesions contain a 50-50 mix of fat and water molecules.
4. Which of the following tissue interfaces would not be expected to show an India ink artifact?
   A. Proteinaceous cyst and retroperitoneal fat
   B. Lymph node and mesenteric fat
   C. Proteinaceous cyst and renal parenchyma
   D. Renal parenchyma and perirenal fat
5. What is the most likely diagnosis?
   A. Simple cyst
   B. Hemorrhagic cyst
   C. AML
   D. Oncocytoma

FIG. 7.C6. Axial T1-weighted, out-of-phase image. There is a large, predominantly hyperintense mass in the left kidney extending into the renal sinus (*arrow*). An India ink artifact is present between the mass and renal parenchyma, with little to no India ink artifact between the mass and retroperitoneal fat. Also note the presence of several foci of signal loss within the mass.

FIG. 7.C7. Axial T1-weighted, out-of-phase image from a different patient. An exophytic lesion is seen arising from the anteromedial aspect of the left kidney (*arrow*). The India ink artifact extends along the outer margin of the lesion (on the border with the retroperitoneal fat), but not along the inner margin (on the border with the kidney).

Angiomyolipoma and Hemorrhagic Cyst

The most likely diagnosis in Case 7.6 is an AML. AMLs are the most common benign solid renal neoplasms and are almost always diagnosed based on the presence of large amounts of fat. Typical AMLs are triphasic neoplasms characterized by varying amounts of mature adipose tissue, dysmorphic blood vessels, and smooth muscle components.[8] Although these were once thought to be hamartomas, we now know AMLs to be a diverse group of neoplasms considered among the family of perivascular epithelioid cell tumors. Although most often sporadic, 20% of AMLs are associated with tuberous sclerosis complex. Note that renal cell carcinoma may also contain fat; therefore the mere presence of fat does not exclude malignancy.[9] The lesion in Case 7.7 is a hemorrhagic cyst.

Using the India Ink Artifact

The patients in Cases 7.6 and 7.7 both have renal lesions that are hyperintense on T1-weighted images. In general, strong T1-shortening identified within abdominal lesions is usually secondary to the presence of fat, blood products, proteinaceous debris, or gadolinium-based contrast agents. Fortunately, the India ink artifact can be used to help better characterize the content of these lesions, helping establish the correct diagnosis. If we know what type of tissue is immediately adjacent to a T1-hyperintense lesion, we may be able to infer some information about the content of the lesion using an understanding of the type 2 chemical shift artifact (in- and out-of-phase imaging).

AMLs (see Case 7.6) often contain areas composed entirely or predominantly of fat, which makes them hyperintense on T1-weighted images. Unfortunately, hemorrhagic cysts and hemorrhagic renal cell cancers are also hyperintense on T1. The India ink artifact can sometimes help differentiate these lesions.[10] Remember, this artifact occurs only on out-of-phase images at fat-water interfaces. When the India ink artifact is identified between the renal parenchyma and a lesion (as in Case 7.6), that part of the lesion must contain fat because the renal parenchyma is composed almost entirely of water. In contradistinction, if the India ink artifact extends only along the interface between the lesion and the retroperitoneal fat, and not along the interface with the kidney (as in Case 7.7), the fat-water interface is on the outside of the lesion only. This implies a predominantly water component to the lesion, which may represent solid tissue or, in this case, a hemorrhagic cyst.

CASES 7.6 AND 7.7 ANSWERS

1. **B. Fat**
2. **B. Angiomyolipoma (AML)**
3. **A. Voxels contain predominantly fat molecules**
4. **C. Proteinaceous cyst and renal parenchyma**
5. **B. Hemorrhagic cyst**

CASE 7.8

FIG. 7.C8

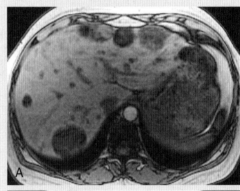
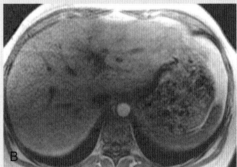

1. Which of the following is the most likely diagnosis?
   A. Hemangiomas
   B. Multiple hepatic adenomas
   C. Multiple focal nodular hyperplasia
   D. Metastatic disease
2. If the lesions in Case 7.8 were siderotic nodules, what would be the expected appearance on in- and out-of-phase images?
   A. Signal loss on out-of-phase image relative to in-phase image
   B. Signal loss on in-phase image relative to out-of-phase image
   C. No signal loss on either phase
   D. Equal signal loss on both in-phase and out-of-phase images

FIG. 7.C8. (A) Axial T1-weighted, out-of-phase image. Multiple low signal masses are seen throughout the liver. (B) Axial T1-weighted, in-phase image of a normal-appearing liver.

Hepatocellular Adenoma

Hepatic adenomas are benign lesions of the liver that have traditionally been associated with oral contraceptive and steroid use.[11] These lesions are typically solitary (70%–80%) and are often discovered incidentally at the time of imaging performed for other purposes.[12] Multiple adenomas may be sporadic or encountered in the setting of glycogen storage disease.[13] Small solitary adenomas are typically managed conservatively, whereas larger lesions may be resected due to the risk of hemorrhage and rare malignant degeneration.[14] Many hepatic adenomas contain large amounts of lipid interspersed within their tissues, which results in significant signal loss on the out-of-phase images compared with in-phase images. If hemorrhage is present, however, these lesions may have a heterogeneous signal on all sequences.

In Case 7.8, the lesions demonstrate signal loss on out-of-phase images, suggesting the presence of intracellular fat. Of the answer choices in question 1, option B (multiple hepatic adenomas) is most correct because adenomas are the most common fat-containing lesion in a noncirrhotic liver. Focal nodular hyperplasia can uncommonly contain fat, and other fat-containing liver lesions (e.g., lipoma, AML, teratoma, liposarcoma) are relatively rare. In a cirrhotic liver, hepatocellular carcinoma is an important consideration for a fat-containing liver lesion.

In the case of siderotic nodules, iron within the nodules results in accelerated T2* decay. As discussed previously, this manifests as signal loss on the in-phase images, which are acquired later (longer TE).

CASE 7.8 ANSWERS

1. **B. Multiple hepatic adenomas**
2. **B. Signal loss on in-phase image relative to out-of-phase image**

CASE 7.9

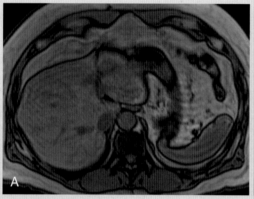
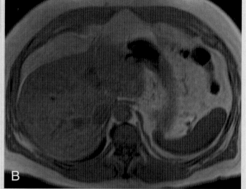
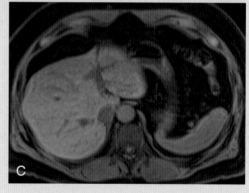

FIG. 7.C9. (A) Axial T1-weighted, out-of-phase image of a normal abdomen. (B) Axial T1-weighted, in-phase image of a normal abdomen. (C) Water-only image using the two-point Dixon technique.

Dixon Technique

Initially described by Tom Dixon in 1984, the two-point Dixon technique adds and subtracts the data from the in- and out-of-phase images to create two additional images. The signal intensity in one of these additional images will be theoretically entirely from water protons (the so-called water-only image), and the signal intensity from the other will be entirely from fat protons (the fat-only image).[15] It is important to note that the water-only image will still have the weighting of the original GRE image (usually T1-weighted or proton density), so bulk water will not appear bright, as it would in a T2-weighted image. Remember that the in-phase image is essentially a water + fat image and that the out-of-phase image is a water − fat image. By adding the two, the fat cancels out, and the resulting image is composed only of water signal:

$$(\text{Water} + \text{Fat}) + (\text{Water} − \text{Fat}) = 2 * \text{Water} + 0 * \text{Fat}$$

Examining the water-only image more closely, it is not simply the result of adding the in- and out-of-phase magnitude images. For example, the subcutaneous fat is bright on both the in- and out-of-phase images, but it is dark on the water-only image. Remember, a pixel displays the absolute value of the signal intensity, not the vector value. However, when the two original vector values are used, there is cancellation of the two fat signals.

What is the benefit of the two-point Dixon technique? This can be used to create a T1-weighted image with signal only from water protons (and no signal from fat protons)—in other words, a fat-suppressed, T1-weighted image. Therefore this technique adds a third method for the generation of fat-saturated images in addition to using a fat saturation prepulse or inversion recovery. The fat suppression in water-only images is typically more homogeneous than the fat suppression achieved using a fat saturation prepulse and does not incur the scan time or signal-to-noise penalty associated with the inversion recovery technique. As a result, it is the preferred method for fat suppression in some scenarios. It is important to note that creating this sequence does not add additional scan time beyond the acquisition of the in- and out-of-phase sequence because the images are simply generated by a computer using the same equation as above, with a small phase adjustment. This can replace the precontrast fat-saturated, T1-weighted sequence to decrease overall scanning time.

One of the problems encountered with the two-point Dixon technique is an artifact termed *fat-water swapping.* Practical implementation of the two-point Dixon technique includes an algorithm that assigns the two data points from the Dixon calculation to the water-only or fat-only image. However, those assignments are based on assumptions that may be incorrect, which may result in some of the signals

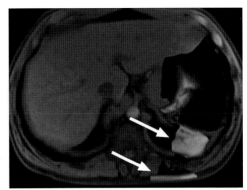

FIG. 7.2. Example of fat-water swapping. A water-only image created using the two-point Dixon technique demonstrates areas of incorrect water signal assignment to the subcutaneous and retroperitoneal fat *(arrows).*

from water being incorrectly assigned to the fat-only image, and vice versa (Fig. 7.2). Improvements in those algorithms, as well as improvements in shimming techniques, have reduced the occurrence of this artifact, leading to a resurgence of interest in the Dixon method. Currently, it is used clinically for fat suppression in a variety of different applications.

CASE 7.10

FIG. 7.C10

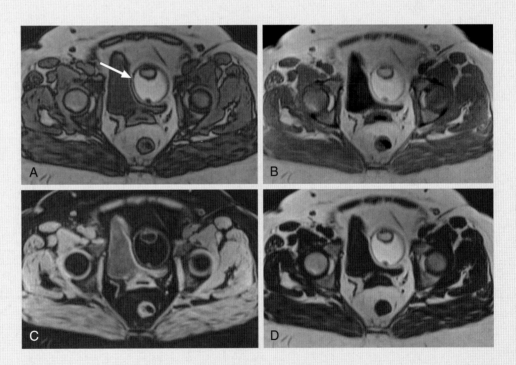

1. What is the diagnosis?
   A. Hemorrhagic cyst
   B. Ovarian mucinous cystadenoma
   C. Uterine fibroid
   D. Mature cystic ovarian teratoma (dermoid cyst)
2. The water-only (Fig. 7.C10C) and fat-only (Fig. 7.C10D) images show a region of fat within this ovarian lesion.

Why does this area still appear hyperintense on out-of-phase imaging?
   A. This is caused by a fat-water swapping artifact.
   B. Voxels contain predominantly fat molecules.
   C. Voxels contain predominantly water molecules.
   D. The out-of-phase sequence was mistakenly acquired after the in-phase sequence.

FIG. 7.C10. (A) Axial T1-weighted, out-of-phase image demonstrates a left pelvic mass *(arrow)* with intrinsic high signal intensity internally. Note the appearance of the peripheral low signal about the margins of the mass. (B) Axial T1-weighted, in-phase image. The left pelvic mass exhibits persistent intrinsic high signal intensity internally. (C) Axial T1-weighted, water-only image demonstrates near-complete signal intensity loss of the mass centrally. (D) Axial T1-weighted, fat-only image demonstrates high signal centrally within the mass.

Mature Cystic Ovarian Teratoma (Dermoid Cyst)

Mature cystic ovarian teratomas (or dermoid cysts) are the most common type of germ cell neoplasms. They are benign, slow-growing lesions that contain mature elements from at least two of the three germ cell layers—ectoderm, endoderm, mesoderm. They are typically asymptomatic; however, a minority of patients will present with abdominal pain from ovarian torsion or rupture or after the tumor has grown to a large size.[16] Most cystic ovarian teratomas are composed of a unilocular cyst containing sebaceous material and are lined with epithelium. The wall of the cyst may contain variable amounts of muscle, hair follicles, glands, fat, bone, cartilage, and teeth, as well as gastrointestinal and bronchial epithelium. Up to 75% of these lesions contain adipose tissue on gross pathology, and the presence of fat within the tumor on imaging is diagnostic.[17]

Using Fat-Water Separation Imaging

Case 7.10 demonstrates the utility of water-only and fat-only images derived from the Dixon method. Note that the region of fat within this dermoid cyst appears hyperintense on in- and out-of-phase images—that is, the fat does not cancel out on the out-of-phase images. Why is this the case? Recall that a type 2 chemical shift artifact (fat-water cancellation) occurs on the out-of-phase sequence when voxels contain a mix of fat and water molecules, with maximum cancellation (signal loss on the out-of-phase image) occurring when that ratio is 1:1. In the case of mature adipose tissue, such as in an ovarian dermoid (or subcutaneous fat), the voxels contain predominantly fat molecules, and thus cancellation (signal loss) on out-of-phase images will be minimal. However, macroscopic fat will still lose signal on the water-only image (Fig 7.C10C) and will appear hyperintense on the fat-only image (Fig 7.C10D). All these findings confirm the presence of fat in the mass in Case 7.10, a frequent finding in an ovarian dermoid, thereby establishing the diagnosis. Nonetheless, the diagnosis could also have been suggested based on identification of the India ink artifact surrounding the margins of the central fat on the out-of-phase image, which provides indirect evidence of a fat-containing lesion because this artifact occurs at fat-water interfaces.

CASE 7.10 ANSWERS

1. **D. Mature cystic ovarian teratoma (dermoid cyst)**
2. **B. Voxels contain predominantly fat molecules**

TAKE-HOME POINTS

Physics

1. There is a slight difference between the resonance frequencies of protons found in fat and those found in water due to differences in their respective electromagnetic microenvironments.
2. Fat and water protons are in and out of phase with one another at regular intervals (time points).
3. Setting the TEs to these time points in a multiecho GRE sequence provides the in- and out-of-phase images.
4. A type 2 chemical shift artifact, or chemical shift cancellation artifact, is present only on out-of-phase images when there is a substantial proportion of both fat and water signal in a pixel.
5. The negative value of fat and the positive value of water in a pixel partially cancel each other out on the out-of-phase image, resulting in signal intensity loss and the lesion appearing darker.
6. The characteristic India ink artifact surrounds the abdominal organs on the out-of-phase sequence and occurs because signal from the water protons in the organs and signal from the fat protons cancel each other.
7. Voxels that contain solely fat do not lose signal on out-of-phase images because there is no water signal within the pixel to provide a canceling effect.
8. The size of the India ink artifact depends on the pixel and voxel size only. It is independent of the magnetic field strength (in contradiction to the type 1 chemical shift artifact).

Clinical Considerations

1. In- and out-of-phase sequences are extremely helpful in abdominal imaging for detecting small proportions of fat.
2. The presence of both fat and water protons in an adrenal lesion confirms the diagnosis of adrenal adenoma and makes malignancy highly unlikely. The presence of bulk fat and very little water in all or portions of a renal lesion strongly suggests an AML.
3. Hepatic steatosis results in signal loss within the liver on out-of-phase images and is caused by abnormal hepatic triglyceride deposition.
4. In hepatic steatosis, normal areas of liver can appear as hyperintense lesions on the out-of-phase sequence because of the signal loss in the surrounding fatty liver.
5. Because the India ink artifact occurs at water-fat interfaces, it can demonstrate the chemical composition of a lesion based on how it outlines a lesion.
6. The liver and spleen can appear darker on in-phase images in the setting of hemosiderosis as a result of increased T2* effects, as long as the in-phase images are acquired with a longer TE than (i.e., after) the out-of-phase images.
7. The two-point Dixon technique can be used to obtain a water-only image, which is used as a fat-suppressed, T1-weighted sequence.
8. This water-only image can be used as the precontrast T1-weighted, fat-saturated sequence, decreasing overall scan time.

References

1. Blake MA, Cronin CG, Boland GW. Adrenal imaging. *AJR Am J Roentgenol.* 2010; 194:1450–1460.
2. Hood MN, Ho VB, Smirniotopoulos JG, Szumowski J. Chemical shift: the artifact and clinical tool revisited. *Radiographics.* 1999;19:357–371.
3. Brateman L. Chemical shift imaging: a review. *AJR Am J Roentgenol.* 1986;146:971–980.
4. Merkle EM, Dale BM. Abdominal MRI at 3.0 T: the basics revisited. *AJR Am J Roentgenol.* 2006;186:1524–1532.
5. Merkle EM, Nelson RC. Dual gradient-echo in-phase and opposed-phase hepatic MR imaging: a useful tool for evaluating more than fatty infiltration or fatty sparing. *Radiographics.* 2006;26:1409–1418.
6. Earls JP, Krinsky GA. Abdominal and pelvic applications of opposed-phase MR imaging. *AJR Am J Roentgenol.* 1997;169:1071–1077.
7. Kawashima A, Sandler CM, Ernst RD, et al. Imaging of nontraumatic hemorrhage of the adrenal gland. *Radiographics.* 1999;19:949–963.
8. Jinzaki M, Silverman SG, Akita H, et al. Renal angiomyolipoma: a radiological classification and update on recent developments in diagnosis and management. *Abdom Imaging.* 2014;39:588–604.
9. Wasser EJ, Shyn PB, Riveros-Angel M, et al. Renal cell carcinoma containing abundant non-calcified fat. *Abdom Imaging.* 2013;38:598–602.
10. Israel GM, Hindman N, Hecht E, Krinsky G. The use of opposed-phase chemical shift MRI in the diagnosis of renal angiomyolipomas. *AJR Am J Roentgenol.* 2005;184:1868–1872.

11. Edmondson HA, Henderson B, Benton B. Liver-cell adenomas associated with use of oral contraceptives. *N Engl J Med.* 1976;294:470–472.

12. Faria SC, Iyer RB, Rashid A, Whitman GJ. Hepatic adenoma. *AJR Am J Roentgenol.* 2004;182:1520.

13. Labrune P, Trioche P, Duvaltier I, et al. Hepatocellular adenomas in glycogen storage disease type I and III: a series of 43 patients and review of the literature. *J Pediatr Gastroenterol Nutr.* 1997;24:276–279.

14. Charny CK, Jarnagin WR, Schwartz LH, et al. Management of 155 patients with benign liver tumours. *Br J Surg.* 2001;88:808–813.

15. Glover GH. Multipoint Dixon technique for water and fat proton and susceptibility imaging. *J Magn Reson Imaging.* 1991;1:521–530.

16. Outwater EK, Siegelman ES, Hunt JL. Ovarian teratomas: tumor types and imaging characteristics. *Radiographics.* 2001;21:475–490.

17. Caruso PA, Marsh MR, Minkowitz S, Karten G. An intense clinicopathologic study of 305 teratomas of the ovary. *Cancer.* 1971;27:343–348.

CHAPTER 8

Susceptibility Artifact

Neal K. Viradia, Elmar M. Merkle, Allen W. Song, and Wells I. Mangrum

OPENING CASE 8.1

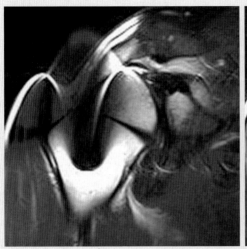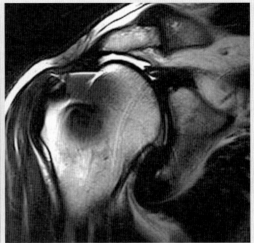

1. The figure at left is distorted by significant artifact. What imaging parameters can the technologist alter to decrease this artifact?
   A. Change the sequence to a gradient recalled echo
   B. Decrease echo train length
   C. Increase receiver bandwidth
   D. Decrease receiver bandwidth

OPENING CASE 8.1

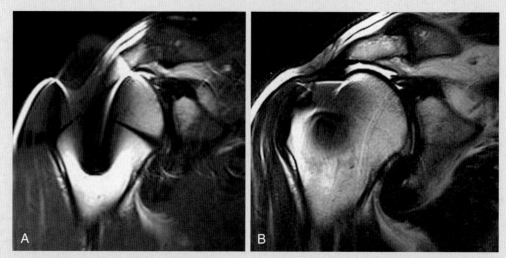

FIG. 8.C1. (A) Coronal T2-weighted, fast spin echo (FSE) sequence of the right shoulder. There is low signal centrally within the humeral head, with surrounding high signal. Note that the image distortion is greater in the craniocaudal direction (frequency-encoding direction) than in the mediolateral (phase-encoding) plane. The artifact limits evaluation of the rotator cuff. (B) Modified coronal T2-weighted, FSE sequence. In an effort to reduce the susceptibility effects, the echo train length was increased from 9 to 23, and the receiver bandwidth was increased from 130 to 435 kHz. Note the significant decrease in susceptibility artifact. The low-signal rotator cuff tendons end abruptly at the level of the acromioclavicular joint. T2 bright signal, consistent with fluid, is seen between the humeral head and acromion.

1. The figure at left is distorted by significant artifact. What imaging parameters can the technologist alter to decrease this artifact?
   C. Increase receiver bandwidth

Discussion

Metal in the proximal humerus is causing susceptibility artifact. The susceptibility artifact results in geometric distortion in spin echo imaging and signal loss in gradient recalled echo (GRE) imaging. Susceptibility artifacts are less pronounced in spin echo imaging compared with GRE imaging due to the 180-degree refocusing pulse used in spin echo imaging. To reduce susceptibility artifact, one would increase both the receiver bandwidth and the echo train length (see discussion below).

Susceptibility Artifact

The magnetic susceptibility of a substance is defined by the effect of the substance on the local magnetic field. If the material increases the local magnetic field, then the material has a positive magnetic susceptibility; if it decreases the local magnetic field, then it has a negative magnetic susceptibility. Substances that have positive magnetic susceptibilities are considered ferromagnetic or paramagnetic, depending on how much they increase the local magnetic field. Iron is a ferromagnetic substance because it significantly increases the local magnetic field and is magnetized, even after the removal of the magnetic field. Hemosiderin and deoxyhemoglobin are examples of paramagnetic substances that also increase the local magnetic field. However, paramagnetic substances are different from iron in that they do not increase the magnetic field to the same degree as iron, and they do not retain permanent magnetism. Diamagnetic materials have a negative magnetic susceptibility and thus decrease the local magnetic field. Free water and most human soft tissues are predominantly diamagnetic. Cortical bone is even more diamagnetic than soft tissue.[1]

Susceptibility artifact occurs when two substances of different magnetic susceptibilities are within proximity to one another. The substance with the higher magnetic susceptibility will increase the local magnetic field, whereas the adjacent substance with the lower magnetic susceptibility decreases the local magnetic field. The net result is that the local magnetic field is heterogeneous, with high strength next to the paramagnetic or ferromagnetic substance and low strength next to the diamagnetic substance. The susceptibility artifact increases as the difference between the magnetic susceptibilities increases.

Susceptibility artifacts can cause both signal loss and geometric distortion. The signal loss caused by susceptibility artifact is best seen on T2*-weighted sequences (GRE sequences). Recall that protons dephase in the transverse plane because of local magnetic field differences (see Chapter 2). When the local magnetic field is highly heterogeneous (e.g., when metal is in the field), this dephasing can result in significant signal loss. *The longer the time to echo (TE), the longer the protons have to dephase and the greater the susceptibility-induced* *signal loss will be. This effect can be nullified by using the 180-degree refocusing pulse used in spin echo imaging.* The refocusing pulse allows rephasing of the protons.

The second manifestation of susceptibility artifact is geometric distortion of the image. *Geometric distortion is the dominant manifestation of susceptibility artifact in spin echo imaging.* (Geometric distortion also occurs in GRE imaging, but its recognition is often masked by the dominant signal loss from proton dephasing.) To understand geometric image distortion, first recall that in the ideal situation, the MRI scanner creates a relatively uniform main magnetic field and three sets of linear spatial gradient fields across the body. These fields are required for spatial encoding. Susceptibility effects cause local heterogeneity in these fields, resulting in deviations in the spatial-encoding gradients and distortions in the final image. *The size of the geometric distortion is inversely related to the receiver bandwidth.*[2,3] The direction of the geometric distortion depends on the imaging sequence. For most conventional imaging, in which phase encoding is achieved in separate excitations, the geometric distortion occurs in the frequency-encoding direction. However, in most single-shot acquisitions (e.g., echo-planar imaging [EPI]), the distortion is predominant in the phase-encoding direction because the sampling rate (hence, the received bandwidth) is much lower in this direction.

A strategy to reduce susceptibility-induced image distortion is to reduce the length of readout windows for individual spin echoes (i.e., by effectively reducing the accumulated phase errors during the readout window). This can be achieved by increasing the receiver bandwidth and/or echo train length. This is the strategy used to reduce the geometric distortion in Case 8.1.[2,3] To uproot the distortion problem altogether, one can measure the magnetic field using a dual-echo sequence and apply the field correction in the reconstruction process to restore spatial fidelity.

CASES 8.2, 8.3, AND 8.4

FIG. 8.C2

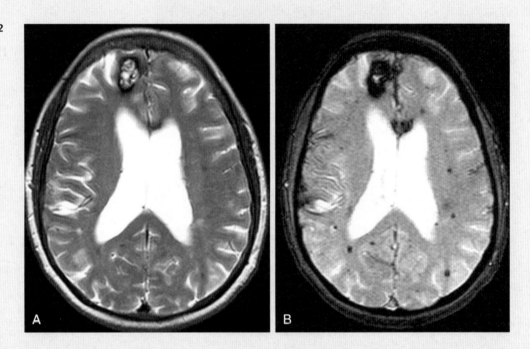

1. What is the most likely diagnosis?
   A. Metastatic disease
   B. Multiple cavernomas
   C. Multiple sclerosis
   D. Multifocal glioblastoma

FIG. 8.C2. (A) Axial T2-weighted FSE image of the brain. A high T2 signal lesion with a low T2 signal rim is identified in the right frontal lobe. The other scattered punctuate foci of low T2 signal in the bilateral cerebral hemispheres are difficult to appreciate. (B) Axial T2-weighted GRE sequence of the brain. The lesion in the right frontal lobe is again identified. The low T2 signal rim of the lesion is more pronounced. Additionally, multiple punctuate low T2 signal foci are distributed diffusely throughout the brain.

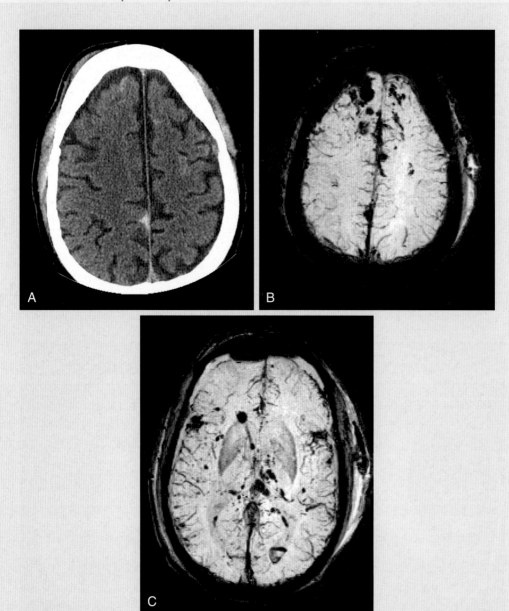

FIG. 8.C3

2. A 35-year-old man was found lying on the side of the road. He was the unbelted passenger in a motor vehicle collision. Images from his admission CT scan and subsequently performed MRI are provided. Which of the following accounts for the dark signal seen on the MRI images in the frontal lobes?
   A. Hyperostosis frontalis
   B. Pneumocephalus
   C. Frontal lobe contusion
   D. Epidural hematoma

3. In addition to the SWI sequence shown above, which of the following other MRI sequences could have been performed to demonstrate this finding?
   A. GRE
   B. Spin echo
   C. Diffusion
   D. Proton density

FIG. 8.C3. (A) Axial noncontrast helical CT of the brain. Focal triangular extraaxial hyperdensity is along the posterior flax. Small scattered hyperdense foci are in the cortex of the bilateral frontal lobes. (B) T2-weighted susceptibility-weighted (SWI) images. This image corresponds to the same level as the CT image in Fig. 8.C3A. (C) This image is lower, at the level of the lateral ventricles. Multifocal areas of low signal (blooming) are seen involving the bilateral frontal more than the parietal lobes. These lesions are predominantly centered at the gray-white junction. The dominant lesion is in the right frontal lobe. In addition, there is low signal along the falx.

FIG. 8.C4

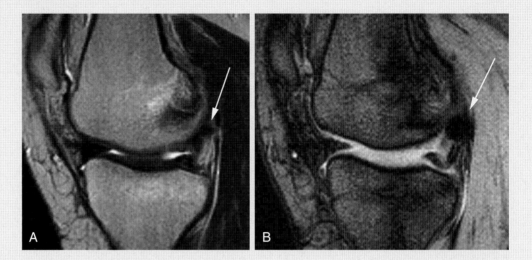

4. What is the best diagnosis?
   A. Status post–anterior cruciate ligament reconstruction
   B. Loose body in the knee joint
   C. Meniscal cyst
   D. Avian spur

FIG. 8.C4. (A) Sagittal T2-weighted FSE image of the knee. A subtle low T2 signal focus *(arrow)* is identified in the posterior knee joint. (B) Sagittal T2-weighted GRE image of the knee. The low T2 signal focus *(arrow)* "blooms" and is much more evident.

Discussion

Question 1: The T2 bright lesion with a low T2 signal rim in the right frontal lobe has the appearance of a cavernoma. Cavernomas have chronic recurrent bleeds that result in the characteristic hemosiderin ring. Cavernomas can be multiple, as shown in this case.[4]

Questions 2 and 3: The history of trauma and the location of the dominant lesions in the anterior aspect of the frontal lobes lead to the conclusion that these are areas of hemorrhage related to contusion of the frontal lobes. The additional foci at the gray-white junction are small foci of hemorrhage related to diffuse axonal injury. Diffuse axonal injury usually occurs at the gray-white junction, corpus callosum, basal ganglia, dorsolateral brainstem, and cerebellum.[5]

Question 4: Loose bodies in the knee joint can come from detached cartilage or bone. Free loose bodies within a joint can cause intermittent joint locking and pain. This case shows a classic location for a loose body.

CASES 8.2, 8.3, AND 8.4 ANSWERS

1. **B. Multiple cavernomas**
2. **C. Frontal lobe contusion**
3. **A. GRE**
4. **B. Loose body in the knee joint**

Susceptibility in Gradient Recalled Echo and Susceptibility-Weighted Image Sequences

In Cases 8.2 to 8.4, the pathology results in susceptibility artifact. In Cases 8.2 and 8.3, paramagnetic blood products increase the local magnetic field. In Case 8.4, the calcified loose body is diamagnetic and decreases the local magnetic field. Despite their opposite effects on the local magnetic field, both paramagnetic and diamagnetic substances share the property of causing susceptibility artifact.

The loose body and blood products are difficult to detect on the spin echo sequences but are readily apparent on the GRE sequences. Spin echo sequences have a 180 degree refocusing pulse that corrects for the dephasing caused by the magnetic field heterogeneity. Consequently, *spin echo sequences are favored when susceptibility effects need to be minimized. Conversely, GRE sequences can be helpful when susceptibility effects need to be enhanced.* The dephasing caused by the local changes in the magnetic field is more pronounced with GRE imaging and results in greater degrees of signal loss. Sometimes this susceptibility-induced signal loss associated with GRE imaging is colloquially referred to as "blooming."

SWI is often used in neuroradiology. *SWI is a three-dimensional, high–spatial resolution image that is a completely velocity-corrected GRE MRI sequence.[6,7] Following acquisition, postprocessing takes place, which includes application of a phase map. The phase images are multiplied with the magnitude images to accentuate the directly observed signal loss from the magnetic susceptibility differences.[6,7]*

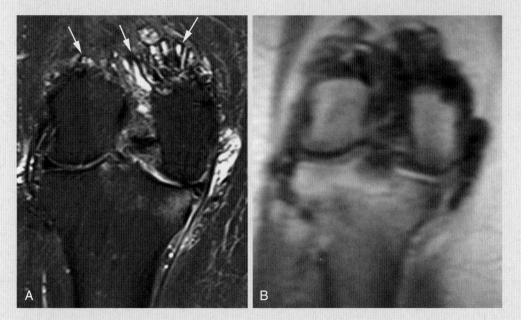

FIG. 8.C5

1. Given the imaging findings, what is the most likely diagnosis?
   A. Amyloid arthropathy
   B. Hemophilia-related arthropathy
   C. Pigmented villonodular synovitis (PVNS)
   D. Synovial sarcoma

FIG. 8.C5. (A) Coronal fat-saturated, T2-weighted FSE image of the posterior aspect of the knee joint. Curvilinear low T2 signal intensity is identified within the left knee joint *(arrows)*. (B) Coronal GRE localizer sequence. The signal-to-noise ratio is low on this sequence because it was obtained for localizing purposes and not for diagnostic purposes. The low signal structures within the knee joint bloom on this GRE image.

Discussion

The hemosiderin deposition in PVNS result in the susceptibility artifact shown in this case. Amyloid arthropathy should not demonstrate the "blooming" artifact seen in PVNS and can be essentially ruled out.[8] Hemophilia can be ruled out by history and by the lack of hemophilia-associated bony abnormalities.[8]

Further Considerations Regarding Susceptibility in GRE and SWI Sequences

As discussed in Cases 8.2, 8.3, and 8.4, paramagnetic or diamagnetic substances can cause susceptibility artifact that is more readily detected on GRE or SWI sequences. However, GRE and SWI images are not always obtained. A crude substitute for a routine GRE or SWI sequence is the localizer sequence. A GRE sequence can be used for a localizer sequence. The resolution of the localizer sequence is poor, but the localizer can confirm the presence or absence of susceptibility artifact, as shown in Case 8.5.

CASE 8.5 ANSWER

1. **C. Pigmented villonodular synovitis (PVNS)**

FIG. 8.C6

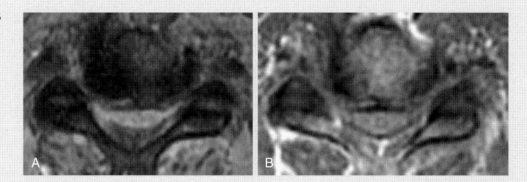

1. Why does the degree of neuroforaminal stenosis vary between the two MRI images?
   A. There is no difference; the degree of stenosis is the same.
   B. Susceptibility from bone exaggerates the degree of stenosis.
   C. There is a chemical shift artifact between cortical bone and intrathecal fat.
   D. Maximum intensity projection postprocessing is used.

FIG. 8.C6. (A) Axial T2-weighted GRE image of the cervical spine shows canal and bilateral neuroforaminal stenosis. Ossification of the posterior longitudinal ligament and ligamentum flavum hypertrophy results in severe canal stenosis. In addition, uncovertebral and facet degenerative changes result in neuroforaminal stenosis. (B) Axial T1-weighted FSE image of the cervical spine. The canal stenosis and foraminal stenosis are less pronounced on the FSE image.

Blooming Due to Susceptibility

Case 8.6 shows how susceptibility artifact in GRE imaging can be problematic. Cortical bone and the bone formed by degenerative changes are diamagnetic and cause susceptibility artifact. Consequently, cortical bone and degenerative osteophytosis bloom on GRE imaging, making them appear thicker than they really are. As a result, canal and foraminal stenosis can be overdiagnosed on GRE imaging.

CASE 8.6 ANSWER

1. **B. Susceptibility from bone exaggerates the degree of stenosis.**

CASES 8.7 AND 8.8

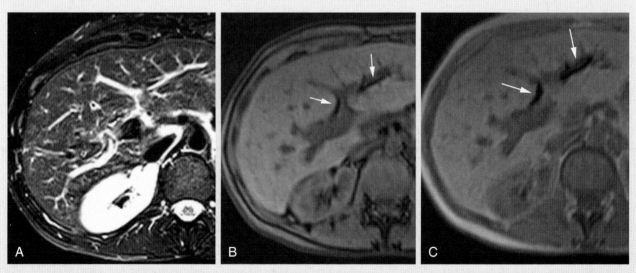

FIG. 8.C7

1. What is the cause of the low linear signal seen in Figs. 8.C7B and 8.C7C?
   A. Pneumobilia
   B. Portal venous gas
   C. Dilated bile ducts
   D. Flow void in the portal veins

FIG. 8.C7. (A) T2-weighted FSE image of the liver. No abnormality is identified. (B) T1-weighted, out-of-phase image of the abdomen (TE = 2.38 ms). A branching low signal structure is identified centrally within the liver, adjacent to the portal veins *(arrows)*. (C) T1-weighted, in-phase image of the abdomen (TE = 4.76 ms). The branching low signal structure is more pronounced *(arrows)*.

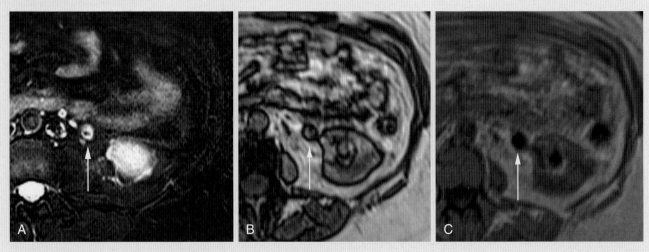

FIG. 8.C8

1. What is the most likely cause of the abnormality in the proximal left ureter?
   A. Transitional cell carcinoma
   B. Flow void artifact
   C. Ureteral stricture
   D. Ureteral stone

FIG. 8.C8. (A) Axial fat-saturated, T2-weighted FSE image of the left hemiabdomen. A small filling defect is identified in the left proximal ureter *(arrow)*. (B) Axial T1-weighted, out-of-phase image (TE = 2.38 ms). A low signal filling defect *(arrow)* is seen within the left ureter. (C) Axial T1-weighted, in-phase image of the abdomen (TE = 4.76 ms). The low signal filling defect *(arrow)* is more prominent on the in-phase image.

Discussion

Portal venous gas is another differential consideration for a low signal branching structure in the liver that is most evident on the longer TE sequence. However, in this case, the low signal branching structures are seen adjacent to the portal veins and not within the veins.

The leading differential considerations for a ureteral filling defect include a blood clot, transitional cell carcinoma, and renal stone. Transitional cell carcinoma would be expected to enhance.[9] Also, it is rare for transitional cell carcinoma to calcify. In this case, calcification in the ureteral stone is causing susceptibility artifact.

Susceptibility Effects in Relation to Time to Echo

Air and liver have widely disparate magnetic susceptibilities and result in susceptibility artifact when adjacent to one another. To see these effects best, a GRE sequence should be obtained, such as in-phase and out-of-phase imaging.[10] As previously described, the lack of a refocusing pulse makes GRE imaging more prone to susceptibility effects. Comparing the in-phase to out-of-phase image also demonstrates the effects of TE on susceptibility artifacts. The in-phase image has a longer TE. *The longer TE allows the susceptibility-induced dephasing of the protons to have a greater effect.* This results in more susceptibility artifact on the in-phase sequence than on the out-of-phase sequence.

CASES 8.7 AND 8.8 ANSWERS

1. A. Pneumobilia
2. D. Left ureteral stone

FIG. 8.C9

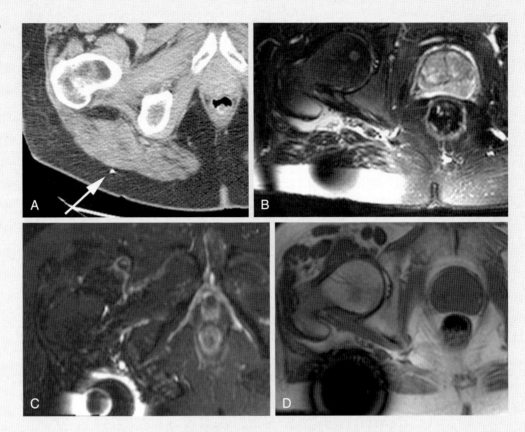

1. A patient has a small piece of metal embedded in the gluteal subcutaneous fat from a prior gunshot injury. Which sequence would result in the most optimum fat suppression?
   A. MRI should not be performed; bullet fragments are never safe.
   B. T1-weighted, in-phase GRE
   C. STIR
   D. Fat-saturated FSE

FIG. 8.C9. (A) CT scan of the pelvis. A tiny piece of metal is noted in the posterior subcutaneous tissues *(arrow)*. (B) Axial fat-saturated FSE image of the pelvis. Susceptibility artifact results in signal loss at the site of the metal. The size of the signal loss is much larger than the size of the metal. Chemical-selective fat saturation is insufficient in the immediate surroundings due to metal-induced local alterations of the magnetic field. (C) Axial short tau inversion recovery (STIR) image of the pelvis. Signal loss is again seen at the site of the metal. The size of the signal loss is roughly equivalent to the signal loss on the FSE image. The bright circle of incomplete fat saturation is smaller on the inversion recovery sequence than on the FSE chemical-selective fat saturation sequence. Although some bullets are not safe in MRI, not all bullet fragments are MRI incompatible. (D) T1-weighted, in-phase GRE image of the pelvis. The area of signal loss is much larger than the signal loss seen on the FSE or STIR images.

Susceptibility and Fat Suppression

In Fig. 8C.9, the small metal foreign body has a high magnetic susceptibility and results in a significant distortion of the magnetic field, despite its small size. The susceptibility effects are pronounced, in part because this MRI was performed on a 3-T magnet. *The higher the magnetic field strength, the greater the susceptibility effects.*[1] The greatest signal loss is seen in the in-phase GRE sequence. This is in keeping with the discussions from the previous cases.

Another teaching point from this case is how susceptibility artifact affects fat saturation. As discussed in Chapter 5, homogeneous fat suppression via frequency-selective saturation is dependent on protons within the fat having a uniform precession frequency. However, *the magnetic field heterogeneity caused by susceptibility effects changes the precession frequency of adjacent fats.* Consequently, the fat saturation preparatory pulse may miss the fat that has an altered precession frequency. Inversion recovery imaging, in contrast, is not as affected by local changes in the magnetic field because it depends purely on the T1 relaxation time. Consequently, inversion recovery fat suppression techniques work better in the presence of susceptibility artifacts.

CASE 8.9 ANSWER

1. C. STIR

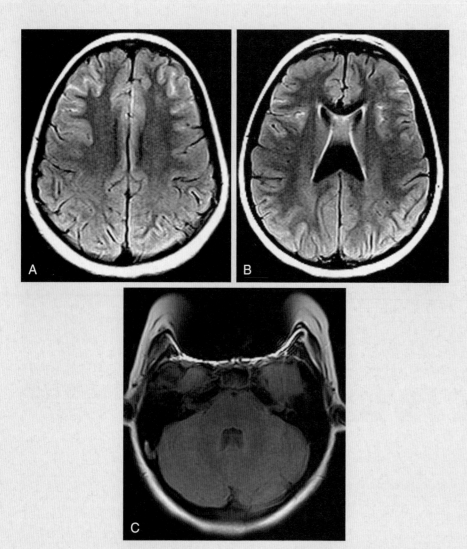

FIG. 8.C10

1. What is the most likely diagnosis?
   A. Pseudosubarachnoid hemorrhage
   B. Subarachnoid hemorrhage
   C. Meningitis
   D. Leptomeningeal spread of tumor

FIG. 8.C10. (A–B) Axial fluid-attenuated inversion recovery (FLAIR) images demonstrate increased signal in the region of the leptomeninges of the bilateral frontal lobes. (C) Axial FLAIR image through the level of the cerebellum. Loss of signal is seen in the anterior half of the face, with surrounding hyperintense signal and image distortion.

Discussion

At first appearance, the findings are worrisome for abnormal signal in the leptomeninges, possibly from infection, hemorrhage, or neoplasm. However, the more inferior image showing the characteristic signal loss in the region of the mouth (see Fig. 8.10C) is a finding that is characteristic of orthodontic hardware.

Susceptibility With Flair Imaging

Orthodontic hardware disrupts the local magnetic field. Consequently, the protons in the cerebrospinal fluid of the frontal lobes have a magnetic field that is altered by the orthodontic hardware. This alteration in signal is enough to cause incomplete fluid suppression by the FLAIR sequence, resulting in a pseudosubarachnoid hemorrhage appearance. Note that the CSF adjacent to the parietal lobes is farther away from the orthodontic hardware and experiences normal fluid suppression. This pseudosubarachnoid hemorrhage is not an uncommon finding in patients with orthodontic braces.

CASE 8.10 ANSWER

1. **A. Pseudosubarachnoid hemorrhage**

FIG. 8.C11

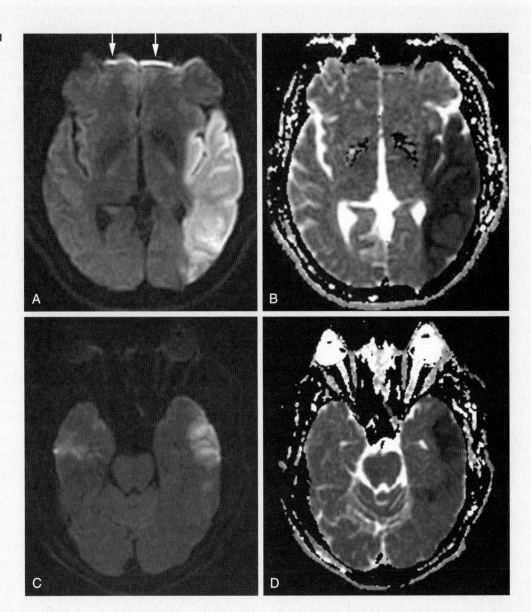

1. What vascular territory supplies the regions of infarction?
   A. Bilateral anterior cerebral artery (ACA) and left MCA
   B. Bilateral ACA and right MCA
   C. Left MCA
   D. Right MCA
   E. Bilateral MCA
   F. Bilateral ACA

FIG. 8.C11 (A) Axial diffusion-weighted image of the brain. High signal is noted in the left temporal, frontal, and parietal lobes in the middle cerebral artery (MCA). An additional thin rim of high signal is seen adjacent to the frontal sinuses bilaterally (arrows). (B) Apparent diffusion coefficient (ADC) map. Low ADC signal in the left temporal, parietal, and frontal lobes confirms the restricted diffusion in the left MCA distribution. No thin rim of low signal is seen adjacent to the frontal sinuses. (C) Axial diffusion-weighted image of the brain. High signal is seen in the lateral aspect of the temporal lobe bilaterally, greater in the left than in the right. (D) ADC map. Low ADC values are identified in the lateral left temporal lobe. The right temporal lobe is normal.

Discussion

Areas of high signal adjacent to the frontal sinuses and in the right temporal lobe are normal on the ADC map and are due to susceptibility artifact from the cortex of the adjacent bone and the air in the frontal sinuses. A high diffusion-weighted imaging (DWI) signal with a corresponding low ADC signal in the left MCA territory is concerning for an acute infarct.

Susceptibility With Diffusion Imaging

Diffusion images are frequently obtained with EPI. EPI typically is acquired with a single-shot technique, a technique with a long readout window. This causes DWI to be highly sensitive to susceptibility effects.[1] The differences in magnetic susceptibilities between air in the paranasal sinuses and brain and between cortical bone and brain cause susceptibility effects. This is seen as high signal in the brain adjacent to the sinuses on DWI. The ADC maps of these areas will be normal (as shown in this case). Functional MRI is another technique that uses EPI, and consequently is also highly sensitive to susceptibility effects (see Chapter 17).

CASE 8.11 ANSWER

1. **C. Left MCA**

CASES 8.12, 8.13, AND 8.14

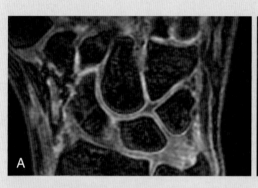
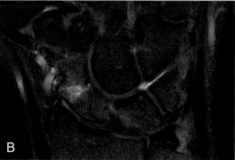

FIG. 8.C12

1. Which sequence is optimal in diagnosing subtle fractures?
   A. Fat-suppressed, T2-weighted GRE
   B. Non–fat-suppressed, T2-weighted GRE
   C. Fat-suppressed T2-weighted FSE
   D. SWI

Diagnosis

This is a scaphoid waist fracture.

FIG. 8.C12. (A) Coronal fat-suppressed, T2-weighted GRE image. There is questionable linear distortion of the trabeculae in the waist of the scaphoid. No increased T2 signal is seen in the scaphoid. (B) Coronal fat-suppressed, T2-weighted FSE image. Linear and wedge-shaped increased T2 signal is noted in the waist of the scaphoid.

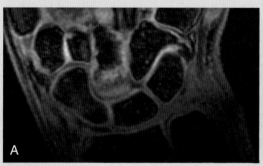
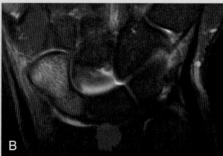

FIG. 8.C13

Diagnosis

This is a scaphoid waist fracture with marked surrounding bone marrow edema.

FIG. 8.C13. (A) Coronal fat-suppressed, T2-weighted GRE image. There is slightly increased T2 signal with associated trabecular distortion in the waist of the scaphoid. (B) Coronal fat-suppressed, T2-weighted FSE image. Linear low T2 signal is noted through the waist of the scaphoid. High T2 signal is noted in the bone marrow of the scaphoid.

FIG. 8.C14

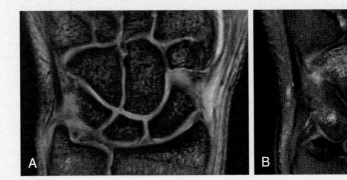

Diagnosis

There is contusion of the hamate and triquetrum. A hook of hamate fracture was shown on other images.

FIG. 8.C14. (A) Coronal fat-suppressed, T2-weighted GRE image. No abnormality is identified. (B) Coronal fat-suppressed, T2-weighted FSE image. Increased T2 signal is noted in the distal half of the hamate and in the distal tip of the triquetrum.

Susceptibility With T2-Weighted Imaging

Trabecular and cortical bone are diamagnetic substances with low magnetic susceptibilities that can result in susceptibility artifact.[11] Case 8.6 showed an example of how blooming from cortical and degenerative bone can exaggerate canal stenosis. Cases 8.12, 8.13, and 8.14 show how the susceptibility artifact from cortical and trabecular bone can mask bone marrow edema on GRE images. The diamagnetic bone alters the local magnetic field, causing increased dephasing of protons and signal loss. This signal loss hides the signal gain that results from the bone marrow edema. Note that the bone marrow edema is readily apparent on the spin echo sequences because the refocusing pulse rephases the dephasing protons.

CASES 8.12, 8.13, AND 8.14 ANSWER

1. **C. Fat-suppressed T2 FSE**

TAKE-HOME POINTS

Defining Susceptibility

1. Magnetic susceptibility is defined as the relative ability of a substance to become magnetized when exposed to a magnetic field.
2. Materials can be defined by their magnetic susceptibility to be ferromagnetic, paramagnetic, or diamagnetic.
3. Susceptibility artifact occurs when tissues of widely different magnetic susceptibilities are adjacent to one another, such as metal adjacent to soft tissue.

Methods to Reduce Susceptibility Artifact

1. Spin echo or FSE imaging
2. Long echo train length
3. Shortened TE
4. Increased receiver bandwidth
5. Decreased magnetic field strength (1.5 T has less artifact than 3 T)

Clinical Utility of Susceptibility Artifact

1. When looking for air: pneumobilia
2. When looking for metal: to detect evidence of surgical changes
3. When looking for blood products: cavernomas, diffuse axonal injury, PVNS
4. When looking for calcification: loose body in the joint, renal stone

Susceptibility Artifact Interference With Diagnosis

1. Geometric distortion and signal loss from metal hardware can obscure the image.
2. Susceptibility artifact can create false signal, such as pseudosubarachnoid hemorrhage caused by orthodontic braces and signal adjacent to the sinuses in DWI.
3. Susceptibility artifact can hide true bone marrow edema, such as scaphoid fracture and hamate edema.
4. Susceptibility artifact can exaggerate stenosis from degenerative changes.

Sequences Sensitive to Susceptibility Effects

1. GRE, and particularly SWI sequences, are highly sensitive to susceptibility artifact.
2. In-phase imaging is more sensitive to susceptibility effects than out-of-phase imaging because of the longer TE.
3. EPI in DWI or functional MRI is sensitive to susceptibility effects.

References

1. Runge VM, Nitz WR, Schmeets SH, et al. *The Physics of Clinical MR Taught Through Images*. New York: Thieme; 2005.
2. Harris CA, White LM. Metal artifact reduction in musculoskeletal magnetic resonance imaging. *Orthop Clin North Am*. 2006;37:349–359.
3. Stadler A, Schima W, Ba-Ssalamah A, et al. Artifacts in body MR imaging: their appearance and how to eliminate them. *Eur Radiol*. 2007;17:1242–1255.
4. Maraire JN, Awad IA. Intracranial cavernous malformations: lesion behavior and management strategies. *Neurosurgery*. 1995;37:591–605.
5. Parizel PM, Özsarlak Ö, Van Goethem JW, et al. Imaging findings in diffuse axonal injury after closed head trauma. *Eur Radiol*. 1998;8:960–965.
6. Roberto G, Pinelli L, Liserre R. New MR sequences in daily practice: susceptibility weighted imaging. A pictorial essay. *Insights Imaging*. 2001;2(3):335–347.
7. Haacke EM, Xu Y, Cheng YC, Reichenbach JR. Susceptibility weighted imaging (SWI). *Magn Reson Med*. 2004;52:612–618.
8. Garner HW, Ortiguera CJ, Nakhleh RE. Pigmented villonodular synovitis. *Radiographics*. 2008;28:1519–1523.
9. Leyendecker JR, Barnes CE, Zagoria RJ. MR urography: techniques and clinical applications. *Radiographics*. 2008;28:23–46.
10. Merkle EM, Nelson RC. Dual gradient-echo in-phase and opposed-phase hepatic MR imaging: a useful tool for evaluating more than fatty infiltration or fatty sparing. *Radiographics*. 2006;26:1409–1418.
11. Majumdar S, Thomasson D, Shimakawa A, Genant HK. Quantitation of the susceptibility difference between trabecular bone and bone marrow: experimental studies. *Magn Reson Med*. 1991;22:111–127.

CHAPTER 9

Motion, Pulsation, and Other Artifacts

Phil B. Hoang, Steven Y. Huang, Allen W. Song, and Elmar M. Merkle

OPENING CASE 9.1

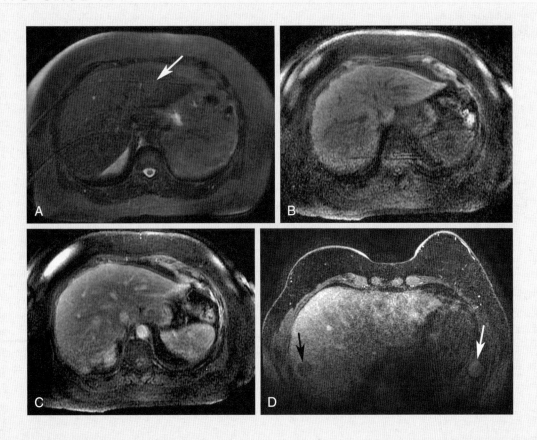

1. In the above figure, parts A–C are from a liver MRI of
   patient 1, and part D is from a breast MRI of patient 2.
   The lesions depicted by the arrows in A and D represent
   pulsation artifacts. Which of the following is true regarding
   the phase-encoding direction during image acquisition?
   A. Patient 1, *y*-axis; *y*-axis for patient 2
   B. Patient 1, *x*-axis; *z*-axis for patient 2
   C. Patient 1, *x*-axis; *y*-axis for patient 2
   D. Patient 1, *y*-axis; *x*-axis for patient 2

OPENING CASE 9.1

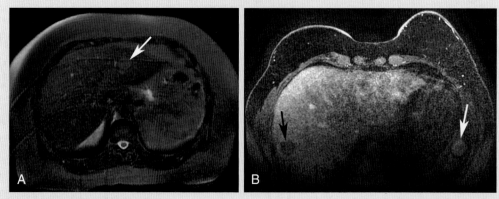

FIG. 9.C1. (A) Fat-suppressed, T2-weighted axial image of the upper abdomen demonstrates a round high signal intensity lesion in the left hepatic lobe *(arrow)*. This lesion is not seen on the precontrast and postcontrast fat-suppressed, three-dimensional (3D) gradient recalled echo (GRE) axial T1-weighted sequences. (B) Fat-suppressed axial, 3D GRE T1-weighted sequence from a dedicated breast MRI (different patient) demonstrates a round low signal lesion in the right hepatic lobe *(black arrow)* and a round high signal lesion in the region of the spleen and abdominal wall *(white arrow)*.

1. Which of the following is true regarding the phase-encoding direction during image acquisition?
   D. Patient 1, *y*-axis; *x*-axis for patient 2

Discussion

Patient 1 has a T2 bright lesion in the left hepatic lobe (Fig. 9.C1A) without corresponding abnormality on the precontrast (Fig. 9.C1B) and postcontrast (Unn. Fig. 9.C1C) fat-suppressed 3D, GRE axial T1-weighted sequences. Patient 2 has a low signal lesion to the right of the aorta in the right hepatic lobe and a corresponding high signal lesion to the left of the aorta within the spleen. These artifacts in patients 1 and 2 are referred to as *ghosting artifacts*. Ghosting artifacts appear as replicas of the moving structure from which they arise but are in abnormal locations. They are observed in the phase-encoding direction and can be the result of any periodic motion, such as respiration, arterial pulsation, or cerebrospinal fluid (CSF) pulsation. Unn. Figs. 9.C1A–C were obtained from an abdominal MRI, during which the phase-encoding direction was oriented vertically; therefore the artifact is also seen along the *y*-axis. Unn. Fig. 9.C1D was obtained from a breast MRI in which the phase-encoding direction was horizontal; thus the artifact appears along the *x*-axis. Incidentally, the regular repeating stripes in Fig. 9.C1A (one of which goes through the left hepatic lobe pseudolesion) are caused by respiratory motion. Patient breath-holding, respiratory triggering, and the use of faster imaging sequences can help mitigate this artifact.

Motion and Pulsation Artifact

Motion is a very common cause of artifacts in MRI scans. Motion artifacts are the result of movement during the data acquisition period. More specifically, when motion is present, tissues excited at a specific location during the radiofrequency (RF) pulse are erroneously mapped to a different location or often to different locations (in cases of motion artifacts) during detection. Motion is often divided into two categories, gross body movement and physiologic motion, such as cardiac and respiratory cycles or blood or CSF flow. In most conventional imaging methods, motion artifact is predominantly manifested in the phase-encoding direction.

Gradients in Image Formation and Their Implication in Motion Artifacts

Why are gradients necessary? If an RF pulse were broadcast without gradients, then every proton within the main magnetic field would be excited. The receiver coil would receive signals from the protons all resonating at the same frequency and with the same phase-making spatial localization, so a coherent MR image would be impossible to obtain.[1] The three magnetic field gradients required to form an image are the slice selection, frequency-encoding, and phase-encoding gradients. The primary purpose of these gradients is to assign spatial localization to the resultant MRI scan. Typically, for an axial image, the slice selection gradient assigns location in the z direction, the frequency-encoding gradient or readout gradient assigns location in the x direction, and the phase-encoding gradient assigns location in the y direction.

The purpose of a slice selection gradient is to expose protons along the z-axis to different magnetic fields inducing the protons to precess at a wide range of frequencies; at the same time, an RF pulse with a very narrow range of frequencies is administered, which results in excitation of only a thin slice of tissue along the z-axis. That is, only those protons along the z-axis gradient that have frequencies corresponding to the RF pulse are excited.[1] The range of frequencies transmitted by the RF pulse is termed the *transmitter bandwidth*. The slice thickness can be made thicker or thinner by adjusting the gradient strength or the transmitter bandwidth. Increasing the gradient strength or reducing the transmitter bandwidth results in a thinner slice. Decreasing the gradient strength or increasing the transmitter bandwidth results in a thicker slice.

The frequency-encoding gradient is critically important for spatial localization along the x-axis. Unlike the slice selection gradient, which is applied at the same time as the RF excitation pulse, the frequency-encoding gradient is applied concurrently with echo sampling. The frequency-encoding gradient induces protons along the x-axis at different locations to precess at different frequencies. For example, the protons on the right side of the body will precess a little faster than protons on the left side of the body. With use of the Fourier transformation, these differences in frequency can be translated into differences in signal at each spatial location to create the MRI scan.

The frequency-encoding gradient is also important in the generation of an echo. Over time, proton spins in the presence of a spatial gradient would accumulate phase shifts. The generation of MR signal is dependent on the protons being in phase at just the right time during echo sampling. Gradients' dephasing properties are manipulated in a controlled fashion so that phase coherence can be achieved and an echo generated. This is accomplished by applying a gradient with two lobes that have opposite polarity. The first lobe of the gradient is the dephasing lobe. A second gradient is then applied with opposite polarity and typically twice the duration, called a rephasing lobe. Thus at the midpoint of this rephasing lobe, the sampled protons are most in phase, and an echo is generated. This is referred to as

a gradient echo. If a 180-degree refocusing pulse is applied prior to the rephasing lobe and after a 90-degree excitation pulse, the generated echo is referred to as a spin echo. Pulse sequences are usually timed so that the gradient echo and the spin echo occur at the same time. In the case of a spin echo acquisition, the rephasing lobe should be applied with the same polarity (rather than the opposite polarity) as the dephasing lobe because the 180-degree refocusing pulse results in a complete reversal of phase. The direction of the frequency-encoding gradient is almost always applied along the axis with the widest dimension (e.g., right to left in the abdomen and anterior to posterior in the head).[2]

Finally, a phase-encoding gradient is used for spatial localization along the y-axis. In contrast to the frequency-encoding gradient, the phase-encoding gradient is applied right before data acquisition, but also after the slice excitation. As such, the protons would have already experienced the gradient and accumulated certain controlled phase shifts. Because the phase-encoding gradient is turned off before the data readout, these phase shifts would remain fixed to ensure the same amount of phase encoding. To complete the coverage for a two-dimensional (2D) image, for example, different phases are assigned with different phase-encoding gradient amplitudes before the data acquisition window. A subsequent Fourier transformation can then be used to resolve the image spatially along the phase-encoding direction. It is worth noting that a rephasing gradient (e.g., like that used in slice selection) or a dephasing gradient (e.g., like that used in frequency encoding) is not usually needed for phase encoding. Spatial localization is encoded from differences in phase rather than frequency by applying the phase-encoding gradient after the initial excitation pulse and before echo sampling.[1]

Spatial encoding along the frequency-encoding direction can be performed in its entirety with a single RF excitation pulse. Along the phase-encoding axis, spatial localization usually (except for single-shot imaging techniques such as echo-planar imaging) requires the application of numerous phase-encoding gradients, each with a different strength with each new RF excitation. The number of phase-encoding steps required determines the extent of the MR image along the y-axis and, along with the time to repetition (TR), is an important contributor to image acquisition time. Strong phase-encoding gradients create larger differences in phase and allow better discrimination of objects that are close together (better spatial resolution) in the resultant MR image. The downside of a stronger gradient is that because the protons are more out of phase, there is reduced signal and contrast. Weaker gradients result in better signal and contrast. This principle has important implications in how k-space is filled. By convention, the center of k-space is the high-contrast region, and the periphery contributes to the fine detail and spatial resolution of the image. Therefore the center of k-space is filled first with echoes resulting from the weaker phase-encoding gradients; the gradient strength increases gradually as the k-space is filled from central to peripheral.[1]

The extensive use of spatial gradients often complicates and amplifies the motion artifacts because stronger gradients would induce larger phase shifts from motion. Although some gradient combinations can be made insensitive to motion (e.g., the flow-compensated gradients; see below for more details), many of the imaging gradient pulses are not. As such, the inconsistent nature of motion can induce different phase shifts during the image readout period. When viewed from the phase-encoding direction in the final data space, these inconsistencies introduce local deviations, which would result in ghosting artifacts in the image space as the result of Fourier transformation. For example, a pulsatile effect in one of the data lines (along the frequency-encoding direction) would be viewed as a spike along the phase-encoding direction, which would then result in a streaking line artifact along the phase-encoding direction. More severely, several inconsistent data lines would result in more extensive ghosting artifacts.

In short, motion artifacts are predominantly manifested along the phase-encoding direction. More specifically, random motion results in smearing or blurring in the phase-encoding direction, and periodic motion (cardiac motion and blood vessels) results in ghosting artifacts. Ghosting artifacts appear as replicas of the moving structure at specific intervals along the phase-encoding axis. The motion artifact patterns are dependent on how repeatable the phase shifts were along the phase-encoding direction in k-space. For example, if only one line deviates, then the artifact will be a solid line across the MR image. If it repeats every other line, then the artifact will be a displacement over half of the field of view. If all the lines deviate the same way (e.g., after excessive averaging), the artifact will not be apparent.[3]

Why does flowing blood cause motion artifacts? After application of the dephasing lobe of the slice selection and frequency-encoding gradients, blood moves to a different location and experiences a rephasing gradient of a different strength. The phase shift induced by the dephasing lobe cannot be reversed by a gradient of a different strength, and the phase difference persists as ghost artifacts.[2]

Numerous methods can be used to reduce motion artifacts. Increasing the sampling bandwidth is a simple method to reduce motion artifact at the expense of signal to noise. In general, increasing the gradient strength or the time in which the gradient is applied will increase susceptibility to motion artifact. Increasing the strength of the frequency-encoding gradient is an exception; however, the sampling bandwidth increases with increasing gradient strength, which decreases the sampling time.[2]

Another method to reduce motion artifact is termed *gradient moment nulling*. When motion occurs during the dephasing or rephasing lobe of the gradient, there is incomplete phase cancellation, which leads to a net accumulation of phase, referred to as the gradient moment. This phase accumulation can be the result of protons moving with constant velocity motion (first-order motion), acceleration (second-order motion), or pulsatile or jerk motion (third-order motion). In its simplest form, an applied gradient without motion correction is a unipolar gradient. Application of additional gradient pulses, such as in the form of a bipolar gradient, can rephase the phase shift from stationary and moving tissues and significantly reduces first-order or constant velocity motion. Application of more complex gradient pulses can also reduce second- and third-order motion; however, gradient moment nulling works best for first-order motion. Gradient moment nulling requires a longer echo time (TE). With first-order nulling, the increase in TE is negligible, but with second- or third-order nulling, the longer TE can be problematic.[3]

Switching the direction of the frequency and phase-encoding gradients is a simple way to manipulate motion artifact. Motion artifact is not eliminated with this method but is displaced along another axis. This method can be very helpful in trying to distinguish whether a finding represents true pathology or is due to motion artifact.

A **presaturation pulse** is another method that is often used to reduce the effects of motion artifact. This technique is preferred if the signal to be nulled is not necessary for image interpretation. A presaturation pulse can be used to null fat if its signal is contributing to the motion artifact. It can also be used to saturate the protons in flowing blood before it enters the volume of tissue being imaged, and is a frequently used technique in time-of-flight (TOF) imaging.[2]

Averaging is a motion reduction technique that is often used to eliminate ghosting artifacts due to respiratory motion. This method takes advantage of the fact that on average, normal tissue stays in a relatively constant location with each respiratory cycle while the location of the ghosting artifacts varies much more with each breath. Averaging is typically accomplished by acquiring more than one signal with each phase-encoding step. The average signal of tissue is much more coherent and contributes more to the overall appearance of the image when compared with the signal produced from the ghosting artifacts.[2]

Respiratory triggering is a method used to decrease respiratory motion artifact. This is accomplished with a bellows on the upper abdomen, which tracks the motion of the respiratory cycle, or with a so-called navigator technique, which produces a signal that indicates the position of the diaphragm. Typically the signals are acquired during end-expiration with each cycle. Image acquisition takes longer with this technique because signal acquisition is restricted to end expiration. Cardiac gating synchronizes image acquisition with the electrocardiogram, which is very useful for eliminating cardiac motion artifact.

Perhaps the most effective method to reduce respiratory motion is respiratory suspension. With patients who are capable of doing this, single breath-hold techniques with 2D multislice or 3D acquisitions can be performed. With patients who have difficulty holding their breath, ultrafast imaging techniques can be helpful in producing diagnostic images.[2]

CASE 9.2

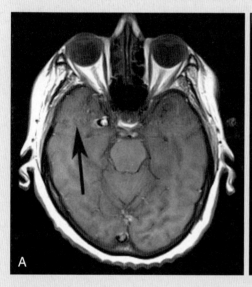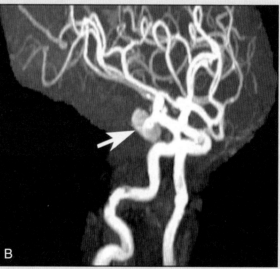

FIG. 9.C2

1. What is the artifact depicted by the arrow in Fig. 9.C2A?
   A. Ghosting artifact
   B. Chemical shift artifact
   C. Aliasing artifact
   D. Entry slice phenomenon artifact

FIG. 9.C2. (A) Axial T1-weighted image of the head demonstrates a focal lesion along the medial aspect of the right temporal lobe, with a central high T1 signal and peripheral low T1 signal. Ghosting artifact is seen on both sides of the lesion extending in the phase-encoding direction *(arrow)*. (B) Maximum intensity projection (MIP) image of the circle of Willis from a TOF magnetic resonance angiography scan. There is a saccular outpouching seen adjacent to the right supraclinoid internal carotid artery *(arrow)*.

Discussion

It is extremely important to consider the diagnosis of an aneurysm when developing a differential for an extraaxial parasellar mass. Cerebral aneurysms classically demonstrate a central flow void, with circumferential rings of varying signal intensity extending peripherally, secondary to partial thrombosis with blood products of different ages. The diagnosis is clinched with recognition of a pulsation artifact in the phase-encoding direction, which is due to pulsatile blood flow in the aneurysm. However, lack of artifact does not exclude an aneurysm, because completely thrombosed aneurysms will not produce pulsation artifact. The protons in the moving blood experience a rephasing gradient of a different strength and accumulation phase, which results in the ghosting artifact seen.

A chemical shift artifact arises because fat protons precess slower than water protons during frequency encoding. This misregistration causes artificial boundaries to be created at fat-water interfaces, resulting in the chemical shift artifact. An aliasing artifact occurs when the scanned body part is larger than the field of view, resulting in mapping of the body part outside the field of view into part of the image within the field of view. An entry slice phenomenon artifact occurs when unsaturated protons enter into an observed slice. The protons emit a strong signal because they are unsaturated, resulting in flow-related enhancement.

CASE 9.2 ANSWER

1. **A. Ghosting artifact**

CASE 9.3

FIG. 9.C3

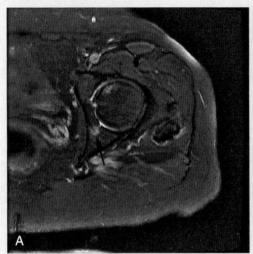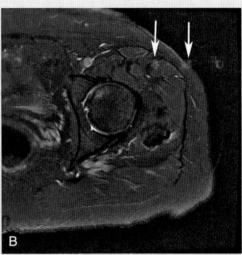

1. The round high T2 signal focus in the posterior acetabulum in Fig. 9.C3A is an example of pulsation artifact. This image was obtained after Fig. 9.C3B. Which of the following was done before acquiring Fig. 9.C3B?
   A. Administration of a saturation band
   B. Switching the directions of the frequency and phase encoding
   C. Increasing the acquisition matrix from 320 × 192 to 320 × 240
   D. Asking the patient to do a better job of keeping still

FIG. 9.C3. (A) High signal focus is identified in the left posterior acetabulum *(arrow)*. (B) Axial fat-suppressed T2-weighted image, same patient. The high signal acetabular focus seen in A is no longer identified. Note the vascular pulsation artifact arising from the left femoral artery *(arrows)*.

Discussion

A vascular pulsation artifact can be a source of confusion because it can frequently be mistaken for a true focal lesion, which is evident in this case. If an artifact is a possibility, a simple way to resolve this is to swap the phase- and frequency-encoding directions. Although this does not eliminate the artifact, it does shift it into another direction in the image, enabling more accurate evaluation. The phase-encoding direction is shifted from a vertical to a horizontal direction, clearly confirming the lesion to be outside the bone, which is consistent with a ghosting artifact.

CASE 9.3 ANSWER

1. **B. Switching the directions of the frequency and phase encoding**

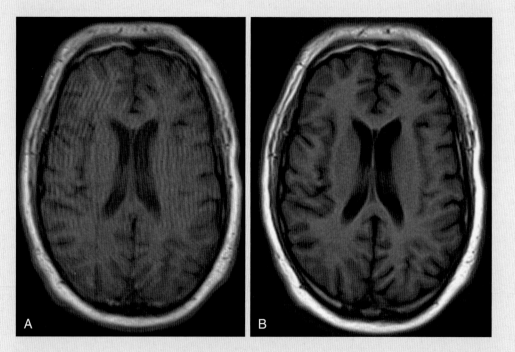

FIG. 9.C4

1. What can be done to reduce the patient motion artifact seen in Fig. 9.C4A to produce the image seen in Fig. 9.C4B?
   A. Apply a presaturation pulse prior to the RF pulse
   B. Apply gradient moment nulling
   C. Use a multishot turbo spin echo sequence
   D. Increase the strength of the phase-encoding gradient

FIG. 9.C4. (A) Axial T1-weighted image through the brain, which is severely degraded by motion artifact. (B) Axial BLADE sequence with T1 weighting, with significant reduction in the motion artifact.

Discussion

Another way of overcoming motion degradation is to use a multishot turbo spin echo (TSE) sequence. BLADE (Siemens) is a TSE sequence that uses a nonrectilinear sampling of k-space to reduce motion sensitivity. As in a traditional TSE sequence, for every TR, one group of parallel lines of k-space is acquired. However, unlike a traditional TSE sequence, each group surrounds the center of k-space, and each group is rotated relative to the other groups rather than being shifted in the phase-encoding direction relative to the others. This reduces motion sensitivity in two ways. First, motion artifacts get distributed throughout the image and thus appear more like an increase in random noise than coherent ghosting. Second, by repeatedly sampling the k-space center, it is possible to detect in-plane rigid body motion and correct for it in the reconstruction. However,

because of the redundant sampling of the k-space center, it takes longer to acquire a BLADE image than to acquire a traditional TSE image.

Administration of a presaturation pulse would render part of the image nondiagnostic, which did not occur in this case. Gradient moment nulling is a motion correction technique best used for artifacts arising from constant velocity. Gradient moment nulling requires a longer TE, which is negligible for constant velocity nulling. For random motion, the technique is difficult to use because of unacceptable increases in TE. Increasing the gradient strength will increase susceptibility to motion artifact.

CASE 9.4 ANSWER

1. **C. Use a multishot turbo spin echo sequence**

FIG. 9.C5

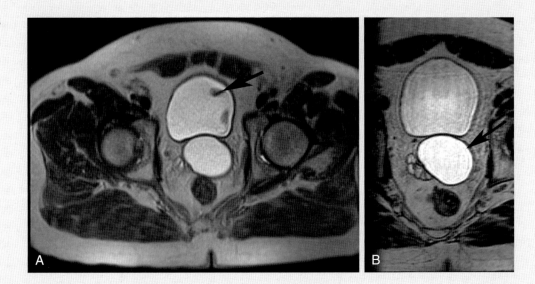

1. Fig. 9.C5A was obtained from an axial HASTE sequence and demonstrates a flow-related artifact from a left ureteral jet *(arrow)*. Fig. 9.C5B was obtained from a 3D TSE sequence. Which of the following is true regarding 3D TSE sequences?
   A. Images are obtained using nonisotropic voxel sizes.
   B. Flow-related artifacts are reduced by filling in k-space over a single TR.
   C. These sequences use short, nonspatially selective RF pulses and variable flip angles.
   D. There is limited clinical application due to long image acquisition times.

FIG. 9.C5. (A) Axial HASTE (half-Fourier acquisition single-shot turbo spin echo) image demonstrates curvilinear low signal *(arrow)* in the left aspect of the bladder. (B) Axial SPACE (**s**ampling **p**erfection with **a**pplication-optimized **c**ontrasts using different flip angle **e**volutions) image at the same level through the bladder. The curvilinear area of low density is no longer present. There is a second cystic structure *(arrow)* posterior to the bladder, which was coming from the seminal vesicle. On other images, it was noted that the left kidney was congenitally absent. These findings are consistent with Zinner syndrome.

Discussion

Fig. 9.C5A is an axial HASTE sequence. HASTE is a single-shot, ultrafast imaging technique (acquired in <0.5 seconds), which is very helpful in reducing motion artifact. Single shot means acquiring all the echoes needed to fill k-space after a single excitation pulse. Also, with the HASTE sequence, a little over 50% of k-space is acquired, and the rest is interpolated, which significantly reduces acquisition time. HASTE is a T2-weighted sequence. There is no repetition of the excitation (no TR), which eliminates T1 weighting.[2] Although the HASTE sequence is very useful in avoiding the effects of motion, it is still a flow-sensitive sequence, as seen in Fig. 9.C5A, with the femoral blood vessels appearing dark. The turbulent flow from the left ureteral jet in the left aspect of the bladder creates a curvilinear-appearing signal void. This can also be found when there is a large amount of ascites in the abdomen; it results from the motion of fluid between

excitation and readout. The SPACE sequence, on the other hand, is a multishot sequence. Here k-space if filled over multiple TRs, and the inconstant flow effects of ureteral jets cancel each other out, making the urinary bladder appear homogenously bright. To mitigate the issue of long acquisition times, 3D TSE sequences use short, nonspatially selective RF pulses to shorten the echo spacing and variable flip angles to lengthen the usable echo train. 3D TSE is useful for imaging the brain, spine, body, and musculoskeletal system. The sequence acquires high-resolution 3D isotropic data sets that can be reformatted to investigate complex anatomy.

CASE 9.5 ANSWER

1. **C. These sequences use short, nonspatially selective RF pulses and variable flip angles.**

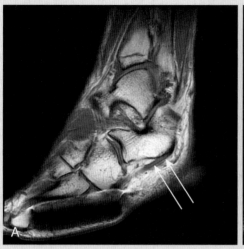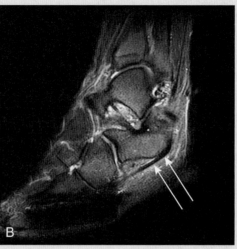

FIG. 9.C6

1. A magic angle artifact is noted in the peroneus brevis tendon on the T1-weighted image (A). Which of the following is characteristic of this artifact?
   A. It resolves with fat suppression
   B. It worsens on long TE sequences
   C. It resolves on long TE sequences
   D. Both A and C are true

FIG. 9.C6. (A) Sagittal T1-weighted image of the lateral ankle demonstrates increased signal involving the peroneus brevis tendon *(arrows)*. Note the signal void related to fifth metatarsal bone hardware. (B) Sagittal T2-weighted image at the same level demonstrates normal low T2 signal of the peroneus brevis tendon.

Discussion

The high signal intensity of the peroneus brevis tendon on the T1-weighted image is due to the magic angle artifact. Tissues composed of ordered collagen fibers (e.g., tendons, ligaments) are normally of low signal intensity on all pulse sequences; this is due to the dipolar interactions of the water molecules in contact with the fibers, which leads to a short T2 relaxation time. If the orientation of the fibers is at a certain angle in relation to the main magnetic field, the dipolar interaction approaches zero, leading to a slight *increase* in the T2 relaxation times. On short TE sequences, such as used in T1- and proton density–weighted sequences, there is inadequate time for T2 decay to take place; this results in a spurious increased signal. Although there is a range of angles at which this artifact appears (45–65 degrees), it is maximal when the tendons are oriented at 54.7 degrees to the main (B_0) magnetic field.[4] The signal abnormality characteristically resolves on longer TE sequences because the increase in T2 relaxation time is still much shorter compared with the TE, which allows adequate T2 decay to take place. Fat suppression techniques (e.g., fat saturation, inversion recovery) do not have any effects on resolving the artifact.

CASE 9.6 ANSWER

1. **C. It resolves on long TE sequences**

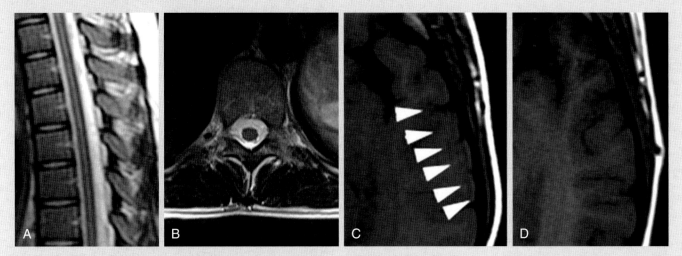

FIG. 9.C7

1. A 27-year-old man presents with midthoracic back pain. What is the most likely cause of the high signal changes present within the thoracic spinal cord in part A? An axial image of the seventh thoracic vertebral body is provided.
   A. Artifact
   B. Demyelination
   C. Edema
   D. Syringomyelia

2. The high signal cord changes represent an artifact. Which of the following is the correct artifact affecting the cord on the sagittal image?
   A. Gibbs artifact
   B. Motion artifact
   C. Pulsation artifact
   D. Wraparound artifact

FIG. 9.C7. (A) Sagittal T2-weighted image of the thoracic spine demonstrates hyperintense signal within the central cord. Also note faint hypointense vertical bands involving the vertebral bodies. (B) Axial T2-weighted image of the midthoracic spine, same patient. The spinal cord is normal. (C) Magnified image of the left temporal lobe demonstrates multiple, peripheral, linear signal abnormalities *(arrowheads)*. Acquisition matrix for this image was 320 × 192. (D) Axial T1-weighted image of the same brain acquired with matrix of 320 × 240. The low signal lines are no longer seen.

Discussion

The truncation (Gibbs ringing) artifact is caused by the limited number of digital samples in k-space and occurs at high-contrast interfaces. Because most examinations undersample in the phase-encoding direction to save time, the highest frequency data are cut off (or truncated); these data represent the sharp-edged interfaces between high-contrast borders. This leads to either an overestimation or underestimation of the signal by the Fourier transform at these boundaries, which is visible as periodic low or high signal intensity lines or bands that form rings on either side of the interface.[5] This ringing characteristically becomes less conspicuous the farther from the interface, which is a differentiating feature from the other artifact for which it is most frequently mistaken (motion artifact).

This artifact is most problematic in spinal cord imaging because of the high-contrast CSF-cord boundary. On T2-weighted images, a band of high T2 signal may be produced in the thoracic spinal cord, which can be seen in a variety of pathologies (e.g., edema, myelomalacia, syringomyelia). However, the axial T2-weighted image of the spinal cord is normal, which verifies the abnormality on the sagittal image as an artifact.

Remedies for this artifact include decreasing pixel size, which can be done by either decreasing the field of view (FOV) or increasing the acquisition matrix in the phase-encoding direction. Of course, the "no free lunch" rule in MRI applies here, with a longer study time and decreased signal-to-noise ratio (due to smaller pixel sizes), which are the consequences of increasing the acquisition matrix.

CASE 9.7 ANSWERS

1. **A. Artifact**
2. **A. Gibbs artifact**

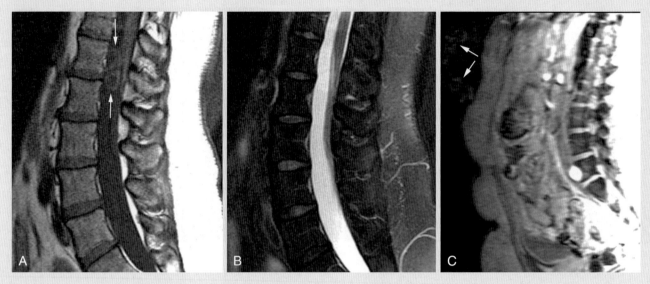

FIG. 9.C8

1. Which of the following represents the artifact *(arrows)* demonstrated on the T1-weighted image (part A)?
   A. Gibbs artifact
   B. Motion artifact
   C. Pulsation artifact
   D. Wraparound artifact

FIG. 9.C8. (A) Sagittal T1-weighted image of the lumbar spine. Unusual round signal abnormalities are identified in the thecal sac, anterior to the conus medullaris *(arrows)*. (B) Sagittal T2-weighted image of the lumbar spine. No focal abnormalities are identified in the thecal sac at the same level. (C) Sagittal GRE localizer image of the lumbar spine. Round foci located anterior to the abdominal wall are noted and appear similar to those seen in Fig. 9.C8A, consistent with the patient's fingers.

Discussion

This is an example of the wraparound artifact, also known as *aliasing*. This is secondary to the use of a small FOV, with signals arising from tissues outside the FOV overlapping onto the opposite side of the image. This is the result of Fourier encoding because the phases of tissues exhibit cyclic behavior in spatial increments that are equal to the FOV. In practice, aliasing is primarily an artifact seen in the phase-encoding direction because the frequency-encoding direction is often oversampled (hence, widening the FOV).

In this case, the patient rested the hand on the abdomen during acquisition of the sagittal T1-weighted sequence.

Together with the small FOV, this resulted in a wraparound artifact, with signals arising from the patient's fingers simulating an abnormality in the spinal canal. This was not seen on the subsequently obtained T2-weighted sequence because the patient moved the hand before acquisition of this sequence. Widening the FOV resolves this artifact, but comes at the expense of decreased image resolution.

CASE 9.8 ANSWER

1. **D. Wraparound artifact**

FIG. 9.C9

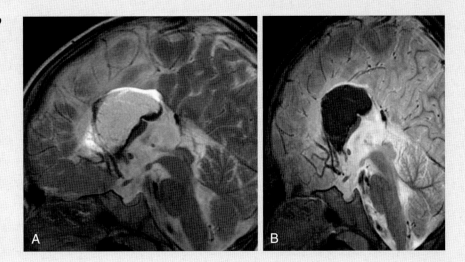

1. This image shows a large pericallosal lipoma. A chemical shift misregistration artifact is present. Which of the following is true about this artifact?
   A. It is most frequently encountered at fat-water interfaces.
   B. It occurs in the frequency-encoding direction on spin echo sequences.
   C. The presence of this artifact can confirm the presence of fat.
   D. All of the above are true.

FIG. 9.C9. (A) Sagittal fast spin echo T2-weighted image of the brain demonstrates a large hyperintense mass involving the corpus callosum. A band of hyperintense signal along the superior margin of the mass is identified. (B) Sagittal proton density–weighted image with fat suppression demonstrates loss of signal within the pericallosal mass, consistent with a lipoma. Note that the band of chemical shift artifact along the superior margin of the mass has decreased.

Discussion

The chemical shift misregistration artifact is one of the more commonly encountered artifacts in MRI. Signals arising from tissues have both frequency and phase components, which are used in the process of spatial encoding during MRI formation. As noted in previous chapters, protons in fat precess at a different frequency compared with protons in water due to differences in molecular environments. Fat and water protons are separated by a chemical shift of 3.5 ppm, which is the equivalent of 224 Hz at a 1.5-T strength magnetic field.

This difference in proton frequencies is erroneously interpreted as a *spatial* difference during image formation and results in a misregistration artifact. The artifact is primarily seen as a linear band of signal abnormality at fat-water interfaces in the body, where the fat-containing voxels are shifted away from their true anatomic positions in the frequency-encoding direction of the image. (Note that this case illustrates a type 1 chemical shift artifact; a type 2 chemical shift artifact, commonly referred to as an India ink artifact, is discussed in greater detail in Chapter 7.) The artifact occurs in the frequency-encoding direction, as covered in this case, and pertains primarily to conventional sequences—spin echo, fast spin echo, and GRE. The misregistration artifact seen in single-shot imaging techniques such as echo planar imaging occurs in the phase-encoding direction, the details of which are beyond the scope of this discussion. Clinically, this artifact is useful because it can confirm the presence of fat within a lesion.

This artifact is most noticeable at 1.5-T field strengths and worsens with increasing field strength as the chemical shift between fat and water protons also increases. Technical adjustments to resolve this artifact include decreasing the pixel size (decreasing the FOV) and increasing the receiver bandwidth. In addition, using fat suppression to decrease the signal contribution from fat will decrease or eliminate the artifact.

CASE 9.9 ANSWER

1. **D. All of the above are true.**

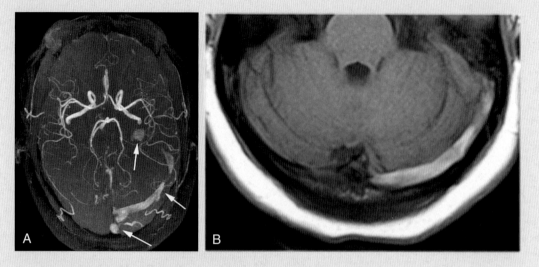

FIG. 9.C10

1. Maximum intensity projection TOF image of the circle of Willis demonstrates a shine-through artifact related to a dural venous thrombus *(arrows)*. What weighting is used in TOF pulse sequences?
   A. Proton density
   B. Noncontrast T1
   C. T2
   D. Postcontrast T1

FIG. 9.C10. (A) TOF maximum intensity projection image of the circle of Willis. The major vessels of the circle of Willis appear patent; signal is present in the region of the left transverse sinus and left jugular foramen *(arrows)*. (B) Axial T1-weighted image of the posterior fossa demonstrates a hyperintense thrombus within the left transverse sinus.

Discussion

Recall that TOF is a noncontrasted angiographic technique that relies on flow-related enhancement from unsaturated, mobile blood cells. This is commonly used to assess vascular patency (see Chapter 12). Case 9.10 illustrates an important pitfall that may occur in the interpretation of TOF images—namely, shine-through artifact related to T1 contamination.

Because the TOF sequence is T1 weighted, tissues with short T1 relaxation times produce signal. This becomes an issue when a subacute hemorrhage or thrombus containing paramagnetic methemoglobin is present.

The TOF MIP image demonstrates normal signal within the circle of Willis, confirming patency. However, the high signal arising from the left transverse sinus and left jugular foramen represents a contamination artifact from subacute venous thrombus. To avoid this potential pitfall, evaluate other sequences—the precontrast and postcontrast T1-weighted and T2-weighted sequences—to verify or exclude an abnormality.

CASE 9.10 ANSWER

1. **B. Noncontrast T1**

FIG. 9.C11

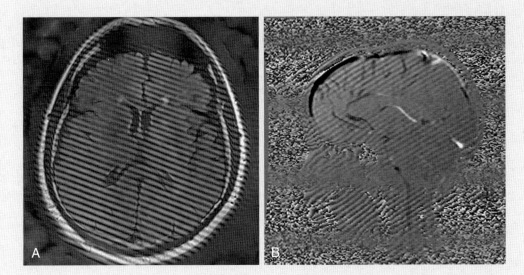

1. A herringbone artifact is demonstrated in two patients in Fig. 9.C11. Which of the following causes this artifact?
   A. Excessively long TR
   B. Excessively short TE
   C. Bad data point in K-space
   D. Excessive echo train length

FIG. 9.C11. (A) Axial fluid-attenuated inversion recovery image at the level of the basal ganglia. Multiple periodic lines obliquely traverse the image; also, a cloudlike signal is noted in the background. (B) Sagittal phase contrast CSF flow study in a different patient. Similar periodic oblique bands are seen throughout the image, although the orientation of the bands is different compared with Fig. 9.C11A.

Discussion

The herringbone, or spike, artifact is due to a transient corruption during the filling of k-space, usually from an electromagnetic spike. The spikes are thought to arise from gradients applied at high duty cycles,[6] which result in a bad data point in k-space. This bad data point is converted into a sinusoidal wave function by the Fourier transform, which is then incorporated into each pixel during image reconstruction. This is manifest as alternating bands propagated across the entire image (Fig. 9.C11A). The artifact severity increases with the intensity of the data spike.

Understanding this artifact requires a basic understanding of the relationship between k-space and the images that are interpreted. Simply put, each individual data point in k-space contains information that represents all voxels in the MR image. This is what we see with the herringbone artifact; the single abnormal spike in k-space has resulted in an artifact that distorts not just a single pixel, but the entire image.

Not only does the presence of a corrupt data point affect the image, but the *location* of the data point in k-space determines its appearance on the image. The lines in the phase contrast CSF flow image (Fig. 9.C11B) propagate from right to left in an inferior to superior orientation; this is the opposite orientation of the bands seen in Fig. 9.C11A. By examining both the angulation and distance between the lines, an estimation of the data spike's location in k-space can be made.

The other answer choices (excessively long TE, excessively long TR, excessive echo train length) would affect tissue contrast and produce a heavily T2-weighted image but would not produce this artifact. Editing (and removing) the bad data point and continuing with subsequent image reconstruction, or simply rescanning the patient if postprocessing capability is limited, are potential ways to resolve this problem.

CASE 9.11 ANSWER

1. **C. Bad data point in k-space**

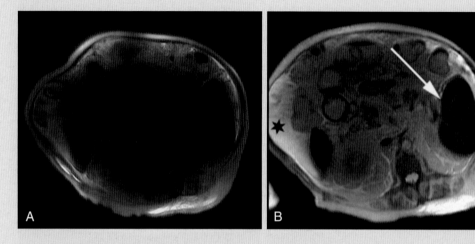

FIG. 9.C12

1. The image in Fig. 9.C12A was obtained on a 3-T magnet, and the image in Fig. 9.C12B (same patient) was obtained on a 1.5-T magnet. Which of the following is most likely responsible for the large artifact present in Fig. 9.C12A?
   A. Ineffective frequency-selective fat saturation
   B. Dielectric effects
   C. Susceptibility artifact
   D. Hemosiderin

FIG. 9.C12. (A) Axial T2-weighted image of the abdomen performed on a 3-T magnet. Marked homogeneous decreased signal intensity is demonstrated in the center of the abdomen. (B) Axial T2-weighted image of the abdomen, same patient, obtained 1 day later on 1.5-T magnet. The diagnostic image quality shows marked improvement; a large volume of ascites is evident in the right hemiabdomen. The spleen is enlarged.

Discussion

Inhomogeneous RF excitation of an imaging volume is due to an assortment of dielectric and conductive properties in tissue.[7] At 3 T, the RF wavelength measures 234 cm in air; the speed and wavelength of the RF field are shortened to 30 cm within the body due to dielectric effects. Actually, 30 cm is also the average FOV for most body imaging examinations; when the RF wavelength approximates the FOV in size, constructive or destructive interference of the RF field occurs. This leads to local areas of signal brightening (usually seen in the brain) or darkening (shading). This artifact has previously been referred to as a dielectric resonance effect, but the terms *standing wave* and *RF interference effects* have also been used.[8]

When a highly conductive medium (e.g., ascites, amniotic fluid) is present in the body, formation of a circulating electrical field is promoted when under the influence of the external RF field. This in turn produces an electrical current; the current acts as its own magnetic field that opposes the main magnetic field. This results in a reduction in the effect of the RF field on the imaging volume and a decrease in signal.

Dielectric effects produce a significant artifact at 3 T.[9] In Fig. 9.C12A the highly conductive ascites promotes signal loss in the central abdomen, rendering the study nondiagnostic. The artifact was immediately recognized and the study subsequently terminated. The examination was completed the next day on a 1.5-T magnet, with a marked reduction in the artifact.

The dielectric effect artifact is an example of an artifact that worsens with increases in magnetic field strength. Other artifacts that are more severe at higher magnetic field strengths include susceptibility and chemical shift artifacts of the first kind.

CASE 9.12 ANSWER

1. **B. Dielectric effects**

TAKE-HOME POINTS

1. Motion is often divided into two categories, gross body movement and physiologic motion, such as cardiac and respiratory cycles or blood or CSF flow.
2. In most conventional imaging methods, motion artifact is predominantly manifested in the phase-encoding direction.
3. When motion is present, tissues excited at a specific location during the radiofrequency pulse are erroneously mapped to a different location or often to different locations (in cases of motion artifacts) during detection.
4. Random motion results in smearing or blurring in the phase-encoding direction, and periodic motion (cardiac motion and blood vessels) results in ghosting artifacts.
5. Many techniques such as gradient moment nulling, switching the direction of the frequency encoding and phase-encoding gradients, presaturation pulses, averaging, respiratory triggering, and cardiac gating can be used to reduce motion artifacts.

6. The Gibbs ringing or truncation artifact is due to the undersampling of k-space and is conspicuous at high-contrast boundaries (CSF-cord, brain-calvarium, cartilage-bone). Decreasing pixel size or increasing the acquisition matrix improves or eliminates the artifact.

7. Although swapping the phase- and frequency-encoding directions does not completely remove the Gibbs ringing artifact, it may remove the artifact from affecting the tissue in question.

8. The magic angle artifact is seen in tendons and ligaments oriented at certain angles to the main magnetic field. It manifests as an artificial high signal on short TE sequences. The artifact is typically not seen on long TE sequences, differentiating this from true pathology.

9. A wraparound artifact represents an error in spatial encoding because signal from tissues located outside the FOV are mapped within the FOV, usually on the opposite side. Widening the FOV to include the entire body part resolves this artifact.

10. Chemical shift misregistration results in an error in spatial encoding of fat voxels due to the differences of resonant frequencies between fat and water. This artifact is most evident at fat-water interfaces in the body and is seen in the frequency-encoding direction of the image on conventional sequences.

11. Because TOF sequences are T1 weighted, tissues with a high T1 signal (e.g., methemoglobin) may appear in the reconstructed MIP image as a T1 contamination artifact. This could mimic patent vessels; evaluation of the source images and other sequences is necessary to prevent this pitfall.

12. Benefits of imaging at higher magnetic field strengths come at the cost of progressively severe artifacts; examples include artifacts related to dielectric, chemical shift, and susceptibility effects.

Suggested Readings

1. Lee VS. *Cardiovascular MRI: Physical Principles to Practical Protocols.* Philadelphia: Lippincott Williams & Wilkins; 2006.

2. Mitchell DG. *Cohen MS. MRI Principles.* 2nd ed. Philadelphia: Saunders; 2004.

3. Brown MA, Semelka RC. *MRI: Basic Principles and Applications.* 3rd ed. New York: John Wiley; 2003.

4. Erickson SJ, Cox IH, Hyde JS, et al. Effect of tendon orientation on MR imaging signal intensity: a manifestation of the magic angle phenomenon. *Radiology.* 1991;181(2):389–392.

5. Czervionke LF, Czervionke JM, Daniels DL, Haughton VM. Characteristic features of MR truncation artifacts. *AJR Am J Roentgenol.* 1988;151(6):1219–1228.

6. Zhuo J, Gullapalli RP. AAPM/RSNA physics tutorial for residents: MR artifacts, safety, and quality control. *Radiographics.* 2006;26(1):275–297.

7. Lee VS, Hecht EM, Taouli B, et al. Body and cardiovascular MR imaging at 3.0 T. *Radiology.* 2007;244(3):692–705.

8. Merkle EM, Dale BM. Abdominal MRI at 3.0 T: the basics revisited. *AJR Am. J. Roentgenol.* 2006;186(6):1524–1532.

9. Lawrence NT. Clinical 3T MR imaging: mastering the challenges. *Magn Reson Imaging Clin N Am.* 2006;14(1):1–15.

CHAPTER 10

Vascular Contrast

Scott M. Duncan

OPENING CASE 10.1

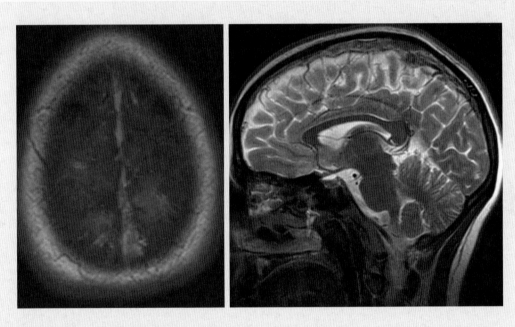

1. What is the cause of the increased signal in or near the superior sagittal sinus?
   A. This is normal flow-related enhancement within the superior sagittal sinus.
   B. This is the normal postcontrast appearance of the superior sagittal sinus.
   C. It is a superior sagittal sinus thrombosis.
   D. It is a subdural hemorrhage near the vertex.
2. Normally, which sequences have flow voids, and which exhibit flow-related enhancement?
   A. Spin echo and gradient echo sequences both demonstrate flow voids.
   B. Gradient echo demonstrates flow-related enhancement only on postcontrast images.
   C. Spin echo sequences have flow voids, and gradient echo sequences have flow-related enhancement.
   D. Both spin echo and gradient echo sequences have flow-related enhancement.
3. Which sequences have the most prominent flow voids?
   A. T1-weighted sequences
   B. T2-weighted sequences
   C. Gradient echo sequences
   D. Diffusion-weighted sequences

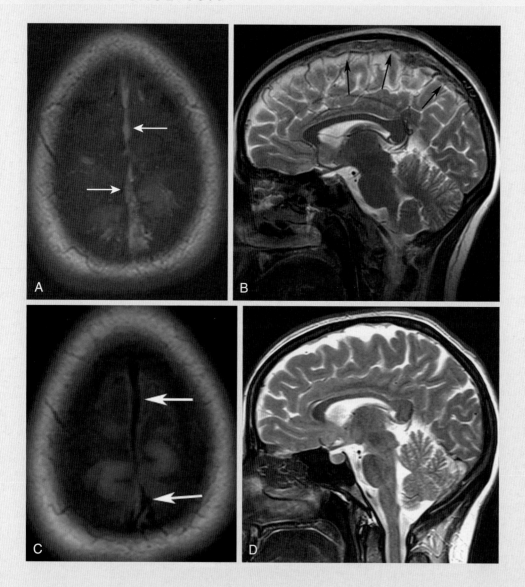

FIG. 10.C1. (A) Axial T1 fast spin echo (FSE) image demonstrates expansion and signal within the superior sagittal sinus and the lack of a flow void *(arrows)*. (B) Sagittal T2 FSE image re-demonstrates the expansion of and signal within the superior sagittal sinus *(arrows)*. (C) Axial T1 FSE image in the same patient 5 months before, demonstrating normal flow void *(arrows)* in a patent superior sagittal sinus. (D) Sagittal T2 FSE image redemonstrates the thin flow void in the superior sagittal sinus *(arrows)*.

1. What is the cause of the increased signal in or near the superior sagittal sinus?
   C. It is a superior sagittal sinus thrombosis.
2. Normally, which sequences have flow voids, and which exhibit flow-related enhancement?
   C. Spin echo sequences have flow voids, and gradient echo sequences have flow-related enhancement.
3. Which sequences have the most prominent flow voids?
   B. T2-weighted sequences

Discussion

Question 1: Spin echo (SE) sequences demonstrate flow voids within the arteries and veins. However, on the initial images, there is increased signal and expansion of the superior sagittal sinus consistent with a superior sagittal sinus thrombosis. Also note the increased signal in the adjacent superficial veins that drain into the superior sagittal sinus, which are also thrombosed. Compare that appearance to the second pair of images, which show the normal appearance of the superior sagittal sinus, where the sinus is completely black and thin.

Flow-related enhancement does not occur on an SE sequence, only on gradient echo sequences, for reasons discussed below. These images are all from T2-weighted sequences and therefore are usually acquired precontrast. Finally, the signal is within the superior sagittal sinus, not adjacent to the sinus, as would be seen in a subdural hematoma.

Question 2: In general, SE sequences have flow voids within a vessel. Gradient echo sequences have flow-related enhancement resulting in a bright signal within the vessel.

Question 3: Sequences with a longer time to echo (TE) result in the most prominent flow voids. As described in detail later in the chapter, protons must experience both the initial pulse and the refocusing pulse to produce signal. Moving protons may not experience both these pulses and thus will not produce a signal. The longer the TE, the more time protons have to move in between pulses and thus may not experience both pulses. Therefore sequences with longer TEs such as T2 have the most durable flow voids; in other words, these sequences will still have flow voids, even in slow-flowing vessels or in vessels with an oblique course through the image.

Vascular Contrast

Perhaps one of the most confusing topics to understand as a novice to MRI interpretation is the differentiation between flow voids and flow-related enhancement. As a first-year resident, I remember the attending physician mentioning the importance of flow voids and then 2 minutes later discussing the bright signal within a vessel on a time-of-flight sequence. I just wanted to know when vessels should be black and when they should be bright.

The answer is actually quite simple. *SE techniques result in flow voids, whereas gradient echo techniques result in flow-related enhancement.* These are, of course, generalizations, and there are exceptions to this rule (see later). However, in most cases this simple generalization holds true.

Flow voids and flow-related enhancement are both based on the same TOF phenomenon. The basis of this phenomenon is that flowing protons within blood do not experience the same radiofrequency (RF) pulses and magnetization as those of stationary protons. Thus the signal obtained from flowing protons is different than that from stationary protons.

Flow Voids

As previously discussed, SE imaging uses two RF pulses to produce a signal. The first is a 90-degree pulse that tips the longitudinal magnetization into the transverse plane. Subsequently, an 180-degree pulse realigns the dephased spins to produce an echo. The proton must experience both RF pulses to create a signal. For example, if a moving proton is hit with the initial 90-degree RF pulse and then moves out of the imaging plane before the 180-degree RF pulse (thereby avoiding the 180-degree pulse), the dephased protons will not be refocused. This absence of refocusing means that all the transverse magnetization will remain dephased, and no signal will be obtained. Alternatively, if the proton is outside the imaging slice when the 90-degree pulse is applied, but then moves into the slice when the 180-degree pulse is applied, the proton's magnetization will be flipped 180 degrees (reversed, or upside down) in the longitudinal direction. In this scenario, there will be no transverse magnetization to provide a signal because the initial 90-degree RF pulse was missed. In both these scenarios, the result is absence of signal, or a flow void.

Although we may think of a flow void as a complete loss of signal, in reality there is a spectrum ranging from full normal signal to a complete signal void. *The degree of the signal void is dependent on several factors, including the velocity of the proton, the slice thickness, the TE, and the course of the vessel.* The higher the velocity of the proton, the quicker it will move out of the imaging slice and the less time it has to experience both the 90-degree and 180-degree RF pulses. Thinner slices mean that there are shorter required distances to traverse the imaging slice, so there is less time to experience both RF pulses and a greater likelihood of a flow void. Longer TEs mean that there is more time between the 90-degree and 180-degree RF pulses; remember that the 90- and 180-degree pulses are separated by 0.5 TE. Therefore there is more time for the moving protons, which have already experienced the initial 90-degree pulse, to be replaced with new protons that have not experienced the first RF pulse before signal acquisition. *Thus sequences with long TEs (e.g., T2 images) have the most prominent and durable flow voids.* This is an important point to remember. If you notice signal in a vessel, and think that it may represent a thrombus or occlusion in a sequence with a short TE, such as a T1-weighted sequence, make sure that you confirm the finding by comparing it with the corresponding T2 sequence because these are less sensitive to slow flow and more specific to the diagnosis of thrombosis.

Finally, the course of the vessel also has implications for the presence or absence of a flow void. The TOF phenomenon only applies to flow that is oriented perpendicular to the imaging plane. (In an axial image, this is flow that is oriented in the

craniocaudal axis.) This makes intuitive sense because when vessels take a course that is parallel to the imaging plane, the protons do not move out of the slice but rather stay within the imaging slice for an extended period, increasing the probability that they will experience both RF pulses and produce signal. *Thus if a vessel courses obliquely or parallel to the imaging plane, an intravascular signal may be seen, despite normal flow within the vessel. This phenomenon is commonly seen in the transverse sinuses of the brain.*

The velocity within the arterial system is usually great enough to result in complete intraluminal signal void, regardless of the obliquity of the vessel (e.g., petrous internal carotid artery, middle cerebral artery). On the other hand, the slower venous flow may not result in a complete signal void, despite patency, especially if the vessel takes an oblique course. As a result, if intraluminal signal is identified within a vein on an SE sequence, the possibility of a thrombus should be raised but should be confirmed with a more flow-sensitive sequence (e.g., phase contrast) or with contrast-enhanced venography.

Flow-Related Enhancement

In gradient echo imaging, the TOF phenomenon has the opposite effect of that seen in SE sequences. Recall that in gradient echo sequences, there is only one RF pulse, not two. Instead, a gradient is applied for phase refocusing rather than a 180-degree refocusing pulse, as in the SE technique. In addition, the time to repetition (TR) in a gradient sequence is very short and is repeated multiple times. Thus the proton's longitudinal magnitude does not fully recover before the next RF pulse is applied. After several TRs are applied, the amount of longitudinal magnetization recovered reaches equilibrium with the amount of magnetization that is tipped into the transverse plane. This is termed *saturation*. *A flowing proton that is entering a slice has not experienced the multiple previous RF pulses and will produce more signal than the adjacent, partially saturated, nonmobile protons. This is the basis of flow-related enhancement* (Fig. 10.1).

Because flow-related enhancement is also a TOF phenomenon, the same variables that determine the flow voids in SE imaging (e.g., velocity, slice thickness) also affect the flow-related enhancement in gradient imaging. For example, increased time between RF pulses also results in an increase in the TOF phenomenon on gradient echo imaging. However, the difference is that the end result is increased flow-related enhancement in gradient echo imaging rather than the increased flow voids

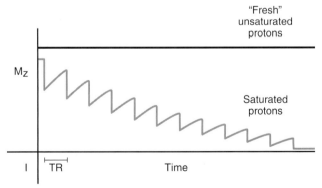

FIG. 10.1. Comparison of magnetization of stagnant and moving protons after multiple RF pulses. The moving unsaturated protons always have maximal signal. However, the stagnant protons are repeatedly hit with RF pulses. The curve shows how the signal progressively decreases after multiple RF pulses. Eventually, a steady state is reached, at which the longitudinal magnetization recovered is equal to the magnitude of magnetization flipped into the transverse plane by the next RF pulse (saturation). M_z, longitudinal magnetization; *TR*, Time to repetition. (Modified from Lee VS. *Cardiovascular MRI: Physical Principles to Practical Protocols.* Philadelphia: Lippincott Williams & Wilkins; 2006:22.)

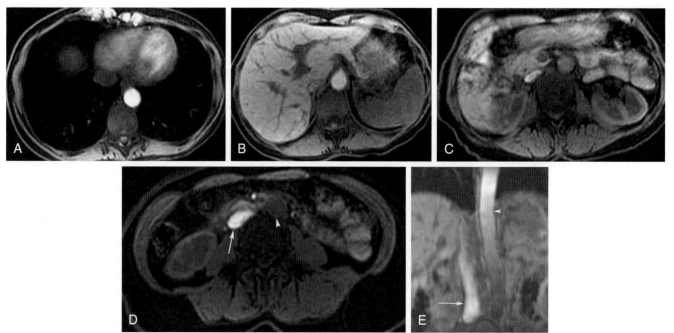

FIG. 10.2. (A) Axial water-only, two-point, Dixon gradient recalled echo (GRE) gyromagnetic ratio, γ (in megahertz). GRE image of the lower chest demonstrates bright signal within the descending thoracic aorta. Note the low signal within the inferior vena cava (IVC). (B) Axial water-only, two-point, Dixon GRE image several centimeters inferior to the first image (at the level of the liver), which demonstrates a slightly darker aorta. The IVC is isointense to the hepatic parenchyma. (C) Axial water-only, two-point, Dixon GRE image even more inferior (at the upper level of the kidneys). There is intermediate signal within the aorta. The IVC is now brighter than the aorta. (D) Water-only, two-point Dixon GRE image at the lower level of the kidneys (most inferior image), which demonstrates a dark aorta *(arrowhead)* and a very bright IVC *(arrow)*. (E) Coronal reformation based on an axially acquired 3D, in-phase, GRE imaging dataset. The aorta becomes progressively darker from superior to inferior *(arrowhead)*; the IVC becomes progressively brighter from superior to inferior *(arrow)*.

seen in SE imaging. Another difference is that because gradient echo sequences make use of only one RF pulse and no refocusing 180-degree echo pulse, the time between RF pulses is represented by the TR rather than by the TE. Therefore the longer the TR in a gradient echo sequence, the more pronounced the enhancement of flowing protons.

Entry Slice Phenomenon

Gradient echo images are often acquired via excitation of a three-dimensional (3D) slab of tissue, rather than excitation of multiple contiguous two-dimensional (2D) slices. With 3D acquisition, a proton must traverse the entire volume of excited tissue to escape the multiple repeated RF pulses. As noted above, if the proton is exposed to multiple RF pulses, it will become progressively more saturated. Thus a proton must travel much farther than with the contiguous, single-slice, 2D acquisition technique to produce high signal. The result is an effect termed the *entry slice phenomenon*. As flowing protons course antegrade through a vessel, they become progressively saturated by the RF excitation pulses sent into the 3D tissue slab. This results in progressive loss of signal within the downstream aspect of the vessel. The images therefore demonstrate bright signal within the vessel at the beginning of the tissue slab, progressive loss of intraluminal vascular signal over the course of the tissue slab, and the least amount of intraluminal signal at the end of the slab.

The entry slice phenomenon is dependent on the direction of flow within the vessel. The images from Fig. 10.2 nicely demonstrate this phenomenon. The axial images, which were reformatted from the acquired 3D dataset, exhibit high signal within the superior aorta because the aorta is receiving fresh (unsaturated) protons from above the imaged tissue slab.[1] These protons are naïve to the saturation pulses and therefore have their full longitudinal magnetization available to provide signal to the image. The axial reformatted images acquired from the central aspect of the imaged slab contain signal from intraluminal protons that have been exposed to

more and more of the excitation pulses and are therefore more saturated. This results in less longitudinal magnetization available to produce signal and accounts for the progressively decreased signal intensity within the inferior aorta. The protons within the most inferior aspect of the aorta are completely saturated and appear dark. The opposite effect occurs within the inferior vena cava (IVC). Within the IVC, the most inferior image has the brightest signal as the IVC receives fresh or unsaturated protons from below the imaging slab. According to the same principle, the superior aspect of the IVC is dark. Flow-related enhancement will extend farther into the imaged volume with higher velocities, longer TRs, and contiguous slices or slabs that are acquired countercurrent to flow.

Gradient Moment Nulling

The TOF phenomenon is the major determinant of vessel contrast in MRI. However, there are several additional factors that attenuate signal within flowing blood, thereby resulting in an accentuation of flow voids in SE sequences and a decrease in flow-related enhancement in gradient echo sequences.

The application of a gradient results in the dephasing of protons secondary to exposure to slightly different magnetic field strengths, which results in slightly different precessional frequencies. This dephasing leads to signal cancelation and an overall decrease in signal. To correct for this signal loss, a bipolar gradient (two equal gradients with opposite polarity) can be applied, which will realign the dephased spins. Bipolar gradients work well for stationary protons but are less successful in the case of mobile protons (e.g., in flowing blood). Flowing protons change their positions between the application of the two lobes of the bipolar gradient—the dephasing and rephasing lobes—and therefore do not experience the equal but opposite gradients. This difference results in the accumulation of a net phase shift for the mobile protons and signal loss, resulting in less flow-related enhancement. The amount of phase shift is dependent on the velocity of the mobile protons (a principle used in phase contrast imaging).

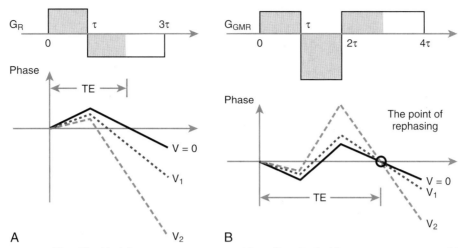

FIG. 10.3. Gradient moment nulling. The *black line* represents protons with no flow. *Dashed lines* represent protons with constant velocity. (A) No flow compensation. The stationary protons do not have a net phase shift at TE but the flowing protons do. (B) However, the application of gradient moment nulling (a trilobed gradient) results in a net 0 phase shift for all protons, regardless of their velocity. Note that this only accounts for protons with a constant velocity. G_{GMR}, Gradient moment nulling gradient; G_R, standard gradient; T, duration of the gradient (equal to one-half the TE).

This signal loss is tolerable for simple anatomic imaging applications, but if the goal is an evaluation of the vasculature, the imaging quality can be improved via utilization of a correction technique, termed a *flow-compensated gradient* or *gradient moment nulling*. *A flow-compensated gradient is a second bipolar gradient, which is a mirror image of the first gradient—that is, the lobes are applied in the opposite order, negative and then positive.* When diagrammed, it appears as a trilobed gradient because the negative lobes are applied back to back (Fig. 10.3). This technique causes mobile protons to acquire a phase shift that is equal and opposite to that acquired during the first bipolar gradient, which results in no net phase shift. Unfortunately, this compensation technique is successful only for flowing protons with a constant velocity.

Higher-order flow, such as pulsatility, can be compensated for by larger, more complex gradient schemes, although these are rarely used because they lengthen the acquisition time.[2] In addition, areas of turbulence cannot be compensated for and always result in decreased signal. The trade-off for the application of gradient moment nulling is that of additional scan time because the TE or TR must be lengthened to allow time for the second bipolar gradient to be inserted into the sequence.

Another way to compensate for flow-related dephasing is by shortening the TE or TR, which reduces the time that protons have to dephase before the signal is acquired. Cardiac imaging uses short TEs and TRs to help compensate for higher-order flow without using more complex and time-consuming gradients.

CASE 10.2

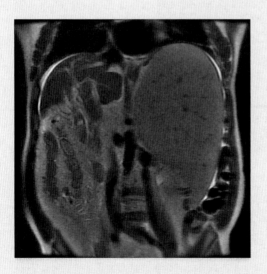

1. What is the diagnosis?
   A. Congenital absence of the portal vein
   B. Hemochromatosis
   C. Portal vein thrombosis
   D. Budd-Chiari syndrome
   E. Primary sclerosing cholangitis

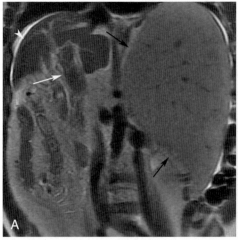

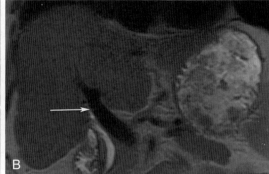

FIG. 10.C2. (A) Coronal T2-weighted half-Fourier acquisition single-shot turbo SE (HASTE) image of the abdomen demonstrating an expanded portal vein containing heterogeneous signal *(arrows)*. Note the small liver and the markedly enlarged spleen. (B) Coronal T2-weighted HASTE image of the abdomen in a normal patient demonstrating the normal size and expected flow void of a patent portal vein *(arrow)*.

Discussion

The expanded portal vein contains heterogeneous signal, is expanded, and lacks a normal flow void, findings consistent with portal vein thrombosis. There are also signs of portal hypertension, including marked splenomegaly *(black arrows)* and trace ascites *(arrowhead)*.

One interesting note is that the portal vein and aorta normally still have flow voids, despite much of the flow remaining

within the plane of the image slice. This is because the portal and arterial flows are fast enough that the protons are able to move out of the imaging slice between the initial pulse and refocusing pulse.

CASE 10.2 ANSWER

1. **C. Portal vein thrombosis**

CASE 10.3

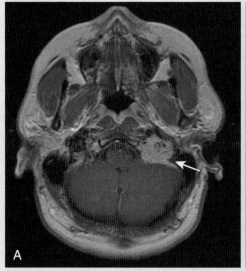

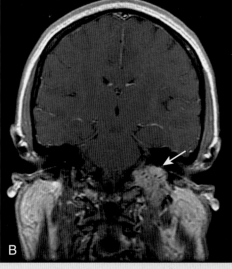

FIG. 10.C3

1. What is the cause of low signal within the mass?
   A. Flow void within a glomus jugulare tumor
   B. Calcifications within a meningioma
   C. Necrotic portions of a petrous bone metastatic lesion
   D. Areas of microhemorrhage within an acoustic schwannoma
   E. Flow void within an arteriovenous malformation (AVM)

2. These masses can occur in all these locations except for which one of the following?
   A. Carotid body
   B. Along the course of the facial nerve
   C. Middle ear
   D. Spine

FIG. 10.C3. (A) Axial T1-weighted, postcontrast image demonstrates an enhancing mass in the region of the left jugular foramen *(arrow)* that contains speckled areas of internal low signal. (B) Coronal T1-weighted, postcontrast image also demonstrates the left jugular foramen mass *(arrow)*. The speckled low signal areas represent flow voids.

Discussion

The glomus tumors (paragangliomas) are extremely vascular. This marked hypervascularity gives them a characteristic salt-and-pepper appearance, which can be identified on either T2-weighted or postcontrast T1-weighted images.[3] The salt (white) portion of the tumor is secondary to the marked enhancement of the lesion (representing hypervascularity) on postcontrast T1 images, as well as the high water content resulting in T2 hyperintensity. The pepper (black) portions of the lesion are a result of prominent internal flow voids, which are fast enough to be seen even on T1-weighted images.

Paragangliomas arise from paraganglion cells and thus can arise wherever paraganglion cells occur. The most common places include the carotid body as a carotid body tumor (chemodectoma), in the middle ear as a glomus tympanicum, and along the vagus nerve as a glomus vagale tumor. There are no paraganglion cells along the facial nerve; therefore they do not occur along the facial nerve. Outside the head and neck, they can occur in the spine and in the adrenal gland as a pheochromocytoma.

CASE 10.3 ANSWERS

1. **A. Flow void within a glomus jugulare tumor**
2. **B. Along the course of the facial nerve**

CASE 10.4

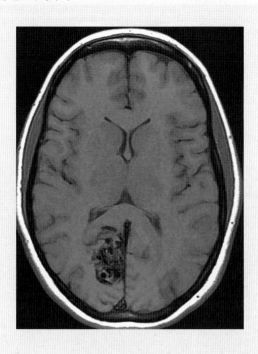

1. What is the diagnosis?
   A. Hypervascular meningioma with calcifications
   B. Hypervascular glioblastoma multiforme with areas of hemorrhage
   C. Cerebral AVM
   D. Venous hemorrhage from sagittal sinus thrombosis
2. Which of the following lesions lack flow voids?
   A. Juvenile angiofibroma
   B. Venous malformation
   C. Peripheral AVM
   D. Glomus tumor
   E. Renal cell osseous metastasis

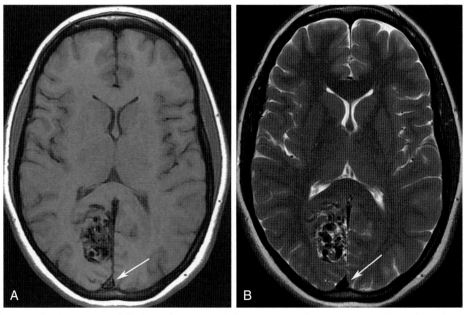

FIG. 10.C4. (A) Axial T1-weighted SE image of the brain (TE = 15 ms) demonstrates a heterogeneous mass in the right occipital lobe in this pediatric patient *(arrow)*. Multiple serpentine flow voids are identified. Note the incomplete flow void within the superior sagittal sinus *(arrow)*. (B) Axial T2-weighted SE image of the brain (TE = 116 ms) redemonstrates a heterogeneous mass in the right occipital lobe. Note that the flow voids are more prominent than those identified on the T1-weighted image. Additionally, note that there is now a complete flow void within the superior sagittal sinus *(arrow)*.

Discussion

The serpentine nature of the low signal confirms that these areas are flow voids and not hemorrhage or areas of calcification. AVMs usually have a nest of prominent vessels that have flow voids. Although there are several hypervascular masses within the brain, no other intracranial mass will have flow voids this large and striking. Even though most masses throughout the body are hypervascular, only a few will have a flow fast enough to produce flow voids.

The signal within the sagittal sinus on the T1 image can be concerning for thrombus, but remember to compare it with the corresponding T2 image, which has a much longer TE and therefore will be more specific for the diagnosis of venous sinus thrombosis. In this case, the T2 image demonstrates a normal flow void.

In Figs.10.C4A–B, the flow voids, including those within the superior sagittal sinus, are more prominent on the T2-weighted image compared with the T1-weighted image. This occurs as a direct result of the longer TE (116 ms vs. 15 ms on the T1-weighted image), which allows more time for the protons to leave the imaging plane and escape the 180-degree echo pulse. Remember that to acquire signal in a SE image, the proton must experience both the initial 90-degree excitation pulse as well as the 180-degree refocusing pulse. Furthermore,

susceptibility artifacts from the iron within blood will be more prominent with longer TEs because there is more time for T2* effects to degrade acquired signal. Sequences with longer TEs (usually T2) are therefore the most sensitive for the evaluation of flow voids and for determining vessel patency.

Identification of flow voids within a lesion can be extremely useful for its characterization, providing clear evidence of hypervascularity and thereby narrowing the differential diagnostic possibilities. Lesions that often contain flow voids include glomus tumors, AVMs (both cerebral and throughout the body), hemangiomas (nonhepatic), juvenile angiofibromas of the nasal cavity, and even renal cell osseous metastases.[4,5] Venous malformations, including hepatic hemangiomas, have a spongy texture, with dilated, poorly formed and organized veins. This results in a relatively stagnant flow and the absence of flow voids. The sluggish flow within the lesion allows the inherent water signal within blood to become pronounced, resulting in high T2 signal.

CASE 10.4 ANSWERS

1. **C. Cerebral AVM**
2. **B. Venous malformation**

CASE 10.5

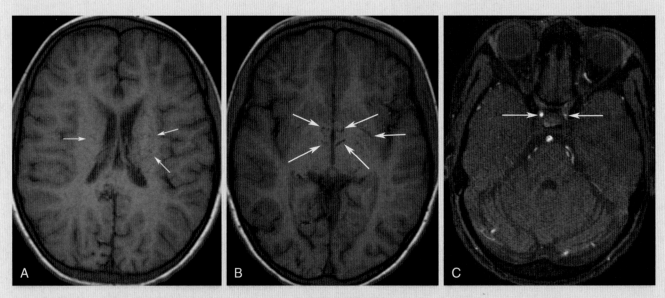

FIG. 10.C5

1. These low signal areas in the corona radiata and thalamus are secondary to which of the following?
   A. Dilated periventricular spaces
   B. Acute thrombosis of the superior saggital sinus, with dilated compensatory draining veins

   C. Microhemorrhage from traumatic brain injury
   D. Chronic narrowing of the distal internal carotid arteries (ICAs), with compensatory dilation of the lenticulostriate arteries

FIG. 10.C5. (A) Axial T1-weighted image at the level of the corona radiata. Multiple curvilinear low signal structures visualized within the periventricular white matter are consistent with flow voids *(arrows)*. (B) Axial T1-weighted image at the level of the thalamus and basal ganglia demonstrating the flow voids *(arrows)*. (C) Axial TOF image at the level of the supraclinoid ICAs demonstrating narrowing of the ICAs, left greater than right *(arrows)*.

Discussion

The serpiginous flow voids in the corona radiata and thalami that are seen are secondary to moyamoya. The term *moyamoya* is Japanese for puff of smoke, a name derived from its characteristic appearance on conventional angiography. When superimposed on each other, the multiple wispy, serpiginous,

dilated lenticulostriate collateral arteries give the appearance of a puff of smoke. These arteries are normally present but dilate and become visible because there has been slow and chronic narrowing of at least one of the terminal ICAs, usually secondary to intimal hyperplasia. The slow and progressive nature of the disease allows for the small lenticulostriate perforating arteries to dilate over time to compensate for the decreased flow from the ICAs. There are several causes of the condition, including idiopathic disease and sickle cell disease. Not surprisingly the idiopathic condition is most prominent in the Japanese population, where the term originated.[4]

CASE 10.5 ANSWER

1. **D. Chronic narrowing of the distal internal carotid arteries (ICAs), with compensatory dilation of the lenticulostriate arteries**

CASE 10.6

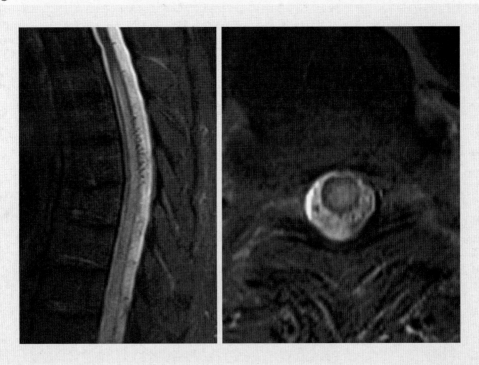

1. What is the cause of the high signal within the cord?
   A. Increased venous pressure and venous ischemia
   B. Hydrosyringomyelia
   C. High-grade canal stenosis in the lower thoracic spine
   D. Contusion
   E. Arterial ischemia from lack of arterial flow as blood is diverted away from the cord

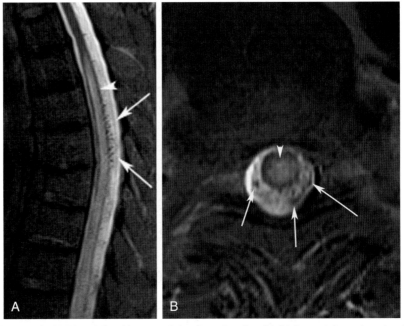

FIG. 10.C6. (A) Sagittal and (B) axial FSE T2-weighted images of the thoracic spine. Multiple serpiginous low signal foci are identified dorsal to the cord, consistent with flow voids *(arrows)*. Note the edema (T2 hyperintensity) and expansion of the cord *(arrowhead)*.

Discussion

High signal in the cord suggests cord injury. The cause of the injury can be difficult to determine. However, in this case, there is a clue that can lead to the underlying cause of the cord damage. The small black dots around the cord are actually dilated dural veins from a spinal dural arteriovenous fistula (SDAVF). The increased flow within the venous system results in dilated veins and flow voids that may exhibit a serpiginous pattern or may manifest as black dots studding the spinal cord.[5]

High signal in the cord is secondary to ischemia. The AV fistula is located inside the dura mater, close to the spinal nerve root, where the arterial blood from a radiculomeningeal artery enters a radicular vein. The increased flow within the veins results in increased spinal venous pressure and decreased drainage of the normal spinal veins. The ischemia that can be induced from the SDAVF is not secondary to lack of arterial flow, but is from venous ischemia due to the increased venous pressure from limited venous drainage. SDAVF can be difficult to diagnose clinically and is an underappreciated cause of myelopathy. Therefore noticing the flow voids and diagnosing an SDAVF can significantly help the referring clinician.[6]

These cases demonstrate how an understanding of MR vascular physics principles can be used to identify pathology and elucidate diagnoses. Flow voids in unexpected locations can signify the presence of collateralization secondary to arterial occlusive disease upstream or can provide the telltale sign of abnormal vascular pathways, as in the case of the SDAVF. One should always include an evaluation for normal and abnormal flow voids in an MR search pattern.

CASE 10.6 ANSWER

1. **A. Increased venous pressure and venous ischemia**

CASE 10.7

1. What is the diagnosis?
   A. Aortitis
   B. Leriche syndrome
   C. Mural thrombus within the aorta
   D. Aortic dissection
   E. Aortic aneurysm rupture

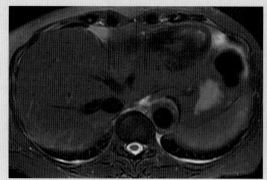
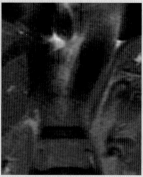

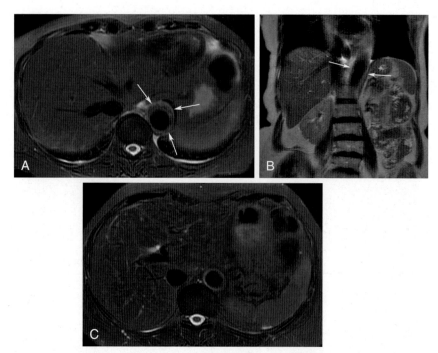

FIG. 10.C7. (A) Axial T2-weighted HASTE image of the abdomen. There is diffuse thickening of the aortic wall *(arrows)*. (B) Coronal T2-weighted HASTE image of the abdomen provides an additional view of the smooth thickening of the aortic wall *(arrows)*. (C) Axial T2-weighted HASTE image of the abdomen 6 months after the initial images. This demonstrates a normal, thin aortic wall. The patient underwent interval treatment with steroids.

Discussion

The increased signal around the aorta suggests an abnormality within the wall of the aorta. There is circumferential thickening of the aortic wall, which is consistent with aortitis. A dissection would not demonstrate a circumferential appearance. This does not represent a thrombus within the aorta because it is uncommon for a mural thrombus to develop in a normal-sized aorta, and the signal is clearly within the wall of the aorta, not the lumen. Leriche syndrome arises from complete aortic thrombosis, usually below the renal arteries. These images do not show any evidence of an occlusion. Finally, the patient has no evidence of an aortic aneurysm.

Flow voids, in addition to providing information about the presence or absence of intraluminal blood flow, also augment the contrast between the lumen and vessel wall, allowing for an excellent evaluation of vessel wall pathology.[7] In this case, the flow void results in improved conspicuity of the diffuse thickening of and heterogeneous signal within the aortic wall, aiding in the diagnosis of aortitis.

CASE 10.7 ANSWER

1. **A. Aortitis**

CASE 10.8

1. What is the cause of enhancing lesion in the first image?
   A. Supraclinoid ICA aneurysm
   B. Cavernous sinus thrombosis
   C. Meningioma
   D. Nerve sheath tumor

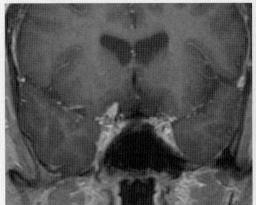 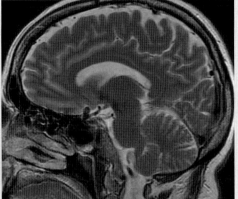

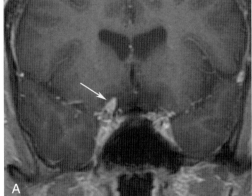 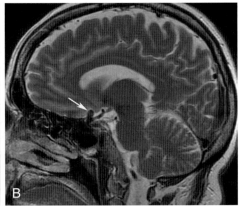

FIG. 10.C8. (A) Coronal T1-weighted, postcontrast image of the brain. There is a small enhancing mass adjacent to the right cavernous sinus *(arrow)*. (B) Sagittal T2-weighted SE image of the brain. A vascular flow void extends superiorly *(arrow)* and corresponds to the mass seen on the coronal T1-weighted image.

Discussion

This is an example of one of the most common ways that flow voids are used in everyday practice. It is uncommon to see dural AV fistulas or moyamoya, but cerebral aneurysms are relatively common. Usually an abnormal flow void on a T2-weighted sequence will be enough to make the diagnosis

and will exclude the multiple other causes of an enhancing mass in the brain.

CASE 10.8 ANSWER

1. **A. Supraclinoid ICA aneurysm**

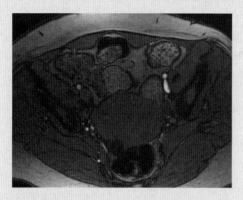

1. What type of sequence is this?
   A. T2 HASTE
   B. T1 FSE
   C. GRE
   D. T1 postcontrast image
2. What is the diagnosis?
   A. Left external iliac AV fistula
   B. Left external iliac artery thrombosis
   C. Left external iliac vein thrombosis
   D. Right external iliac vein thrombosis
   E. Right external iliac artery thrombosis

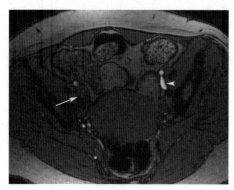

FIG. 10.C9. (A) Axial T1-weighted GRE image of the pelvis demonstrates a filling defect within and expansion of the right external iliac vein *(arrow)*. Compare this with the normal left external iliac vein *(arrowhead)*.

Discussion

Identifying the sequence can be fairly difficult with a single image. The fat is relatively bright, so it could be a T1 or T2 image. The uterus is low signal, meaning that it is not a postcontrast image. However, if you look at most of the vessels, they are bright. That means that this is a gradient sequence because flowing protons have bright signal, not dark signal, as in SE sequences.

Once you realize the type of sequence, the abnormal vessel is much more readily apparent. Clearly, the vessel on the right looks expanded and occluded, suggestive of acute thrombosis. The final piece of the puzzle is determining which vessel is artery and which is vein. Again, this can be difficult with a single image. Remember that the artery is usually smaller than the vein. Also, the iliac veins are usually posteromedial to the accompanying artery.

CASE 10.9 ANSWERS

1. **C. GRE**
2. **D. Right external iliac vein thrombosis**

1. Does this patient need an IVC filter?
   A. Yes, an infrarenal filter
   B. Yes, a suprarenal filter to protect both the iliac thrombus and the thrombus high in the IVC
   C. Unable to tell from these images
   D. No filter needed

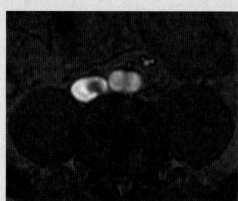

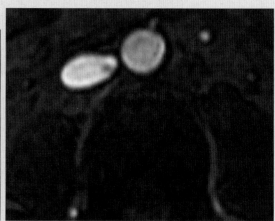

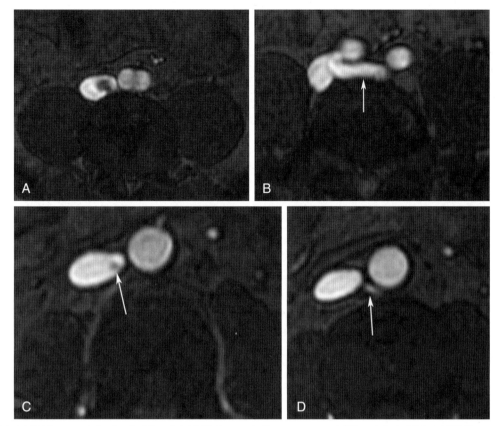

FIG. 10.C10. (A) Axial GRE image at the level of the distal IVC demonstrating an apparent filling defect. (B) Axial GRE image caudal to the first image. There is a transverse course of the left common iliac vein *(arrow)* emptying into the IVC. (C) Axial GRE image more superiorly at the level of the midabdomen. An additional smaller filling defect is identified within the IVC *(arrow)*. (D) Axial GRE image just caudal to the prior image, which demonstrates a transversely oriented lumbar vein emptying into the IVC *(arrow)*.

Discussion

These two images demonstrate inflow artifacts from a horizontal vein. No deep venous thrombosis (DVT) is present on these images, despite the apparent filling defects seen on the two images on the left.

Ultrasound of the bilateral lower extremities is an integral part in the evaluation of DVT, but is limited by its inability to visualize the more central venous structures. MRI has therefore become an important adjunct imaging modality that provides information about the patency of the deep veins within the pelvis and abdomen. MR venography has been proven to be more accurate than traditional contrast venography for diagnosing pelvic thrombus.[8] The inherent flow-related enhancement characteristic of gradient sequences results in a hyperintense appearance to the lumen of patent vessels. A filling defect with associated expansion of the vessel diameter, as seen in Fig. 10.C9, therefore raises the suspicion for a thrombus. However, pitfalls with this technique include slow flow and flow coursing perpendicular to the imaging slice, both of which can mimic a venous thrombus. This commonly occurs in areas of inflow to the IVC such as the confluence of the iliac veins or renal veins. To increase the specificity of the MRV, a T2-weighted fat suppressed TSE sequence is added to assess for edema within the adjacent soft tissues, an expected finding in an acute DVT. Phase contrast images may also be obtained to increase specificity and confidence of interpretation further.[9]

Fig. 10.C10 provides two examples of the lack of sensitivity to in-plane flow on gradient sequences.[10] Evaluated separately, both these filling defects could represent thrombi. However, the images immediately inferior demonstrate the transverse course of the causative vein. This transverse (rather than inferior to superior) course increases the time that the intraluminal protons remain within the imaging slice, which, coupled with the relatively slow flow within the venous system, results in saturation of the protons by the multiple RF pulses sent into the imaging slice. The saturated protons are therefore unable to contribute signal during image acquisition, leading to low signal and apparent filling defects. If there is persistent concern for thrombus, phase contrast images or contrast-enhanced MR venography can be performed to add specificity.

CASE 10.10 ANSWER

1. **D. No filter needed**

TAKE-HOME POINTS

1. Flow voids and flow-related enhancement are both based on the same TOF phenomenon.
2. The TOF phenomenon is based on the fact that flowing protons within blood do not experience the same RF pulses as stationary protons.
3. SE sequences result in flow voids.
4. GRE sequences exhibit flow-related enhancement.
5. Signal loss within flow voids is not binary. Rather, there is a spectrum ranging from full normal signal to a complete signal void.
6. Sequences with long TEs (e.g., T2 images) have the most prominent flow voids.
7. Vessels taking an oblique course through the imaging plane take longer to exit the imaging plane. This increases

the probability that they experience both RF pulses and result in a signal on SE sequences.

8. In GRE sequences, a proton's longitudinal magnitude does not fully recover before the next RF pulse is applied. Multiple repeated TRs in GRE images result in the achievement of an equilibrium between the amount of longitudinal magnetization recovered and the amount of magnetization that is tipped into the transverse plane. This is termed *saturation* and results in decreased signal based on the proton's inherent T1 and T2* properties. Flowing protons moving into a slice are unsaturated. This is the basis of flow-related enhancement.

9. With 3D acquisition, a proton must traverse the entire volume of excited tissue to escape the multiple repeated RF pulses. The result is an effect termed the *entry slice phenomenon*.

10. The entry slice phenomenon results in progressive loss of signal within the downstream aspect of the vessel and is dependent on the direction of blood flow.

11. Bipolar gradients are unable to correct phase shift in moving protons, which results in further signal loss of the flowing protons on GRE imaging.

12. Flow-compensated gradients are a second mirror image bipolar gradient that can account for phase shifts in flowing protons, but are added only if the blood flow is being evaluated.

13. One should always include an evaluation of the vasculature for flow voids on SE-based sequences.

14. Venous thrombosis will manifest as intrinsic signal with the vessel on SE images.

15. Confirmation of flow voids identified on short TE sequences (T1-weighted images) should be made by evaluating long TE sequences (T2).

16. Identifying abnormally positioned or unexpected flow voids can be exceedingly helpful in establishing a diagnosis.

17. T2-weighted images are usually included in evaluating for DVT to look for soft tissue edema, a finding expected in acute thrombosis.

18. The relative lack of sensitivity to in-plane flow on gradient images can result in in-flow phenomena in areas where the vasculature courses parallel to the imaging plane. Common areas where in-flow artifacts are seen include the distal IVC at the intake of the left common iliac vein and at the level of the bilateral renal veins.

References

1. Bradley Jr WG. Carmen lecture. Flow phenomena in MR imaging. *AJR Am J Roentgenol.* 1988;150(5):983–994.
2. Miyazaki M, Lee VS. Nonenhanced MR angiography. *Radiology.* 2008;248(1):20–43.
3. Edelman RR. *Clinical Magnetic Resonance Imaging.* 3rd ed. Philadelphia: Elsevier; 2006.
4. Hasuo K, Mihara F, Matsushima T. MRI and MR angiography in moyamoya disease. *J Magn Reson Imaging.* 1998;8(4):762–766.
5. Krings T, Geibprasert S. Spinal dural arteriovenous fistulas. *AJNR Am J Neuroradiol.* 2009;30(4):639–648.
6. Spain RI, Stuckert E, Sharan A, Skidmore CT. Spinal dural arteriovenous fistula: an overlooked cause of progressive myelopathy. *Hosp Physician.* 2009:33–38.
7. Lee VS. *Cardiovascular MRI: Physical Principles to Practical Protocols.* Philadelphia: Lippincott Williams & Wilkins; 2006.
8. Orbell JH, Smith A, Burnand KG, Waltham M. Imaging of deep vein thrombosis. *Br J Surg.* 2008;95(2):137–146.
9. Spritzer CE, Norconk Jr JJ, Sostman HD, Coleman RE. Detection of deep venous thrombosis by magnetic resonance imaging. *Chest.* 1993;(104):54–60.
10. Glockner JF, Lee CU. Magnetic resonance venography. *Appl Radiol.* 2010;39(6):36–42.

CHAPTER 11

Cardiac Magnetic Resonance Imaging

Scott M. Duncan

OPENING CASE 11.1

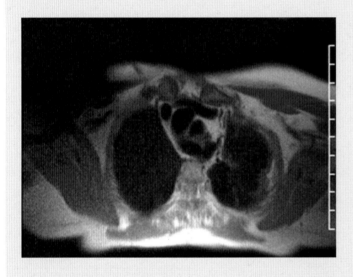

1. Which of the following is true about this entity?
   A. 95% association with other cardiac anomalies
   B. Can lead to dysphagia and wheezing
   C. Must be treated surgically
   D. Associated with left arm weakness

OPENING CASE 11.1

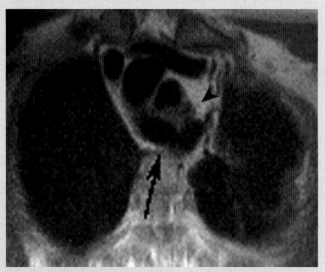

FIG. 11.C1. Axial half-Fourier acquisition, single-shot turbo spin echo (HASTE) image at the level of the aortic arch, which demonstrates a right aortic arch with an aberrant left subclavian artery *(arrow)* coursing posterior to the trachea *(arrowhead)* and esophagus.

1. Which of the following is true about this entity?
   B. Can lead to dysphagia and wheezing

Discussion

The diagnosis on this cardiac MRI is a right-sided aortic arch with an aberrant left subclavian artery. There are two types of right-sided aortic arches, a mirror image aortic arch and a right-sided aortic arch with an aberrant left subclavian artery. Two important differences between these two entities should be noted. First, the right-sided aortic arch with a mirror image branching pattern is almost always (>95% incidence) associated with other cardiac anomalies, most commonly tetralogy of Fallot or a truncus arteriosus. A right-sided aortic arch with an aberrant left subclavian artery is only rarely (5%–10% incidence) associated with other cardiac anomalies. Furthermore, the right-sided aortic arch with an aberrant left subclavian artery results in a vascular ring that is completed by the ductus arteriosus on the left side of the mediastinum. This complete vascular ring can lead to dysphagia and wheezing.[1]

Cardiac MRI

There are two main categories of cardiac sequences, black blood and white blood. The techniques and uses of both these sequences are described in more detail below, but this topic is introduced here by briefly describing how the images are similar to flow void and flow-related enhancement, discussed in the previous chapter (see Chapter 10). *Black blood sequences are spin echo–based sequences that take advantage of flow voids to null signal with the vascular structures. They are primarily used to evaluate anatomy. Conversely, white blood sequences use gradient echo–based sequences designed to take advantage of flow-related enhancement. These series are typically dynamic sequences that are played on a cine loop and provide physiologic information.*

Black Blood Technique

As previously described, black blood images are spin echo–based sequences that take advantage of flow voids to null signal within vascular structures. This allows for better evaluation of the vessel wall and myocardium. Although standard fast spin echo (FSE) techniques are occasionally used to obtain high-resolution images, their lengthy acquisition times preclude routine use in areas of high motion, such as the heart. Therefore most cardiac imaging is performed using a HASTE sequence. As the name implies, this sequence involves a single 90-degree radiofrequency (RF) pulse in combination with a long echo train length (usually >70) to fill k-space. As an additional time-saving measure, only a little more than half of k-space is filled (56%) and the remainder is interpolated via the inherent symmetry of k-space. These two properties allow for very rapid imaging. An acquisition of a single image takes less than 0.5 second.[1] As a result, an entire image series through the thorax can be acquired in a single breath-hold. Although this technique provides increased speed and a reduced motion artifact, it also results in a diminished signal-to-noise ratio because only slightly more than half of k-space is sampled, diminished contrast-to-noise ratio, and decreased spatial resolution.

Black blood cardiac images are acquired during diastole in an effort to reduce motion artifact. However, during diastole, there is reduced blood flow (particularly within the cardiac chambers), resulting in diminished or nonexistent flow voids—no more black blood. *To create the black blood image, a double-inversion recovery technique is added that completely nulls the signal from flowing blood.* An initial inversion recovery pulse is applied to the entire slab of tissue, which inverts all spins. Subsequently, a second inversion recovery pulse is applied only to the slice being imaged. With this technique, all stationary protons within the imaging slice have experienced two 180-degree inversion pulses (for a total of 360 degrees) and have reverted to their normal longitudinal magnetization. They are thereby available to produce signal during the excitation pulse and image acquisition. However, flowing protons (i.e., those within the blood pool) are not located within the imaging slice during the second inversion pulse and therefore do not revert to their normal longitudinal magnetization. Instead, they move into the imaging slice immediately before the excitation pulse and image acquisition. This makes the images much more sensitive to slow-flowing blood.

In addition, the inversion time is set to the null point of blood, further reducing the signal acquired from flowing blood. This combination of techniques provides excellent black blood images.[1]

White Blood Technique

Bright blood imaging is the workhorse of cardiac MRI. It is used in the evaluation of the cardiac lumen, cardiac valves, cardiac defects, and most commonly, cardiac function. In other words, it provides the physiologic information compared to the anatomic information of the black blood technique, although it is also good at delineating some anatomy. Bright blood sequences are usually gated electrocardiographically and displayed in cine form.[1] Unfortunately, this is difficult to illustrate in a text. Functional information, particularly wall motion abnormalities, is much better appreciated and more obvious in the cine form.

As mentioned previously the white blood technique takes advantage of flow-related enhancement with gradient images in much the same way as the black blood technique takes advantage of flow voids in the spin echo (SE) technique. Similar to the black blood technique, the white blood technique has more features to ensure that there is adequate signal intensity from the blood beyond simply relying on flow-related enhancement.

The gradients used in cardiac MRI are very fast, with the time to repetition (TR) shorter than T2* times. The result is residual transverse magnetization that has not decayed when the next RF pulse arrives. This is a significant problem because the residual magnetization will affect and distort the signal of the next acquisition. There are two ways to address this residual magnetization. The first is by spoiling or crushing the residual magnetization using a gradient. The spoiler gradient takes advantage of one of the recurring themes in MRI, that exposing protons to a magnetic gradient will result in rapid dephasing. With gradient imaging, the spins are dephased and then rephased using a bipolar gradient. *The signal acquisition (TE) occurs when the rephasing gradient lobe equals the dephasing gradient lobe. The spoiler gradient works by leaving the rephasing gradient on after the TE, which rapidly dephases the spins again and destroys (spoils or crushes) the residual transverse magnetization. The spoiled gradient is used in time-of-flight imaging.*

In the early 2000s, cardiac imaging used spoiled gradients as the white blood technique. The white blood signal was primarily from flow-related enhancement, as described earlier. That worked fairly well except for two problems. First, because it relies on flow-related enhancement, there is a built-in delay to allow fresh spins to enter the slice. Second, the extra spoiler gradient results in longer acquisition times and longer TRs.

Over the past 15 years there have been technologic advances in gradient manufacturing, which allows them to be switched and adjusted very rapidly. With these fairly recent advances, new and better imaging sequences could be used. Steady-state sequences were based on these advances. *In steady-state imaging, the residual transverse magnetization after the TE is used to obtain more signal in subsequent excitations, rather than being crushed.*

The initial RF pulse tilts the magnetization vector partially into the transverse plane. The subsequent RF pulses knock the magnetization vector back and forth across the z-axis. The process has an appearance similar to a metronome. The result is that both the transverse and longitudinal magnetizations enter a steady state, not just the longitudinal magnetization, as in a spoiled gradient.

There are several advantages to the use of the steady-state technique over the spoiled gradient echo. First, because it uses the residual transverse magnetization instead of wasting it, there is increased signal-to-noise ratio. Second, because the transverse magnetization is added back to the longitudinal magnetization, the steady state is reached more quickly, in as little time as a single TR. Third, the TRs are extremely short, less than 5 ms, allowing for very rapid imaging. For, example a typical four-chamber white blood cine sequence with electrocardiographic gating can be performed in less than 20 seconds—a single breath-hold for most patients.

Another benefit of the steady-state sequence is that the images have both T1 and T2 weighting. In other words, molecules with long T2 and short T1 times will have bright signal (both water and fat). Because blood has long T2 and short T1 times, it is bright on steady-state images. Thus the bright signal in steady-state white blood images is mostly due to inherent signal from the blood, not flow-related enhancement. Therefore the TR does not have to be lengthened to wait for fresh spins to enter the slice, and there will be no signal loss due to slow flow.

Flow-related enhancement does contribute some signal in the steady-state sequence; however, most of the signal is due to inherent bright signal of the blood. Because multiple powerful gradients are being used, and both residual transverse and longitudinal magnetization are being reused, there is increased sensitivity to artifacts from field inhomogeneities and susceptibility.[2]

Most sequences in cardiac MRI, including both the white and black blood images, are electrocardiographically gated. Gating of white blood images allows for the evaluation of dynamic cardiac function and physiology throughout the cardiac cycle (e.g., motion of the myocardium and valve leaflets). The images are typically reviewed in cine form. Gating in black blood images serves to time image acquisition during the diastolic phase of the cardiac cycle, thereby limiting cardiac motion artifact. Electrocardiographic gating has many similarities to gating in nuclear cardiology. However, the detailed technique of electrocardiographic gating is beyond the scope of this text.

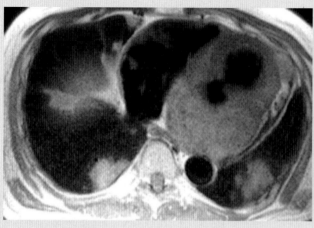
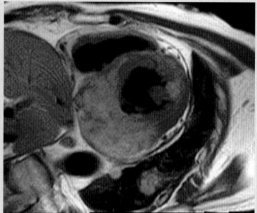

1. What malignancies could cause this appearance?
   A. Metastatic renal cell
   B. Primary angiosarcoma
   C. Primary rhabdomyosarcoma
   D. Lymphoma
   E. All of the above

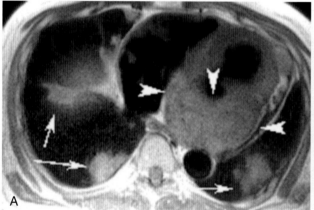
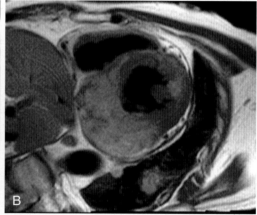

FIG. 11.C2. (A) Axial HASTE image at the level of the left atrium and ventricle. A soft tissue mass involves most of the left atrium (arrowheads). Note the multiple bilateral pulmonary nodules (arrows). (B) Oblique FSE image at the level of the left atrium and ventricle demonstrating the left atrial mass. Note the improved spatial resolution compared with the HASTE image.

Discussion

Malignancy involving the myocardium is relatively rare. Metastatic disease occurs much more frequently than primary tumors.[2] Mesothelioma and melanoma are the two most common tumors to metastasize to the heart, but almost any tumor can metastasize. The incidence of metastatic disease is not as low as would be expected, up to 18% in one postmortem study.[3] Primary malignancies are exceedingly rare in the heart but include angiosarcomas, liposarcomas, and rhabdosarcomas. The patient in Fig. 11.C2 had a history of renal cell carcinoma, and this mass was proven to represent a metastasis via biopsy.

This case juxtaposes the two black blood techniques, HASTE and FSE. There is a marked difference in the spatial resolution between the two images, with the FSE having a much more crisp appearance. Note the increased conspicuity and clarity of the pulmonary nodules on the FSE image. Also, on the HASTE image, the intracardiac mass appears relatively indistinct, whereas on the FSE sequence there is improved differentiation between the normal intermediate-signal myocardium and the hyperintense metastatic lesion; this occurs because of an improved contrast-to-noise ratio. Because of this improved resolution and enhanced discrimination, a second lesion along the anterolateral wall of the left ventricle can be identified.

CASE 11.2 ANSWER

1. **E. All of the above**

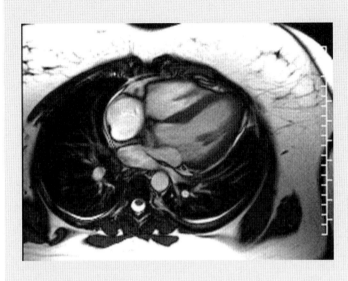

1. What is the diagnosis?
   A. Cor triatriatum
   B. Atrial septal defect (ASD)
   C. Ventricular septal defect
   D. Pulmonary arteriovenous malformation
2. Sequelae of this abnormality results in which of the following physiologic changes?
   A. Right-to-left shunt
   B. Left-to-right shunt
   C. Paradoxic emboli
   D. Pulmonary edema
   E. Left heart failure

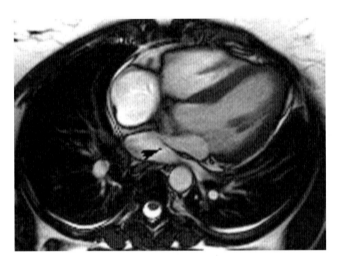

FIG. 11.C3. Balanced steady-state, free precession, four-chamber view of the heart demonstrating a thin septum within the left atrium (arrowhead).

Discussion

This figure demonstrates a septum within the left atrium consistent with cor triatriatum. It causes the left atrium to be partitioned into two chambers,[4] which often results in an obstruction leading to pulmonary venous hypertension and pulmonary edema. More severe forms can cause identifiable right heart failure on a neonatal chest radiograph.

CASE 11.3 ANSWERS

1. **A. Cor triatriatum**
2. **D. Pulmonary edema**

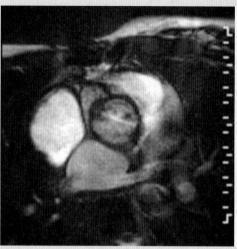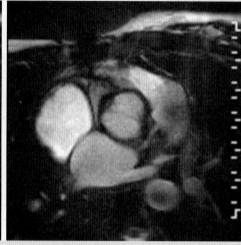

1. Which valve is being imaged?
   A. Aortic
   B. Tricuspid
   C. Mitral
   D. Pulmonic

2. Which of the following is not true about this entity?
   A. Increased risk for aortic aneurysm and dissection
   B. Can result in aortic valve regurgitation
   C. Calcifies more quickly than a normal aortic valve
   D. Results in left atrial dilation
   E. Occurs in 1% of the population

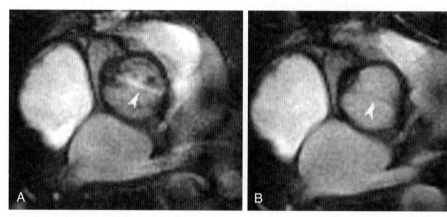

FIG. 11.C4. (A) Steady-state free precession image focused over the aortic valve during systole demonstrating a linear jet of flow *(arrowhead)* consistent with a bicuspid aortic valve. (B) Steady-state free precession image focused over the aortic valve during diastole, confirming the presence of only two aortic valve leaflets *(arrowhead)*.

Discussion

This case demonstrates a bicuspid aortic valve with aortic stenosis and aortic regurgitation. The bicuspid aortic valve is a common congenital cardiac anomaly, with an incidence in the general population of 0.9% to 2.0%. Bicuspid aortic valves are present in 54% of adult patients with aortic stenosis.[5] Aortic stenosis results in turbulent flow, with increased velocities across the valve manifesting as linear heterogeneous signal within the proximal aorta during systole on MR images.

CASE 11.4 ANSWERS

1. **A. Aortic**
2. **D. Results in left atrial dilation**

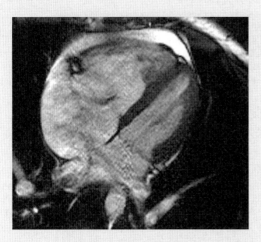

1. What physiologic effects can an ASD have on the cardio-
   pulmonary circulation?
   A. Left heart strain
   B. Pulmonary arterial hypertension
   C. Decreased oxygenation of the blood
   D. Decreased preload on the right heart
   E. All of the above
   F. None of the above

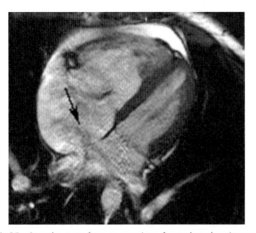

FIG. 11.C5. Steady-state free precession, four-chamber image
demonstrates a large ASD with a turbulent jet of flow across the
defect *(arrow)*. Note the enlarged right atrium and ventricle
secondary to volume overload from the left-to-right shunt.

Discussion

This white blood image nicely demonstrates an ostium secundum ASD. The excellent contrast between the white blood
and dark septum clearly demonstrates the communication
between the right and left atrium and the absence of an intact
septum. Also, the darker turbulent flow extending into the
right atrium provides added conspicuity. The ASD results in
a left-to-right shunt, adding increased volume and preload to
the right heart. This is demonstrated in Fig. 11.C5 by the dilation of the right atrium and ventricle. The increased preload
can result in pulmonary hypertension and Eisenmenger syndrome if not corrected.

CASE 11.5 ANSWER

1. B. Pulmonary arterial hypertension

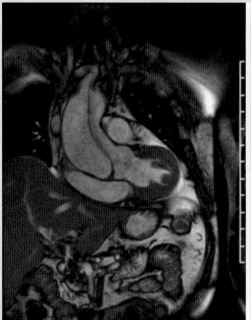
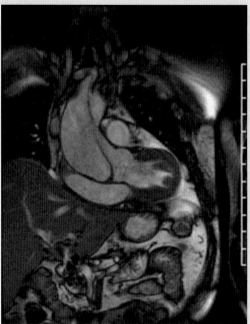

1. Which abnormality is not present on these images?
   A. Aortic stenosis
   B. Aortic regurgitation
   C. Ascending aortic aneurysm
   D. Ascending aortic dissection

2. What is the underlying diagnosis and pathophysiology?
   A. Traumatic aortic dissection status post–malignant ventricular arrhythmia
   B. Marfan syndrome with aortic dissection
   C. Ascending aortic aneurysm from atherosclerotic disease
   D. Dehiscent prosthetic aortic valve post–ascending aorta and aortic valve repair

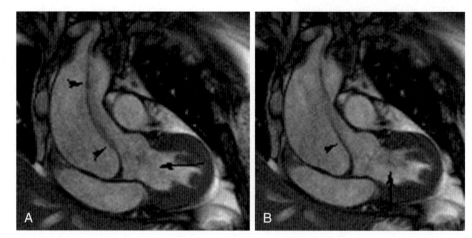

FIG. 11.C6. (A–B) Steady-state free precession image centered over the left ventricular outflow tract. Note the dilated ascending aorta extending into the aortic root as well as a dissection flap within the ascending aorta *(arrowheads)*. A jet of dark signal representing turbulent flow extends retrograde from the aortic valve into the left ventricle, consistent with aortic regurgitation *(arrows)*.

Discussion

Case 11.6 is a good example of Marfan syndrome with annuloaortic ectasia, a dissection of the ascending aorta, and resultant aortic regurgitation. In contradistinction to ascending aortic aneurysms from atherosclerotic disease, aneurysms secondary to Marfan syndrome result in dilation of the aortic root, termed *annuloaortic ectasia*. A defect in the gene that encodes for the glycoprotein fibrillin results in a weakened vascular interstitium and can lead to dissections, as shown in Fig. 11.C6.[6] Aortic insufficiency is a common complication in these patients, occurring secondary to the annuloaortic ectasia and to dissections of the ascending aorta.

White blood images are excellent for evaluation of the cardiac valves. The hyperintense signal from the blood pool provides superb contrast with the low signal cardiac valves. Furthermore, turbulent jets of flow from stenotic or regurgitant valves manifest as conspicuous areas of dark signal on the white blood pool background. Remember that turbulent blood flow results in protons of varying velocities, which therefore acquire differing amounts of phase shift in the setting of a gradient. This phase shift results in cancellation of signal and results in the characteristic dark signal or flow void. Flow-compensated gradients are unable to correct for this dephasing because it is random. Areas of turbulent flow with resultant signal loss are identified in the right atrium adjacent to the ostium secundum ASD in Case 11.5 and in the left ventricle secondary to regurgitant flow in Case 11.6.

On occasion, it can be difficult to determine whether a jet of turbulent flow is secondary to valve regurgitation or to valve stenosis. Intuitively, the direction in which the jet is oriented should help make this determination. To do so, the position of the valve must first be located, which may require several reviews of the cine. Another way to help locate the valve and determine the direction of turbulence is to examine the contour of the jet. Turbulent jets start out from a small point and extend outward from the point in a fan-shaped configuration. Thus the narrower portion of the jet represents the valvular side of the jet, and the broad fan-shaped end represents the direction of turbulent flow. With these two techniques it should be relatively easy to determine the origin of the turbulent flow.

CASE 11.6 ANSWERS

1. **A. Aortic stenosis**
2. **B. Marfan syndrome with aortic dissection**

CASE 11.7

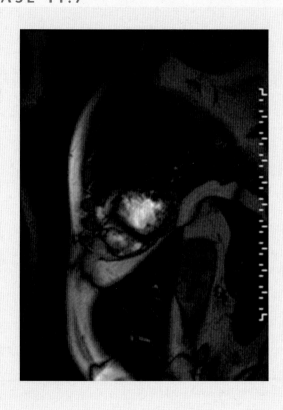

1. The patient had cardiac MRI for restrictive cardiomyopathy. What is the cause?
   A. Amyloid
   B. Sarcoid
   C. Hemochromatosis
   D. Scleroderma
   E. Pericardial effusion

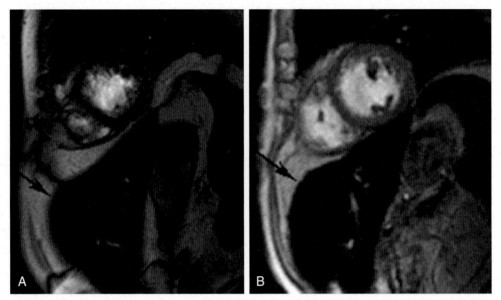

FIG. 11.C7. (A) Steady-state, free precession, short-axis image of the heart and upper abdomen. The myocardium exhibits very dark signal secondary to susceptibility artifact from iron deposition. Also note the black signal within the liver *(arrow)*. (B) Spoiled gradient short-axis image of the heart and upper abdomen demonstrates myocardium with intermediate gray signal. Black signal is again demonstrated within the liver *(arrow)*.

Discussion

Restrictive cardiomyopathy is a relatively rare condition with a limited differential diagnosis that includes amyloid, sarcoid, and hemochromatosis. There is a hint in Fig. 11.C7 that can help lead to the diagnosis. Note that the liver and the spleen are completely black because of hemochromatosis. Therefore the black signal in the left ventricle is from susceptibility artifact caused by iron deposition within the myocardium. In Fig. 11.C7A, there is so much susceptibility artifact in the myocardium that it cannot be evaluated. An astute MR technologist recognized this problem and attempted a spoiled gradient image (Fig. 11.C7B), which successfully decreased the degree of susceptibility artifact in the myocardium. However, note that there remains considerable susceptibility artifact in the liver parenchyma, even on the spoiled gradient images. This is because the iron concentration in the liver is much higher than that in the myocardium.

CASE 11.7 ANSWER

1. C. Hemochromatosis

TAKE-HOME POINTS

1. In cardiac imaging, a white blood technique is a gradient echo–based sequence and a black blood technique is a spin echo–based sequence.
2. Most black blood cardiac imaging is performed using a HASTE sequence. These sequences involve a single 90-degree RF pulse in combination with a long echo train length (usually >70) to fill the k-space.
3. Black blood cardiac images are acquired during diastole to reduce motion artifact.
4. Decreased blood flow during diastole is countered by application of a double-inversion recovery technique that completely nulls the signal from flowing blood.
5. White blood images use steady-state gradient echo sequences to achieve bright signal within the blood.
6. Steady-state images are very sensitive to susceptibility artifacts.
7. Spoiled gradient images provide decreased magnetic susceptibility but take longer to acquire.
8. On white blood cardiac images, look for linear areas of dark signal that represent areas of increased velocity and turbulent flow. These can be seen in valvular stenosis, valvular regurgitation, and septal defects.

References

1. Lee VS. *Cardiovascular MRI: Physical Principles to Practical Protocols.* Philadelphia: Lippincott Williams & Wilkins; 2006.
2. Bussani R, De-Giorgio F, Abbate A, Silvestri F. Cardiac metastases. *J Clin Pathol.* 2007;60(1):27–34.
3. Sparrow P, Kurian J, Jones T, Sivananthan M. MR imaging of cardiac tumors. *Radiographics.* 2005;25(5):1255–1276.
4. Krasemann Z, Scheld HH, Tjan TD, Krasemann T. Cor triatriatum: short review of the literature upon ten new cases. *Herz.* 2007;32(6):506–510.
5. Yener N, Oktar GL, Erer D, et al. Bicuspid aortic valve. *Ann Thorac Cardiovasc Surg.* 2002;(8):26–267.
6. Judge DP, Dietz HC. Marfan's syndrome. *Lancet.* 2005;366(9501):1965–1976.

CHAPTER 12

Time-of-Flight Imaging

Scott M. Duncan

OPENING CASE 12.1

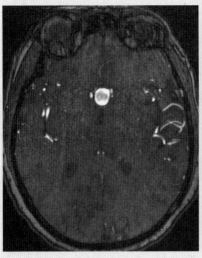 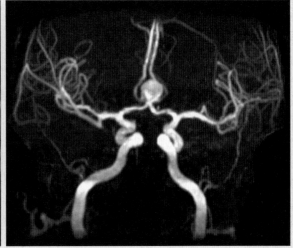

1. These images show a saccular aneurysm of the anterior communicating artery. What is the cause of the low signal in the center of the aneurysm?
   A. Partial thrombosis of the aneurysm
   B. Susceptibility artifact from the calcium in the wall of the aneurysm
   C. Turbulent flow and partial saturation of protons in the aneurysm
   D. Laminar flow artifact

2. What parts of the body are typically imaged with time-of-flight (TOF) angiography?
   A. Circle of Willis, feet, and renal arteries
   B. Thoracic aorta, renal arteries, and circle of Willis
   C. Circle of Willis and feet
   D. Feet, renal arteries, and thoracic aorta

OPENING CASE 12.1

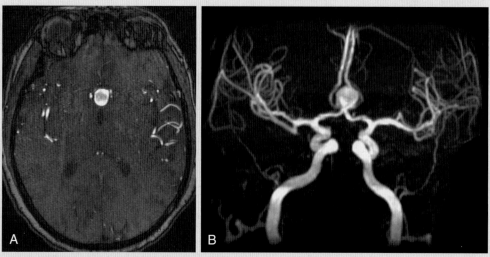

FIG. 12.C1. (A) Axial TOF image. The large high signal lesion anterior to the third ventricle is consistent with an anterior communicating artery aneurysm. (B) Maximum intensity projection (MIP) TOF image of the anterior circulation showing the aneurysm.

1. What is the cause of the low signal in the center of the aneurysm?
   C. Turbulent flow in the aneurysm and partial saturation of the protons within the aneurysm
2. What parts of the body are typically imaged with TOF angiography?
   C. Circle of Willis and feet

Discussion

TOF imaging nicely shows the anterior communicating artery aneurysm because of the high signal-to-noise ratio (SNR) and the lack of venous contamination, which is very common in contrasted MR angiography (MRA) and CT angiography (CTA). TOF is ideal for both the feet and the head for two reasons. First, these areas are more susceptible to venous contamination because they are terminal arteries. Therefore the time when contrast is only in the arteries and has yet to reach the veins is very short and more often nonexistent. Also, there is often enhancement of the more proximal veins before the distal arteries opacify. Second, these areas are not susceptible to breathing motion artifact, and most patients are able to hold these parts of the body still for longer periods.

Although TOF has its benefits, it is also susceptible to many artifacts that can become diagnostic dilemmas without an understanding of the underlying physics. The central low signal in the aneurysm may be alarming to an inexperienced radiology resident or physician. However, with some background of the underlying physics of TOF imaging, a thrombus can be confidently excluded.

Two causes of decreased signal in TOF angiography are turbulent flow and saturation of the protons within blood. As will be discussed in more detail, turbulent flow results in dephasing of the protons that, when summed together, results in partial cancellation of signal.

Protons that do not move out of the plane of imaging become saturated in TOF imaging. Blood does not have a normal linear, unidirectional flow in aneurysms, but rather swirls in the aneurysm, making it susceptible to saturation.

Physics

Much of the physics of TOF angiography is similar to what was discussed in Chapter 10; however, it will also be reviewed here to keep the discussion coherent. TOF angiography is a gradient echo sequence that optimizes certain parameters to produce bright signal within the vessel while suppressing the nonmobile background tissue. The suppression of background tissues is achieved via signal **saturation.** The bright signal within the vessel is a result of inflowing unsaturated (fresh) protons.

Signal Saturation

The suppression of background signal through saturation is performed by applying multiple radiofrequency (RF) pulses in succession to the slice of interest. In TOF imaging, the time to repetition (TR) is so short (usually <30 ms) that longitudinal magnetization of the protons does not completely recover before the next RF pulse. This results in less magnetization available to flip back into the transverse plane, with subsequent RF pulses. *After several repeated RF pulses, the proton reaches a steady state, in which the amount of longitudinal magnetization recovered is equal to the amount flipped into the transverse plane by the next RF pulse.[1] This is called* saturation *or* magnetization equilibrium *and results in significantly decreased signal.* For a more detailed description of this phenomenon, refer Chapter 10, with special attention to Fig. 10.C1.

Saturation is not an all-or-nothing phenomenon; rather, it is a spectrum. Multiple variables affect the degree of saturation, including the flip angle and the TR.[2] Increasing the flip angle means that more longitudinal magnetization is tipped into the transverse plane, which results in less longitudinal magnetization available for the next RF pulse. Therefore the higher the flip angle, the more magnetization that does not return to the longitudinal plane, resulting in less signal. Shortening the TR results in less time for longitudinal magnetization recovery and less magnetization left for the next pulse. Again, decreased signal is the result.

Inflow of Unsaturated (Fresh) Protons

The above-described saturation occurs in nonmoving protons. However, a flowing proton, which is moving perpendicular to the imaging plane, will not have been exposed to the multiple previous RF pulses and will therefore have all of its longitudinal magnetization available when it moves into the imaging plane (i.e., it will not be saturated; Fig. 12.1). Therefore it will have high signal in comparison with the adjacent saturated stagnant spins. This property is known as *flow-related enhancement.* Several variables affect the amount of flow-related enhancement that moving spins will have, including the TR, flip angle, slice thickness, proton velocity, and direction.[2]

The TR and the flip angle are two important parameters that affect the degree of signal saturation and flow-related enhancement.[2] Shortening the TR results in less time for longitudinal magnetization recovery and less magnetization left for the next pulse. The end result of a short TR is improved background signal saturation. Shorter TRs are also beneficial because there will be shorter imaging times and less potential for motion artifact. However, shortening the TR does have a drawback. Shorter TRs may not allow enough time for the flowing saturated spins to exit the slice and new unsaturated spins to enter the slice. *Thus shorter TRs can reduce flow-related enhancement.* One way to improve flow-related enhancement while maintaining a short TR is to obtain thinner imaging slices. Thinner slices mean shorter distances that need to be traversed by the moving protons to exit the image slice, which allows the protons in the vessel to be refreshed more quickly. The net result is improved flow-related enhancement. The use of thinner slices comes at the cost of longer imaging time because more image slices need to be obtained per centimeter of tissue. However, this increased time is offset by the fact that thinner slices allow for shorter TRs. A typical TR for TOF is less than 30 ms, with a slice thickness of less than 1 mm.

The flip angle of the excitation pulse is another parameter that affects the saturation of stagnant spins. Increasing the flip angle means that more longitudinal magnetization is tipped into the transverse plane, which results in less longitudinal magnetization available for the next RF pulse. *Therefore, the higher the flip angle, the more magnetization that does not return to the longitudinal plane, resulting in increased saturation (less signal).* The larger the flip angle, the less residual longitudinal magnetization available

for the next RF pulse and the greater the resultant saturation of stationary protons. For TOF imaging, most flip angles range from 45 to 60 degrees.

Finally, it should be noted that short TRs and large flip angles in gradient echo sequences promote T1 weighting (see Chapter 1). Thus high signal on TOF can be secondary to factors other than flow, including fat or subacute blood products.

Limitations to Time of Flight

There are several factors that decrease flow-related enhancement. Flow-related dephasing, as discussed in Chapter 10, is one such factor. Recall that this can be compensated for by using gradient moment nulling or a short time to echo (TE). A typical TE for TOF angiography is of the magnitude of less than 10 ms. Using a short TE minimizes the need for complex, time-consuming, higher-order flow compensation gradients.[2] Remember that gradient moment nulling compensates for only first-order flow (constant velocity). The major drawback is the increased imaging time required to insert extra gradients.

Flow velocity is not uniform throughout the lumen of the vessel. For example, the normal laminar flow in a vessel results in higher velocities in the center of the vessel and lower velocities at the periphery. Therefore in a normal vessel, signal should be higher centrally and lower at the periphery. In addition, there are also microscopic variations in velocity in a vessel due to turbulence and other factors. These small variations in velocity result in dephasing of spins within a single voxel, termed *intravoxel dephasing.* Signal is lost when protons within the same voxel are out of phase with each other because, when they are summed, their signals are partially canceled. Smaller voxel sizes are used to minimize the amount of dephasing, which has the added benefit of improved spatial resolution. However, like everything else in MRI, this comes at a cost in the form of longer acquisition times and decreased SNR.

One other limitation to TOF is that it detects flow only in a single plane, perpendicular to the imaged slice. This makes sense because if a proton is moving in the plane of the slice, it will still experience all the repetitive RF pulses applied to that slice and will be saturated, like stagnant spins. Therefore when determining a protocol for TOF angiography, the imaging plane should be oriented perpendicular to the direction of flow of the vessel of interest. Most vasculature is oriented vertically, making the axial plane the best for TOF. By extension, tortuous vessels or vessels than run in a transverse or oblique plane (e.g., subclavian or renal arteries and veins) are not well evaluated by the TOF technique.

There are a few more limitations to TOF that need to be noted when formulating a protocol or evaluating a study. First, TOF images will often overestimate the degree of stenosis compared to CTA and conventional angiography for a number

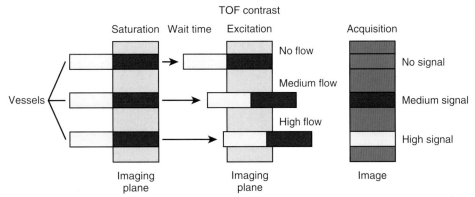

FIG. 12.1. Signal intensity is based on the rate of flow within a vessel. The protons in the imaging plane are saturated. Depending on the velocity of flow within a vessel—high, medium, or none—a certain amount of new nonsaturated protons will enter the imaging plane. When the image is acquired, vessels with high flow will have bright signal because many new nonsaturated protons have entered the imaging plane. Vessels with little or no flow will appear dark because few new unsaturated protons have entered the field.

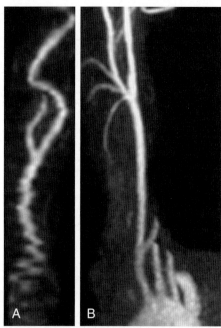

FIG. 12.2. (A) TOF MIP of the right carotid artery showing significant motion artifact at the origin of the carotid, limiting evaluation. The patient could not receive contrast due to acute renal failure. (B) Contrast-enhanced MRA of the right carotid artery—no motion artifact. The aortic arch and proximal great vessels are easily evaluated and normal. Note some venous contamination.

of reasons. First, in general, MRA has less spatial resolution compared with CTA and conventional angiography, making stenosis determination less precise and often overestimated. Second, there is intravoxel dephasing because of magnetic field inhomogeneities experienced by the inflowing protons. The dephasing of spins leads to less signal in the vessel and an apparent increased stenosis. Turbulent flow also leads to rapid dephasing, which cannot be corrected. Thus areas where there is turbulent flow, such as tortuous vessels, aneurysms, or areas of stenosis, will have less signal. In the case of stenosis, this can result in vessels appearing narrower than they really are.[4] Finally, many stenoses are secondary to calcific atherosclerotic disease, and the susceptibility artifact from the calcium will decrease signal. The low signal in aneurysms can give the false appearance of partial thrombosis, as in Case 12.C1.

The major disadvantage of TOF compared with gadolinium-enhanced MRA is time. Gadolinium-enhanced MRA takes only 10 to 15 seconds to be acquired, whereas TOF often takes 4 or more minutes to acquire; this means significantly longer scan times and increased susceptibility to motion. As can be seen in Fig. 12.2, the TOF image is essentially nondiagnostic in the common carotid artery because of its proximity to the chest. *TOF is not an ideal test for imaging close to the chest or abdomen because of respiratory motion artifact.* It can do more harm than good in these areas because the artifact may mask a true lesion, or it may mimic an abnormality that is not present. For this reason, it is generally used to image only a small volume of tissue (usually <10 cm). However, if necessary, it can be used to image larger areas.

However, due to nephrogenic systemic fibrosis, a substantial number of patients are not able to receive gadolinium contrast due to poor renal function. In addition, the risk factors for renal disease (e.g., hypertension, diabetes, smoking, obesity) are the same as those for vasculopathy. The result is that a significant portion of the patients being evaluated for vascular disease cannot undergo CT or contrast MRI. Thus in the past few years, there has been a significant increase in the use of noncontrast MRA using TOF.

Note that as you move farther away from the chest on the TOF MIP, the respiratory motion artifact decreases so that the image distal to the carotid bifurcation is of high quality. This is why it can be used successfully when evaluating the circle of Willis.

There are really only two fundamental ways to decrease acquisition time and, by extension motion artifact, in TOF angiography and in MRA in general. The TR can be decreased or the amount of k-space to fill can be decreased. In recent years, a few techniques have addressed these issues and helped reduce TOF acquisition time. The first is 3-T MRI; this has been around for a while but has become more commonplace, and its use has extended beyond research and academic centers. Because of the higher field strength, 3-T MRI offers several advantages compared with 1.5 T. First, the increased magnet strength results in increased signal and better SNR. The increased signal and strength also mean that the TR is shorter (the TR is usually <20 ms, compared with ≈30 ms at 1.5 T). The shortened TR directly affects and shortens the sequence acquisition time.

The second technique is called the parallel imaging technique. This has been discussed in greater detail in earlier chapters and so will be only summarized here. *Parallel imaging reduces the amount of k-space that is sampled in the phase-encoding direction.* The phase-encoding direction helps determine the spatial resolution. To compensate for the lost spatial information, signal is obtained using an array of independent receivers instead of a large-volume coil. Because these individual receivers are spaced around the patient, they can give information about the spatial location of the signal. Each individual coil receives increased signal from the volume of tissue to which it is closest. A complex algorithm combines the additional spatial information from the various coils with the limited spatial information from k-space to form a complete image.[5] These two advances have significantly improved the acquisition time for TOF imaging, which has allowed an increased range of locations that TOF can image. However, contrast-enhanced MRA is still the much faster and preferred angiographic technique for evaluating carotid bulb and proximal internal carotid artery (ICA) stenosis.[6]

Additional Properties Unique to Time of Flight

In CTAs of the circle of Willis or a CT lower extremity runoff, the MIP images, and even the raw axial data, can be difficult to interpret because there is so much venous contamination that it can be challenging to differentiate artery from vein. One of the major advantages to TOF is the ability to minimize or eliminate venous contamination, resulting in an easier (and more aesthetically pleasing) image to interpret. This is why it is often used in the head and the feet, *even when contrast angiography is available.* I initially thought that MRA took advantage of chemical differences (oxygenation) in venous and arterial blood to remove the signal in veins on TOF angiography. The explanation is not that sophisticated but is still ingenious. *The TOF sequence uses a saturation pulse to null unwanted flow enhancement signal coming from the opposite direction.* A saturation pulse is sent peripherally to the area being imaged (above the circle of Willis for the brain, and in the feet for a runoff examination) to saturate any signal from venous flow coming into the slice (Fig. 12.3). As a corollary, if the venous anatomy were being studied (e.g., for deep venous thrombosis), the saturation ban would be reversed and placed central to the imaging slice to eliminate arterial contamination. In addition, TOF sequences are usually acquired in the reverse order that flow is being detected. For example, in the brain, imaging would commence at the vertex. This ensures that inflowing spins have not been saturated from imaging of the previous slice. If slices were acquired along the direction of flow, the incoming protons would be saturated by the RF pulses that were applied to the preceding slices.

TOF images can be acquired using a two-dimensional (2D) or three-dimensional (3D) technique. The 3D technique has

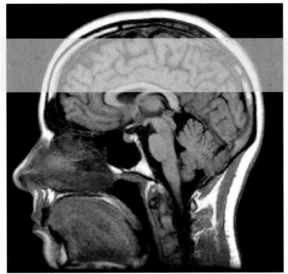

FIG. 12.3. TOF technique uses a saturation band peripheral to the area being imaged to suppress venous contamination that flows into the imaging plane.

several advantages, but it is not appropriate in all cases. The 3D technique has better SNR and is better for evaluating tortuous vessels.[2] However, it can only be used in vessels with high velocities. This makes intuitive sense because a whole slab of tissue is excited for 3D imaging, which means that the proton has to transverse the entire slab instead of a single slice to be refreshed and give signal. If the slab is too thick, there would be bright signal in the vessels of the first slices, with a progressive decrease in signal toward the end of the volume, similar to the entry phenomenon discussed in Chapter 10. To avoid this problem, the flip angles are usually smaller, in the range of 20 to 35 degrees, for 3D TOF. A 3D technique is generally used when evaluating the circle of Willis, the aorta, and the proximal lower extremities. A 2D technique is generally used in the peripheral arteries of the feet and when imaging veins because of the slower flow.

The multiple overlapping thin-slab angiography technique combines 2D and 3D techniques to take advantage of the best features of both. It consists of several thinner 3D slabs, which are overlapped to provide high resolution and high SNR while still maintaining high signal within the vessel because the slabs are thinner. This technique is commonly used for the circle of Willis.

CASE 12.2

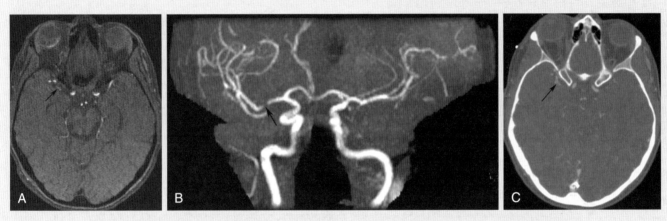

FIG. 12.C2

1. Which image most closely reflects the true degree of stenosis within the right middle cerebral artery (MCA)?
   A Axial TOF image
   B. MIP TOF image
   C. Axial CTA image

2. Which is not a cause of the decreased flow within the right MCA on TOF images compared with CTA images?
   A. Proton dephasing
   B. Turbulent flow
   C. Transverse course of the artery
   D. Laminar flow
   E. All of the above contribute to the decreased flow

FIG. 12.C2. (A) Axial TOF image. Marked narrowing and attenuation of the M1 segment of the right middle cerebral artery (MCA) is seen *(arrow)*. (B) MIP TOF image of the anterior circulation. MIP shows near occlusion of the right MCA *(arrow)*. (C) Axial computed tomographic angiographic image. There is only minimal narrowing of the right MCA.

Discussion

Case 12.2 is a good example of TOF overestimating stenosis. On the MR image, the vessel looks severely attenuated and stenotic, but on the CTA scan it appears almost normal. Note that on the MIP image, the artery looks completely occluded. MIP images exaggerate stenosis because faint vascular enhancement cannot be distinguished from the background by the computer algorithm and is thus suppressed from the image.[4]

One should be careful about determining stenosis using MIP images; always revert to the source images for measurements. This is true for both CTA and MRA.

In regions of stenosis, there is turbulent flow, not laminar flow. Therefore much of the signal loss will be secondary to turbulent flow and the transverse plane of the artery. Although dephasing from laminar flow physiology can cause some signal loss, it is not typically a large component and rarely has a clinically relevant effect on the MR image. It is very common for the proximal MCA to take a transverse and slightly caudal course before its trifurcation. This can result in signal loss because the protons have traveled in the same plane of the image for a prolonged time, making them more susceptible to partial suppression from the multiple repeated pulses. In addition, the slight caudal course of the MCA means that some of the protons are susceptible to saturation from imaging that is more cephalad. Remember that TOF images are acquired from the top down in the brain to minimize saturation of the protons flowing cephalad from the heart.

CASE 12.2 ANSWERS

1. **C. Axial CTA image**
2. **D. Laminar flow**

CASE 12.3

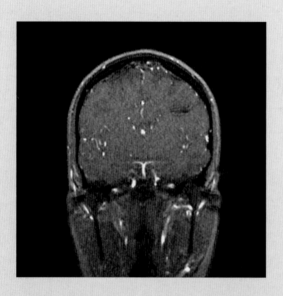

1. A 35-year-old pregnant woman presents to the emergency department with an excruciating headache. What is the diagnosis?
   A. Subarachnoid hemorrhage
   B. Vasospasm
   C. Venous sinus thrombosis
   D. Basilar tip aneurysm
2. Why is there signal within the arteries and veins?
   A. The MR tech forgot to place saturation bands.
   B. A saturation band cannot be placed in the coronal plane.
   C. This sequence used a protocol to image arterial and venous flow simultaneously.
   D. Arterial flow cannot be saturated in the coronal plane because flow is parallel to the imaging plane.

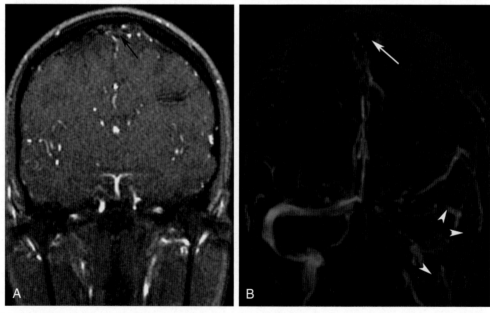

FIG. 12.C3. (A) Coronal TOF image. There is absence of flow in the superior saggital sinus *(arrow)*. Note flow within the basilar artery. (B) TOF MIP. There is absence of flow in the superior saggital sinus *(arrow)*. Also note the absence of flow in the left transverse and sigmoid sinuses along with the left jugular vein *(arrowheads)*.

Discussion

Patients with venous sinus thrombosis often present with nonspecific symptoms. Thus thrombosis is occasionally noticed or suggested on MR examinations that were performed for other reasons. Unfortunately, spin echo techniques are not accurate enough for proper evaluation of the dural sinuses.[7] The TOF sequence is much more sensitive and specific for the detection of thrombosis[7] and should be added to an MR examination whenever there is a question of dural sinus thrombosis.

Venous flow is best imaged by lengthening the TR and decreasing the flip angles to allow time for the slow-flowing venous sinuses to demonstrate flow-related enhancement. The longer TR and flip angle mean that there is less suppression of background tissue.[8] Note that the background tissues have a brighter signal than on other TOF images.

This is one of the few times when coronal slices are used instead of axial slices. This maximizes evaluation of the superior sagittal sinus, which runs in the anteroposterior (AP) plane; in addition, the transverse and sigmoid sinuses have a posteroanterior (PA) direction of flow. Coronal slices are oriented perpendicular to the AP-PA direction, making them ideal to produce flow-related enhancement. Note that institutions have different protocols; some prefer to use the axial plane to evaluate the dural venous sinuses because an arterial saturation band can be used.

Do not be surprised to see arterial flow in this image. Venous sinus flow is both in the AP (superior saggital sinus), and PA (transverse and sigmoid sinus) directions; thus if a saturation band were applied, the flow in one direction would be nulled. Also, the arteries predominantly flow from inferior to superior (parallel to the imaging plane) and have just a small component in the AP or PA direction. Thus minimal flow would be suppressed even if a saturation band were applied.

CASE 12.3 ANSWERS

1. **C. Venous sinus thrombosis**
2. **D. Arterial flow cannot be saturated in the coronal plane because flow is parallel to the imaging plane.**

CASE 12.4

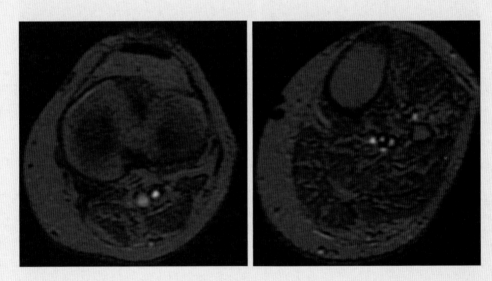

1. What error occurred during this series?
   A. A saturation band was not placed.
   B. The saturation band was inappropriately placed above instead of below the imaged section.
   C. The TR was too long.
   D. The flip angle was too small.

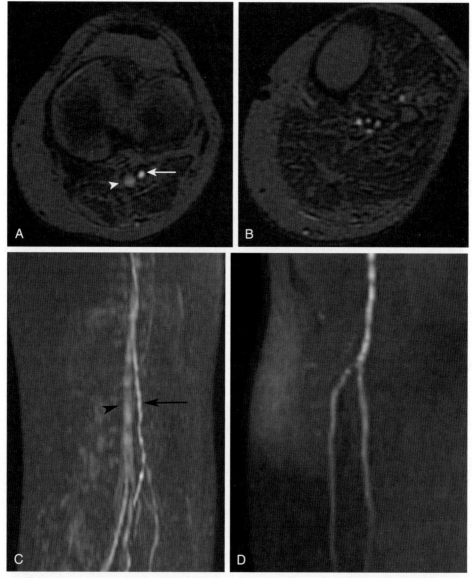

FIG. 12.C4. (A) TOF at the level of the popliteal fossa. Both arterial *(arrow)* and venous *(arrowhead)* signal are identified. (B) TOF at the mid-calf. Multiple high signal vessels are seen, and it is difficult to separate the arteries and veins. (C) TOF MIP of the proximal calf. More superiorly it is relatively easy to separate the popliteal artery *(arrow)* from the popliteal vein *(arrowhead)*. However, the separation is very difficult distally. (D) TOF MIP with venous suppression.

Discussion

What is artery and what is vein? It is difficult to differentiate when the venous saturation band is not applied. The mistake helps illustrate how beneficial venous saturation in TOF can be in regions that have significant venous contamination during contrast angiography (e.g., head, feet).[3] Note that more superiorly, when only a few vessels are present, the artery can be distinguished from the vein by its smaller size and its brightness due to higher velocity and less saturation. More inferiorly, when multiple vessels are involved and the flow is slower, differentiation is not possible.

If a saturation band were placed above and not below the imaged section, then the arterial flow would be suppressed and only veins would be imaged. A longer TR and small flip angles both result in increased signal in the vasculature and the background tissue. In Case 12.4 there is excellent saturation of the adjacent tissue.

CASE 12.4 ANSWER

1. **A. A saturation band was not placed.**

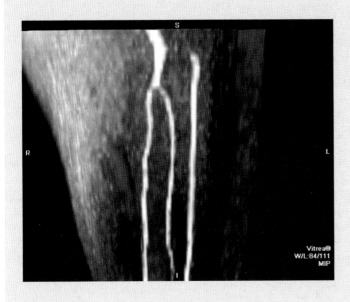

1. A 55-year-old nondiabetic smoker has calf claudication after two blocks. What is the cause of the loss of signal within the anterior tibial artery (AT)?
   A. Saturation of signal because of the transverse orientation of the proximal AT
   B. Short segment occlusion of the proximal AT
   C. High-grade stenosis at the origin of the AT, with resultant turbulent and sluggish flow causing complete absence of signal
   D. None of the above

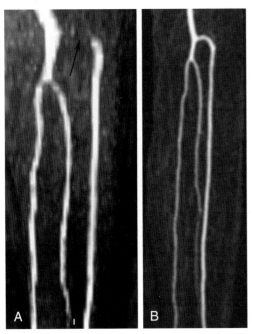

FIG. 12.C5. (A) TOF MIP. There is apparent complete occlusion of the proximal anterior tibial artery (arrow). (B) MIP from contrast-enhanced MRA. The proximal anterior tibial artery is widely patent and normal in appearance.

Discussion

On the initial TOF image, the proximal AT appeared to be completely occluded. However, the peroneal and posterior tibial arteries are widely patent and, more distally, the AT is normal. In addition, the patient is a smoker without diabetes. These patients tend to get proximal disease (aortoiliac or superficial femoral artery [SFA]). In addition, patients with tibial disease do not have calf claudication. The typical understanding is that symptoms occur one level below the level of hemodynamically significant disease. These facts should raise an index of suspicion that the stenosis or occlusion may be artifactual. In this case, contrast was given and temporal resolved images were obtained. The MIP demonstrates a normal-appearing, widely patent, proximal anterior tibial artery.

Similar to Case 12.1, the transverse plane of an artery can result in an artifact. Because the protons remain in the same imaging plane for a prolonged period, they become saturated and lose signal, giving the appearance of an occluded vessel.[4] In addition, this patient had significant aortoiliac inflow disease that resulted in slow flow in the tibial vessels, making them even more susceptible to saturation. Other locations where this can occur are the transversely oriented petrous portion of the ICA and the renal arteries.[3]

CASE 12.5 ANSWER

1. **A. Saturation of signal because of the transverse orientation of the proximal AT**

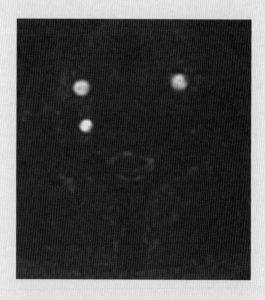

1. A 75-year-old smoker presents with occasional dizziness and syncopal episodes that are affecting his golf game. What is the diagnosis?
   A. Left vertebral artery dissection
   B. Thrombosed left internal jugular vein
   C. Occlusion of the left vertebral artery
   D. Subclavian steal physiology on the left

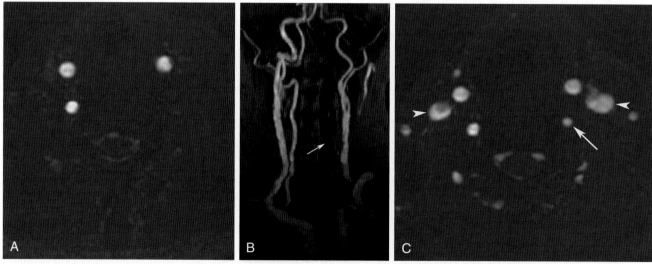

FIG. 12.C6. (A) Axial TOF. There is absence of signal within the left vertebral artery. (B) MIP TOF. There is complete absence of signal in the left vertebral artery *(arrow)* from its origin to the basilar artery. (C) Axial TOF without saturation band applied. There is flow within the right vertebral artery *(arrow)*. Note the venous flow in the jugular veins *(arrowheads)* and other neck veins.

Discussion

On the initial TOF images, there is complete lack of signal within the left vertebral artery along its entire course. Without thinking about how the image was acquired, it would be easy to assume that there is complete occlusion of the vertebral artery. However, a saturation band is applied to saturate venous flow, which will also saturate any arterial flow flowing superior to inferior. This makes subclavian steal with reversal of flow within the vertebral artery a differential possibility.[9] In this case, the TOF sequence was repeated without the saturation band, which shows the flow within the vertebral artery, confirming the diagnosis of subclavian steal. Note that the left vertebral artery is not as bright as the right vertebral artery because of the slower flow. The image acquisition from superior to inferior likely also suppressed some of the signal within the artery.

On a side note, the cerebrospinal fluid appears bright. This is not signal from water—remember that TOF is T1 weighted, not T2 weighted, and water is T1 dark. Instead, it is signal from flow within the cerebrospinal fluid space.

CASE 12.6 ANSWER

1. **D. Subclavian steal physiology on the left**

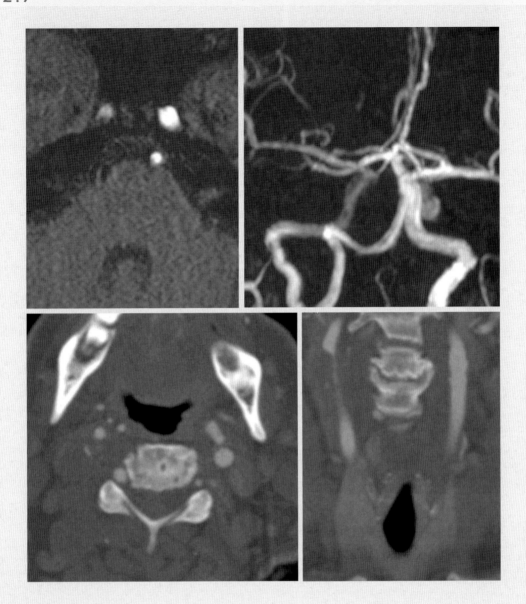

1. A 77-year-old woman presents with a small right MCA distribution acute infarct. What is the cause of the low signal in the right ICA and, to a lesser extent, the right anterior circulation?
   A. Vasospasm
   B. High-grade stenosis of the proximal right ICA
   C. Diffuse atherosclerotic plaque
   D. Susceptibility artifact from metal from prior left-sided facial surgery

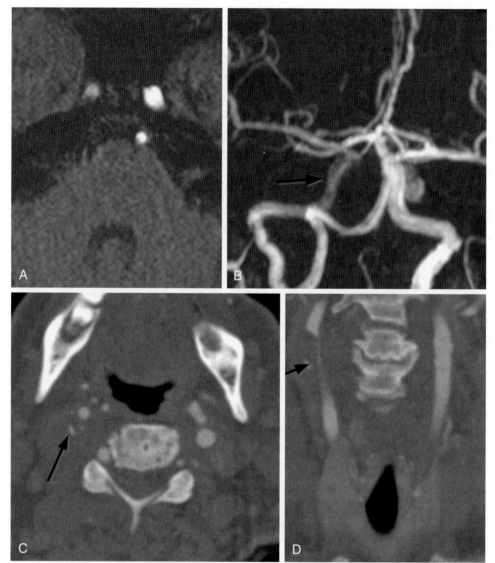

FIG. 12.C7. (A) Axial TOF. There is decreased signal in the petrous right ICA. (B) MIP TOF. There is decreased signal throughout the distal right ICA and, to a lesser extent, the anterior circulation. (Note that the left vertebral artery terminates in the posterior inferior cerebellar artery (a normal variant; *arrow*). (C) Axial CTA scan of the neck. There is severe stenosis in the proximal right ICA *(arrow)*, which is the cause of the slow flow and low signal seen on the TOF images. (D) Coronal CTA scan of the neck showing the severe 3-cm stenosis of the right proximal ICA *(arrow)*.

Discussion

If you guessed A or C, don't be distressed. Even experienced radiologists might think the image showed diffuse atherosclerotic plaque. But even without seeing postcontrast images, a few signs should indicate the correct answer. First, note that the decreased signal is predominantly in the distal ICA, proximal to the anterior or posterior communicating arteries, which can help compensate for the diminished flow. Second, it is extremely uncommon for atherosclerotic disease to have such a long and diffuse appearance in the brain. Also, vasospasm is unlikely to occur this proximally, involving the distal ICA. Susceptibility artifact from metal in the face, proximal to the image, would not have an effect on the arterial signal because the imaging and saturation pulses are all applied distally to the image sequence, not proximally.

This case is interesting and is a good one to finish the chapter because the abnormality on the image is not caused by actual pathology; that is, there is no true narrowing in the distal ICA. Instead, the abnormality reflects a pathology more proximally that is not included in the imaged area and must be inferred. Only by understanding the physics of how TOF images are acquired and produce signal can the correct diagnosis be made. In a case like this one, the knowledge of the underlying physics helps separate the radiologist from other physicians who look at the examination purely for anatomic information.

CASE 12.7 ANSWER

1. **B. High-grade stenosis of the proximal right ICA**

TAKE-HOME POINTS

1. TOF is a gradient echo sequence that suppresses background signal and enhances flow-related contrast to produce angiographic images.
2. Stagnant background tissue is saturated by using short TRs and large flip angles.
3. Flow-related signal is improved by using short TEs, thin slices, and small voxels.
4. One major advantage of TOF is the ability to eliminate flow coming from the opposite direction. This allows for suppression of unwanted venous flow in the head and feet. As a result, TOF is the MR sequence of choice in these areas, even when contrast angiography is available.
5. Limitations to TOF include its overestimation of stenosis and its long acquisition time, making it more susceptible to motion.
6. 3-T MR systems and parallel imaging techniques help reduce the imaging time for TOF, making them more useful in locations closer to the chest, where respiratory motion artifact is a concern.
7. Images can be acquired using a 2D or 3D technique. The 3D technique has better spatial resolution and SNR and is better for evaluating tortuous vessels. However, it takes longer and is not good for evaluating large volumes.
8. The multiple overlapping thin-slab angiography technique combines the 2D and 3D technique to take advantage of the beneficial qualities of each technique.
9. TOF can detect flow in only one dimension, perpendicular to the axis of flow. Because most arterial flow is oriented superior to inferior, or inferior to superior, it is usually acquired in the axial plane. For this reason, it is suboptimal for evaluating tortuous vessels, obliquely oriented vessels, or vessels that course parallel to the imaging plane.

References

1. Edelman RR, Hesselink JR, Zlatkin MB. *Clinical Magnetic Resonance Imaging.* Vol 1. Philadelphia: Elsevier; 2006.
2. Lee VS. *Cardiovascular MRI: Physical Principles to Practical Protocols.* Philadelphia: Lippincott, Williams, & Wilkins; 2005:402.
3. Miyazaki M, Lee VS. Nonenhanced MR angiography. *Radiology.* 2008;248(1):20–43.
4. Kaufman J, McCarter D, Geller SC, Waltman AC. Two-dimensional time-of-flight MR angiography of the lower extremities: artifacts and pitfalls. *AJR Am J Roentgenol.* 1998;171(1):129–135.
5. Weber J, Veith P, Jung B, et al. MR angiography at 3 Tesla to assess proximal internal carotid artery stenoses: contrast-enhanced or 3D time-of-flight MR angiography? *Clin Neuroradiol.* 2015;25(1):41–48.
6. Deshmane A, Gulani V, Griswold MA, Seiberlich N. Parallel MR imaging. *J Magn Reson Imaging.* 2012;36(1):55–72.
7. Vogl T, Bergman C, Villringer A, et al. Dural sinus thrombosis: value of venous MR angiography for diagnosis and follow-up. *AJR Am J Roentgenol.* 1994;162(5):1191–1198.
8. Ayanzen RH, Bird CR, Keller PJ, et al. Cerebral MR venography: normal anatomy and potential diagnostic pitfalls. *AJNR Am J Neuroradiol.* 2000;21(1):74–78.
9. Huston J, Ehman RL. Comparison of time-of-flight and phase-contrast MR neuroangiographic techniques. *Radiographics.* 1993;13(1):5–19.

CHAPTER 13

Time-Resolved Contrast-Enhanced Magnetic Resonance Angiography

Scott M. Duncan

OPENING CASE 13.1

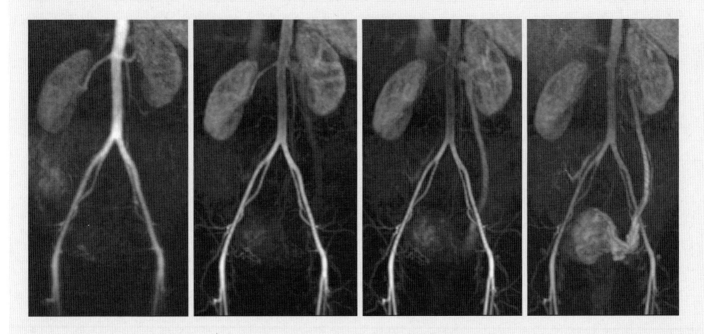

1. What is the cause of the patient's menorrhagia?
   A. Fibroid uterus
   B. Uterine arteriovenous malformation (AVM)
   C. Pelvic congestion syndrome
   D. Endometrial carcinoma

2. What is the best treatment?
   A. Hysterectomy
   B. Uterine artery embolization
   C. Left uterine vein embolization
   D. Uterine artery embolization, including embolization of the left ovarian artery

OPENING CASE 13.1

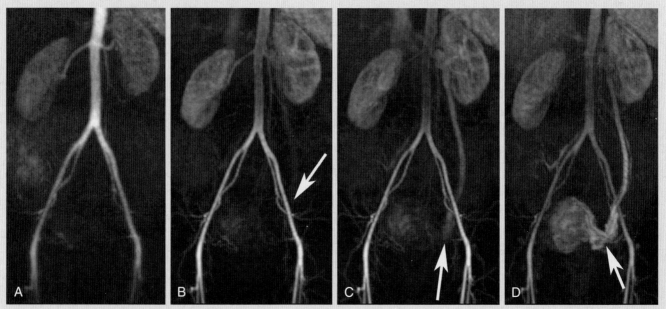

FIG. 13.C1. Time-resolved MR angiography with interleaved stochastic technique sequence. A–D sequentially show how the contrast flows in a retrograde fashion in the left gonadal vein. (B–D) The leading edge of the bolus is annotated with *arrows*.

1. What is the cause of the patient's menorrhagia?
   C. Pelvic congestion syndrome
2. What is the best treatment?
   C. Left uterine vein embolization

Discussion

The images in Fig. 13.C1 are from a time-resolved contrast-enhanced MR angiography (MRA) sequence of the abdomen, which demonstrates contrast opacification that begins at the left renal vein and extends into the left ovarian vein and down to the left ovary and pelvis. These findings suggest pelvic congestion syndrome (PCS). The direction of flow in the gonadal vein is very important in making the diagnosis of PCS; thus static images alone could not provide a diagnosis. Normal flow in the left ovarian vein is from the ovary to the left renal vein. However, if the flow is down the left ovarian vein, toward the pelvis, this can result in PCS. PCS is the result of incompetent valves in the left ovarian vein, which allow venous blood in the left renal vein to flow retrograde into the pelvis, resulting in increased venous pressure, venous pooling, and the development of pelvic venous varicosities, which can lead to PCS. PCS can cause menorrhagia, bloating, pelvic fullness, and dyspareunia. The gold standard for diagnosis and treatment is venography and embolization of the left ovarian vein.[1]

Time-Resolved Magnetic Resonance Angiography

Many of the modalities that are used in radiology, including plain films, CT, and much of MRI, involve static imaging. Static high-resolution images are obviously vital to making many diagnoses. However, the addition of temporal resolution can add physiologic information to help make an accurate diagnosis. Modalities such as ultrasound and fluoroscopy have a high temporal resolution, allowing dynamic imaging to be performed. With the development of time-resolved techniques, MRI now has the capability to perform dynamic imaging. *Time-resolved MRA applies very fast imaging techniques that enable multiple acquisitions during a single-contrast bolus, thereby offering information on the dynamics of contrast enhancement and actual blood flow dynamics.* This is made possible by techniques that have a very rapid image acquisition time while still maintaining sufficient spatial resolution. Time-resolved sequences typically use three-dimensional (3D) sequences that take about 2 to 5 seconds per acquisition.[2]

There are several advantages to time-resolved MRA compared with static CT angiography (CTA) and MRA techniques.

The greatest benefit is that it provides directional information of blood flow, which is beneficial for evaluating reflux and retrograde flow. There are multiple scenarios in which time-resolved techniques can be beneficial, including evaluating AVMs, peripheral vascular disease, and thoracic veins and differentiating between the true and false lumen in aortic dissections.

k-Space Physics

To understand the concepts behind time-resolved MRA, it is important to understand the concept of k-space. k-Space can be a very intimidating subject to understand because it is abstract and very complex. In the simplest terms, k-space is where the raw MR data reside. The raw MR data represent the sum of signals from all voxels under different frequency- and phase-encoding gradients. These can be plotted in a two-dimensional (2D) or 3D format in k-space, where the coordinates are determined by the frequency- and phase-encoding gradients—specifically, the time integrals of these gradients. (Implied in this is that by changing the MR gradients, the location in k-space is also changed.)

An additional consequence is that a single coordinate in k-space does not have a direct correlate on the true image that

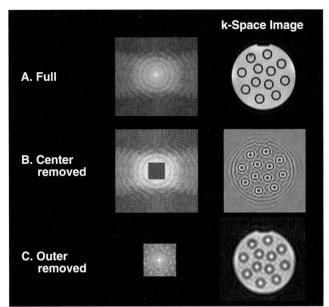

FIG. 13.1. Effects of removing k-space from specific regions. (A) None of k-space has been removed, and the image has good contrast and resolution. (B) The center of k-space has been removed, and the edges and detail of the objects are seen, but there is very little contrast. (C) The periphery of k-space has been removed, and there is good contrast, but the edges appear blurry and lack the fine detail. (From Jacobs MA, Ibrahim TS, Ouwerkerk R. MR imaging: brief overview and emerging applications. *Radiographics.* 2007;27:1213–1229.)

is read. Rather, every coordinate in k-space contributes some information to *every* pixel in the final image. The coordinates of k-space are referred to as kx and ky in two dimensions and kx, ky, and kz in three dimensions. The center of k-space is the main contributor to the signal intensity of the MR image; the periphery of k-space contributes to the fine spatial details. Additionally, the magnitude of k-space data is symmetric from side to side both in the vertical and horizontal directions. The Fourier transform is used to take k-space data and transfer them into an MR image that can be viewed and interpreted. Simply put, the Fourier transform is a mathematical formula that takes complex k-space data and converts them into a spatial image—that is, an MR image.

Because k-space is symmetric and does not have a direct correlate to a physical pixel in the MR image, we can undersample or only partially fill k-space and still have a complete and diagnostic image. Fig. 13.1 demonstrates what happens when the center and periphery of k-space are removed.

k-Space Filling Techniques

As mentioned earlier, changing the encoding gradients will change coordinates in k-space. That means that by changing the gradients, we can fill k-space in any pattern or trajectory that we choose. A linear k-space trajectory fills k-space one line at a time, corresponding to each echo, which is done from one edge of k-space to the next, much like how a conventional printer or typewriter works. Alternatively, the central lines of k-space can be filled first, with the more peripheral lines filled subsequently. This is known as *linear centric k-space filling.*

We can undersample k-space and still get a diagnostic image, and by changing the gradients we can change location within the k-space matrix to fill in k-space however we want. The logical next question is why would we want to only fill portions of k-space? The answer is time. To have dynamic or time-resolved MRA you must be able to produce multiple images in a very short period of time. This is not possible with routine linear filling of the entirety of k-space.

There is a simple formula for determining the acquisition time for a single image (or slab of tissue for 3D imaging):

$$\text{Acquisition time} = \text{TR} \times \text{number of phase-encoding steps} \times (\text{number of acquisitions/echo train length})$$

These four variables—time to repetition (TR), phase-encoding steps, number of acquisitions, and echo train length—can be manipulated to decrease acquisition times. However, this chapter focuses on the methods used to decrease the number of phase-encoding steps and on the undersampling of k-space used in time-resolved MRA.

One of the strategies used to decrease the number of phase-encoding steps and therefore decrease acquisition time is called *partial Fourier k-space acquisition.* This is accomplished by filling only a part of k-space and then by either determining the remainder of k-space from the information already obtained (remember, k-space is symmetric) or simply performing zero filling of k-space. For example, the central portion of k-space can be quickly obtained if the periphery of k-space is filled in with zeroes (as in Fig. 13.1), thereby dramatically reducing the number of phase-encoding steps. Also, because all of k-space is filled (central actual data and periphery zeroes), the desired matrix size is still acquired and the spatial resolution interpolated.[2]

Other methods of k-space filling have been developed that enable faster imaging techniques. Most of these techniques are faster because they preferentially fill the center of k-space over the periphery. One of these approaches to filling k-space is termed *keyhole imaging.* Keyhole imaging typically starts by filling the full extent of k-space in the first acquisition. On later acquisitions of k-space, only the central portion of k-space is filled, and the peripheral parts of k-space are copied from the prior acquisition. This technique increases the temporal resolution significantly in the later acquisitions because it not only samples the center of k-space, but also maintains spatial resolution in the latter acquisitions by copying lines of the peripheral k-space from the initial k-space acquisition. This technique can also be modified by sampling several lines of the periphery of k-space at different time points, along with the central portion of k-space, rather than just copying them from the initial acquisition. This improves the spatial resolution of the data acquired from the periphery of k-space along the different time points.[2,3]

View sharing is another technique used primarily in cardiac cine imaging to increase temporal resolution while maintaining the acquisition time. In cardiac cine imaging, numerous frames or images of the cardiac cycle are obtained with every heartbeat. The filling of k-space with this technique is referred to as *segmented* because only a portion of k-space is filled in every frame during one heartbeat. With the next heartbeat, another few lines of k-space are filled in every frame, and so on, until all k-spaces are filled over numerous heartbeats. View sharing significantly increases the number of frames acquired with each heartbeat and therefore increases temporal resolution. This is accomplished by acquiring a limited number of lines of k-space from every other frame and copying the remainder of the needed k-space lines from the other acquired images.[2]

Parallel Imaging

Parallel imaging uses multiple receiver coils at different locations to reduce the number of phase-encoding steps, thereby reducing image acquisition time. A distinct advantage of parallel imaging is that it does not sacrifice spatial resolution because some of the spatial data are based off the location of the multiple different receivers. Parallel imaging can be used in concert with the above techniques to perform time-resolved imaging.[2]

Two different techniques for parallel imaging are commonly used, **sens**itivity **e**ncoding (SENSE) and **si**multaneous **a**cquisition of **s**patial **h**armonics (SMASH). Undersampling k-space by decreasing the number of phase-encoding steps results in a phenomenon known as *wraparound artifact* or *aliasing*. Essentially, this occurs when the field of view is smaller than the body part being imaged. With wraparound artifact, part of the image on one side is folded over to the other side. With SENSE, this wraparound artifact is eliminated during image processing in the image space. This is accomplished by being able to distinguish the difference in signals contributing to the true image and those signals contributing to the aliased portion of the image, based on the known spatial sensitivity profile of individual coils at different locations. Once the correct signals are distinguished and calculated, each voxel can be reassigned its appropriate signal intensity, whether it is in the aliased portion of the image or in the true

image. Then the image can be reconstructed with a full field of view, without any aliasing. Similar to SENSE, SMASH takes advantage of differing sensitivity profiles of individual receiver coils to restore the image, but all operations are carried out in k-space domain.[2]

The most commonly used sequences currently applied in contrast-enhanced MRA are as follows:
- Time-resolved angiography with interleaved stochastic technique (TWIST)—Siemens
- Time-resolved imaging of contrast kinetics (TRICKS)—GE Healthcare
- Time-resolved angiography using keyhole (TRAK)—Phillips Healthcare

All these sequences use various proprietary combinations of the techniques described above to decrease acquisition times and increase temporal resolution while maintaining adequate spatial resolution.

CASE 13.2

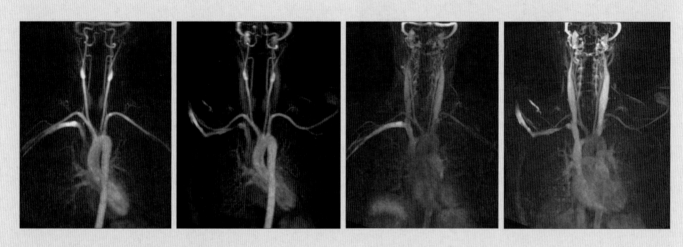

1. Which is the most common system affected by thoracic outlet syndrome?
   - A. Subclavian artery
   - B. Subclavian vein
   - C. Brachial plexus
   - D. Lymphatic system

2. What shoulder position is the most sensitive for detection of thoracic outlet syndrome?
   - A. Abduction
   - B. Internal rotation
   - C. External rotation
   - D. Adduction
   - E. Neutral

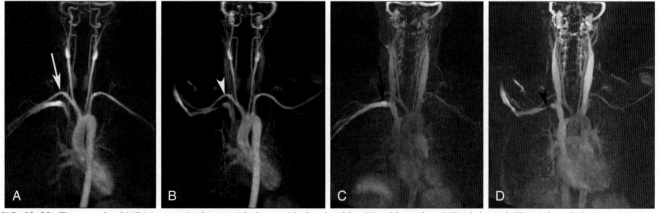

FIG. 13.C2. Time-resolved MRA images in the arterial phase with the shoulder (A) adducted and (B) abducted. The right subclavian artery retains its normal caliber with the arms down (*arrow,* A) and up (*arrowhead,* B). Images taken during the venous phase with the shoulder (C) adducted and (D) abducted. In D, the *arrowhead* demonstrates narrowing of the right subclavian vein that occurs when the patient's arms are up versus the normal-appearing caliber when the arms are down (*arrow,* C).

Discussion

Thoracic outlet syndrome refers to abnormal compression of the brachial plexus, subclavian artery, or subclavian vein as they travel between the clavicle and the first rib. Compression can have both bony and soft tissue causes. The symptoms depend on which part of the neurovascular bundle is affected. Clinically, symptoms can sometimes be elicited or exacerbated with abduction of the shoulders.[4] Time-resolved MRA can be very helpful in determining whether the symptoms are due to compression of the artery or the vein. In this case, there is marked narrowing of the right subclavian vein when the arms are elevated. If thrombus forms within the vein, this is referred to as *effort thrombosis* or *Paget-Schroetter syndrome.*[5]

CASE 13.2 ANSWERS

1. **B. Subclavian vein**
2. **A. Abduction**

CASE 13.3

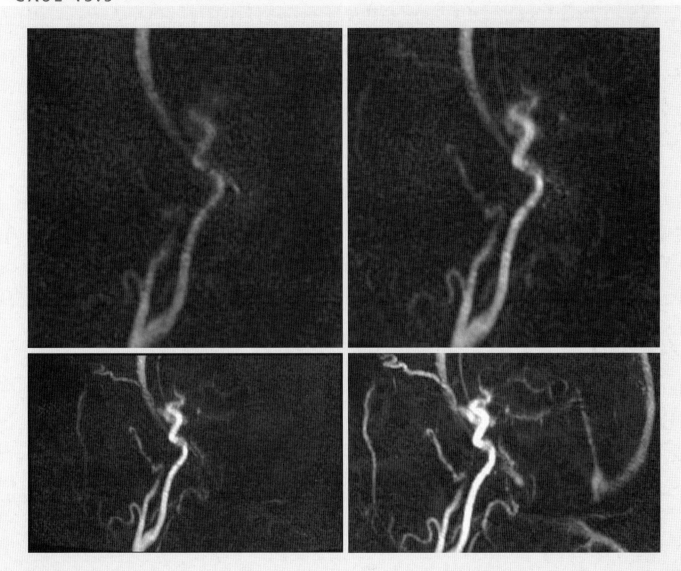

1. Which is not a common cause of carotid cavernous (CC) fistulas?
   A. Trauma
   B. Atherosclerotic disease
   C. Ruptured aneurysm
   D. Congenital

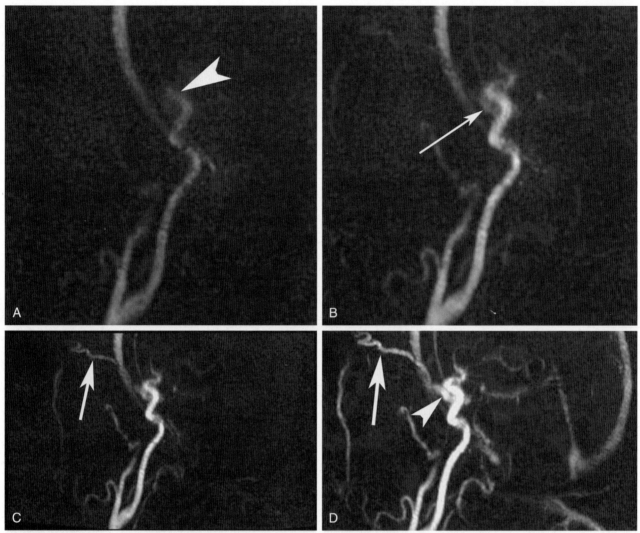

FIG. 13.C3. Sequential sagittal time-resolved MRA of the internal carotid artery. (A) Early arterial phase image. The *arrowhead* in A is the cavernous portion of the internal carotid artery. (B) Slightly later time point with almost immediate ipsilateral filling of the cavernous sinus *(arrow)*. (C) Late arterial phase image shows retrograde filling of the superior ophthalmic vein *(arrow)*. (D) Early venous phase image demonstrates increased prominence of the cavernous sinus *(arrowhead)* and superior ophthalmic vein *(arrow)*.

Discussion

Fig. 13.C3 portrays how time-resolved imaging can be extremely helpful in making the diagnosis of a CC fistula. The high temporal resolution, particularly throughout the arterial phase, allows very good visualization of the early-filling cavernous sinus, which confirms the diagnosis. CC fistulas are most commonly due to trauma but can also be due to ruptured aneurysms and atherosclerotic disease. The patient often presents with proptosis, chemosis, and an orbital bruit from venous congestion. Findings on static MR and CT images include asymmetric enlargement of the superior ophthalmic vein, proptosis, and extraocular muscle enlargement.

CASE 13.3 ANSWER

1. **D. Congenital**

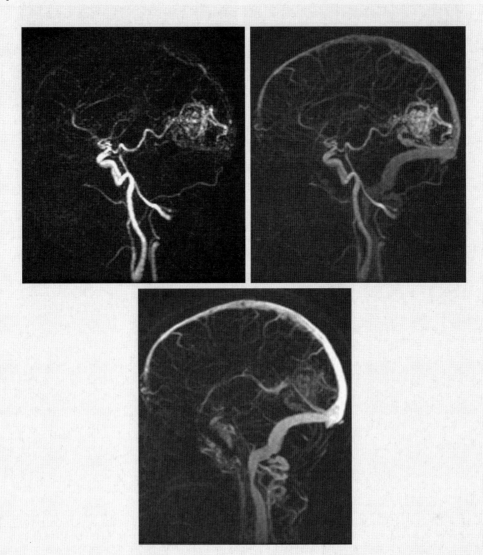

1. What is the diagnosis?
   A. Cerebral AVM
   B. Developmental venous anomaly
   C. Cavernoma
   D. Glioblastoma
2. Sequelae of this lesion include which of the following?
   A. High output cardiac failure
   B. Stroke
   C. Hemorrhage
   D. Drop metastases

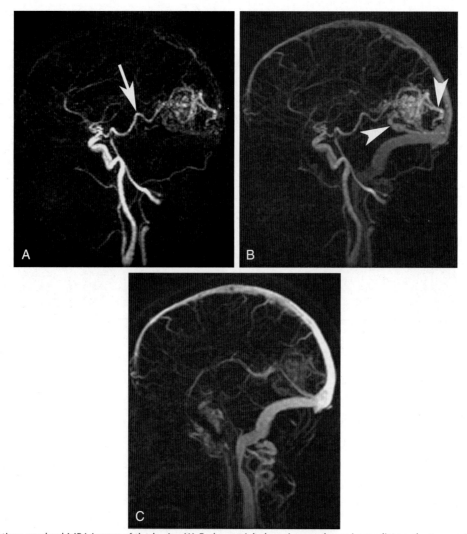

FIG. 13.C4. Sagittal time-resolved MRA image of the brain. (A) Early arterial phase image shows immediate enhancement of a tangle of vessels in the occipital region of the brain. The *arrow* denotes an enlarged posterior cerebral artery feeding the tangle of vessels. (B) Early venous phase image demonstrates venous drainage from this vascular abnormality via the superficial cortical and tentorial branches that drain into the distal superior sagittal sinus and proximal right transverse sinus *(arrowheads)*. (C) Midvenous phase image demonstrates some degree of washout from vascular abnormality.

Discussion

A cerebral AVM is a direct shunt between one or more large feeding arteries and one or more draining veins, with an intervening vascular nidus. These lesions are developmental in origin. There is approximately a 1.5% to 3% overall yearly risk of hemorrhage of AVMs, which include a risk of death with the first bleed of approximately 10%.[6] The Spetzler-Martin criteria are most commonly used to grade these lesions from 1 to 6. The lesions are graded on size (1–3 cm, 3–6 cm, >6 cm), venous drainage (either deep or superficial), and whether or not they involve eloquent cortex. The higher the number, the more difficult they are to resect. Conventional high-resolution MRA is somewhat limited in the evaluation of these lesions because it can be difficult to sort out arteries from veins. Contrast-enhanced time-resolved MRA is especially helpful in diagnosing and characterizing AVMs because the high temporal resolution of this technique enables the differentiation between AVMs and venous malformations, based on the timing of the enhancement of the abnormal vessels. Furthermore, this technique helps distinguish the arterial supply and draining veins.

CASE 13.4 ANSWERS

1. **A. Cerebral AVM**
2. **C. Hemorrhage**

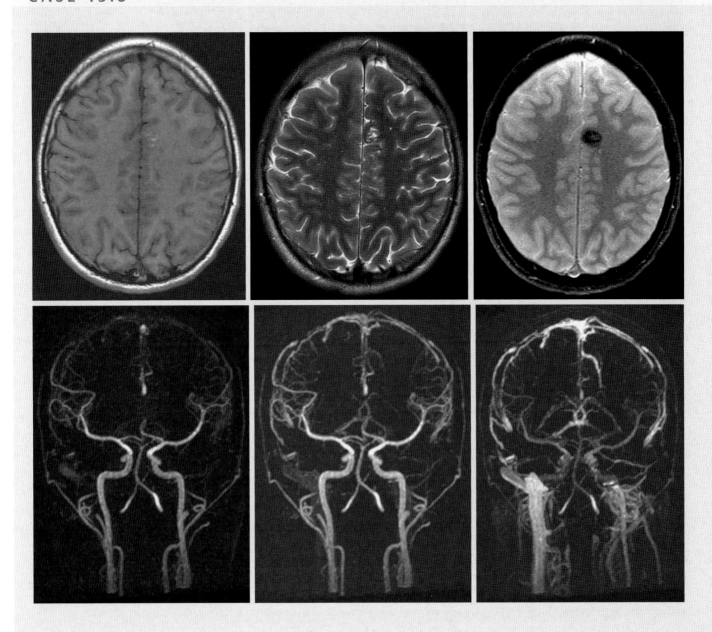

1. With which other cerebral vascular abnormality are these
   lesions associated?
   A. Developmental venous anomaly
   B. Cerebral AVM
   C. Stroke
   D. Venous sinus thrombosis

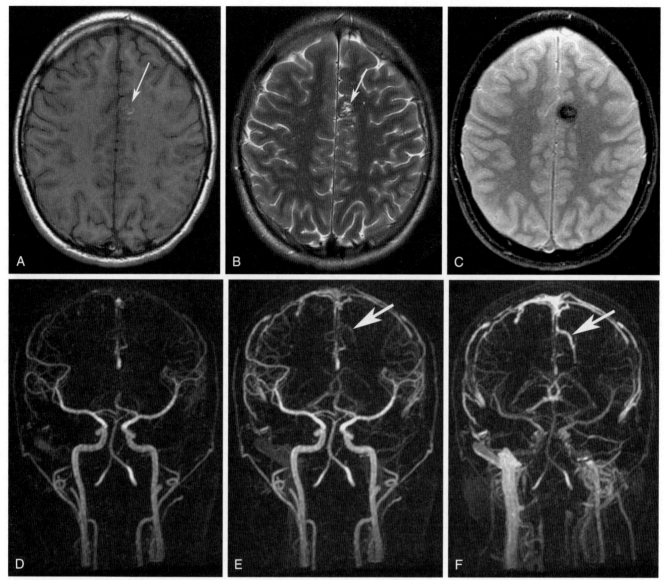

FIG. 13.C5. (A) Axial T1-weighted, (B) T2-weighted, and (C) gradient recalled echo (GRE) sequences that demonstrate a lesion in the left medial frontal lobe, with increased signal centrally on the T1- and T2-weighted images. On the T2-weighted image, there is a subtle low signal rim *(arrow)* surrounding the lesion. This low signal rim blooms on the GRE sequence. Coronal time-resolved MRA images in the (D) early arterial phase, (E) late arterial phase, and (F) early venous phase. The contrast-filled structure in E *(arrow)* becomes more apparent on the venous phase image *(arrow, F)*. There is no large artery feeding this structure, and it appears to be draining toward the dural surface.

Discussion

The noncontrast images (see Figs. 13.C5A–C) demonstrate the classic findings of a cavernous hemangioma. The increased signal within the lesion on the T1- and T2-weighted images is due to methemoglobin. The low peripheral T2 signal surrounding the lesion, which becomes even darker on the GRE image, is a result of susceptibility artifact from hemosiderin deposition. Developmental venous anomalies (DVAs) are often associated with cavernous hemangiomas. Dynamic imaging is helpful in establishing the diagnosis of a DVA and excluding an AVM (Figs. 13.C5D–F).

The difference is that AVMs have both abnormal supplying arteries and draining veins interspersed with abnormal brain. In contradistinction, DVAs just have abnormal venous drainage of normal brain. It is important to distinguish a DVA from an AVM because DVAs are incidental findings, and their removal can result in a venous infarct.

CASE 13.5 ANSWER

1. **A. Developmental venous anomaly**

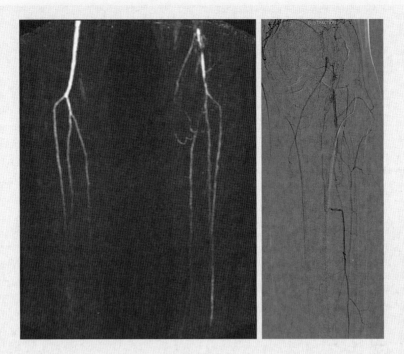

1. What symptoms would be expected with the peripheral vascular disease in this distribution?
    A. Thigh claudication
    B. Calf claudication
    C. Nonhealing foot wounds
    D. Acute cold foot

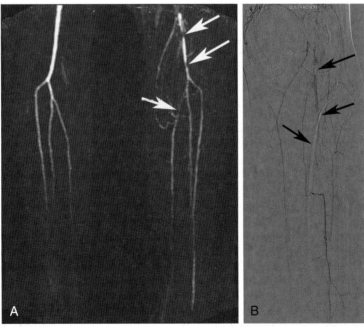

FIG. 13.C6. (A) Time-resolved MRA in the arterial phase of both lower extremities. (B) Subtracted angiographic image of the left leg in the same patient. The *arrows* in both images denote stenosis of the popliteal artery, tibioperoneal trunk, and posterior tibial artery.

Discussion

Peripheral vascular disease below the knee typically affects wound healing in the foot. This is most typically seen with diabetics, who often have a combination of microscopic angiopathy with superimposed calf disease, resulting in poorly healing or nonhealing wounds that can lead to amputation.

Evaluation of the calf vasculature can be very difficult on static CTA and MRA for several reasons. First, there is often asymmetric disease in the legs. Thus the contrast bolus often reaches the calves at different times, making it difficult or impossible to time the bolus correctly to image the distal arterial flow. Second, because it is distal vasculature, there is often venous contamination, which can make interpretation difficult. Again, time-resolved MRA can be beneficial in this scenario because the imaging can be repeated multiple times to ensure that the contrast bolus is well seen, with little or no venous contamination.

CASE 13.6 ANSWER

1. **C. Nonhealing foot wounds**

CASE 13.7

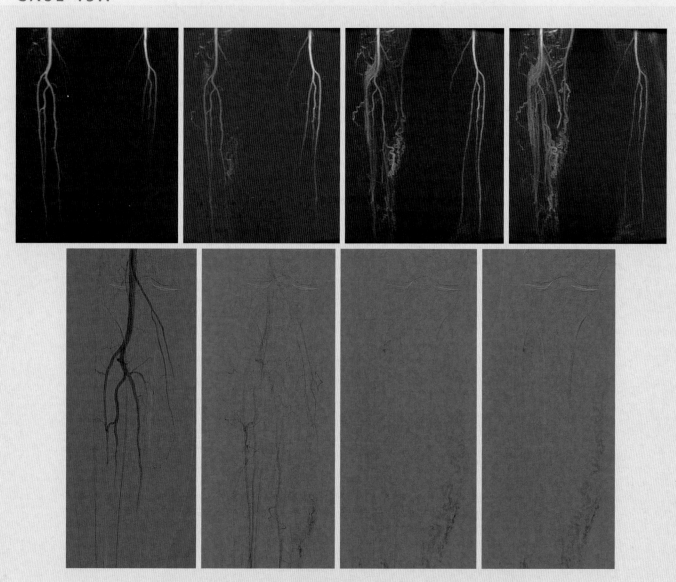

1. What is the diagnosis?
   A. AVM
   B. Venous malformation
   C. Capillary malformation
   D. Soft tissue metastatic lesion

156

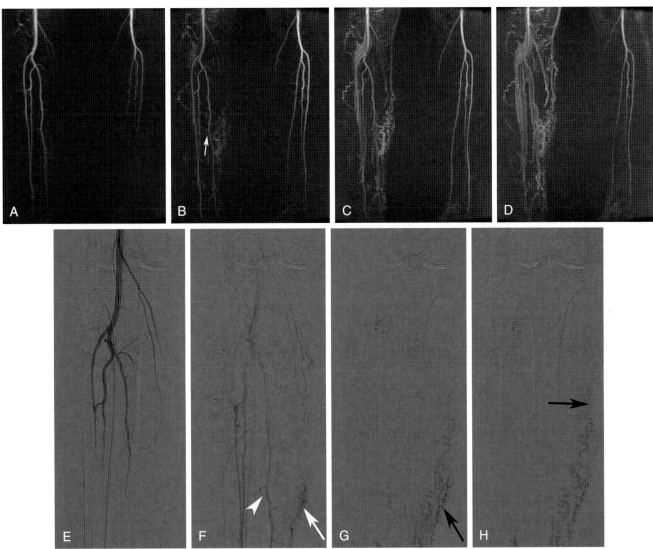

FIG. 13.7. Time-resolved MRA images. (A) Image demonstrating earlier filling and enlargement of the tibial arteries on the right compared with the left. (B) The *arrow* denotes the supplying artery (posterior tibial artery) with filling of a tangle of vessels in the medial calf. (C–D) Images demonstrating progressive enhancement of extensive venous structures, making it more and more difficult to distinguish vein from artery. Digitally subtracted images from an arteriogram. (E) Normal early arterial phase. (F) A late arterial phase image that shows early filling of a tangle of vessels in the left calf *(arrow)* and a dominant feeding artery off the posterior tibial artery *(arrowhead)*. (G–H) Progressive filling of the dilated venous channels *(black arrows)*.

Discussion

This case and Case 13.6 both demonstrate how time-resolved MRA compares very favorably with angiography in diagnosing certain conditions without the radiation and invasiveness of angiography. It is clear both on the angiogram and the time-resolved MRA scan that dynamic imaging is helpful not only in making the diagnosis, but also in identifying the feeding arteries of the lesion for treatment planning.

CASE 13.7 ANSWER

1. **A. AVM**

TAKE-HOME POINTS

1. Although static images with high resolution are obviously vital to making many diagnoses, temporal resolution is sometimes helpful or necessary to make certain vascular diagnoses accurately.
2. Modalities such as ultrasound and fluoroscopy have a high temporal resolution and allow dynamic imaging to be performed. With the development of time-resolved techniques, MRI now has the capability to perform dynamic imaging.
3. Time-resolved MRA requires obtaining multiple MR images rapidly to obtain dynamic information.
4. Decreasing acquisition times to perform time-resolved imaging is primarily achieved by decreasing the number of phase-encoding steps through k-space undersampling, as well as parallel imaging.
5. Time-resolved MRA takes advantage of limited k-space filling techniques to obtain images rapidly.
6. Some examples of the use of time-resolved techniques include evaluating AVMs, peripheral vascular disease, deep vein thrombosis, thoracic outlet syndrome, CC fistulas, and PCS.

References

1. Kim CY, Miller MJ Jr, Merkle EM. Time-resolved MR angiography as a useful sequence for assessment of ovarian vein reflux. *AJR Am J Roentgenol.* 2009;193:W458–W463.
2. Lee VS. *Cardiovascular MRI: Physical Principles to Practical Protocols.* Philadelphia: Lippincott Williams & Wilkins; 2006.
3. Edelman RR, Hesselink JR, Zlatkin MB, Crues III JV. *Clinical Magnetic Resonance Imaging.* 3rd ed. Philadelphia: Saunders Elsevier; 2006.
4. Kim CY, Mirza RA, Bryant JA, et al. Central veins of the chest: evaluation with time-resolved MR angiography. *Radiology.* 2008;247:558–566.
5. Kaufman JA, Lee MJ. *Vascular and Interventional Radiology: The Requisites.* 2nd ed. Philadelphia: Saunders Elsevier; 2014:154–155.
6. Hadizadeh DR, von Falkenhausen M, Gieseke J, et al. Cerebral arteriovenous malformation: Spetzler-Martin classification at subsecond-temporal-resolution four-dimensional MR angiography compared with that at DSA. *Radiology.* 2008;246:205–213.

CHAPTER 14

Phase Contrast

Nancy Pham, Ari Kane, and Timothy J. Amrhein

OPENING CASE 14.1

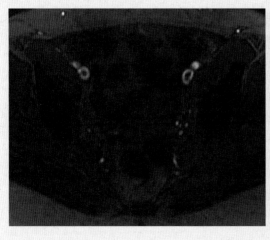 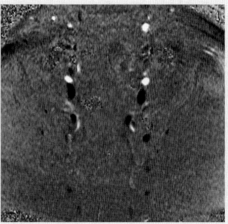

1. What is the cause for the low signal intensity in the bilateral external iliac veins on the gradient recalled echo (GRE) image?
   A. Thrombus
   B. Slow flow artifact
   C. Pulsation artifact
   D. Tumor invasion
2. What is the most sensitive MR sequence for detecting slowly flowing blood?
   A. Spin echo T2
   B. Proton density
   C. Spin echo T1
   D. Phase contrast

3. Why do the arteries and veins have opposite signal intensities on the phase contrast image (i.e., why do the arteries appear hyperintense or white and the veins appear hypointense or black)?
   A. Same flow direction
   B. Opposing flow direction
   C. Difference in flow velocities
   D. Difference in size of the vessels

OPENING CASE 14.1

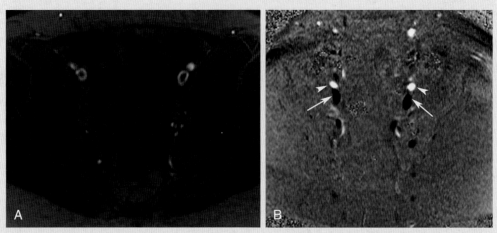

FIG. 14.C1. (A) Axial T1-weighted GRE image. There are filling defects in the bilateral external iliac veins. (B) Axial phase contrast image, with a hyperintense signal in the bilateral external iliac arteries *(arrowheads)*. There is hypointense signal in the bilateral external iliac veins *(arrows)*.

1. What is the cause for the low signal intensity in the bilateral external iliac veins on the GRE image?
   B. Slow flow artifact
2. What is the most sensitive MR sequence for detecting slowly flowing blood?
   D. Phase contrast
3. Why do the arteries and veins have opposite signal intensities on the phase contrast image (i.e., why do the arteries appear hyperintense or white and the veins appear hypointense or black)?
   B. Opposing flow direction

Discussion

The central areas of low signal within the external iliac veins on the GRE image are concerning for bilateral venous thrombosis (Fig. 14.C1A). However, this finding could also be secondary to slowly flowing blood. Phase contrast images through the concerning level were obtained for further clarification. On the phase contrast images, there is hypointense signal within the bilateral external iliac veins, confirming flow within the vessel and excluding a thrombus (Fig. 14.C1B). This case is an excellent example of *phase contrast imaging's superior sensitivity for the detection of slowly flowing blood.*

The labeling of flow direction is arbitrary on phase contrast imaging. Hyperintense (white) signal signifies flow in one direction, whereas hypointense (black) signal signifies flow in the opposite direction. In this case, the hyperintense signal represents craniocaudal flow and the hypointense signal represents caudocranial flow.

CASE 14.2

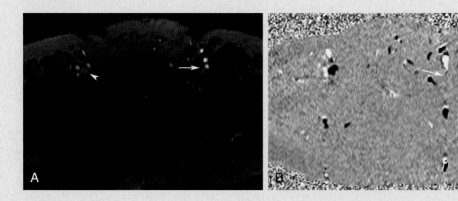

FIG. 14.C2

1. Phase contrast operates on which of the following principles?
   A. Moving protons experience a static magnetic field, and stationary protons experience a changing magnetic field.
   B. Both moving protons and stationary protons experience a changing magnetic field.
   C. Stationary protons experience a static magnetic field, and moving protons experience a changing magnetic field.
   D. Both stationary protons and moving protons experience a static magnetic field.

2. An acquired phase contrast image demonstrates aliasing. Which is the appropriate value to change to obtain an accurate measurement?
   A. Increase the *velocity* *enc*ode value (VENC).
   B. Decrease the VENC.
   C. Increase the applied gradient.
   D. Decrease the applied gradient.

3. Phase contrast sequences apply to which of the following?
   A. 180-degree refocusing pulse
   B. Anisotropy calculations to determine phase
   C. Spoiler gradients to maximize contrast
   D. Bipolar gradients with both dephasing and rephasing lobes

FIG. 14.C2. (A) Axial T1-weighted GRE. There is flow-related enhancement in the right femoral vein *(arrowhead)*. There is no flow-related enhancement in the left femoral vein *(arrow)*. (B) Axial phase contrast image. A hypointense (black) signal is seen at the confluence of the right superficial and deep femoral veins. Only gray signal is seen on the left *(arrow)*. Hyperintense (white) signal is seen in the bilateral femoral arteries laterally.

Thrombus

In this case, the phase contrast image (Fig. 14.C2B) supports the findings on the GRE image (Fig. 14.C2A) and confirms a left femoral vein deep venous thrombosis (DVT). Given phase contrast's increased sensitivity to slow flow, the absence of signal within the left femoral vein means that the diagnosis of a DVT can be made with greater confidence.[1,2]

Phase Contrast Imaging
Conventional Two- and Three-Dimensional Phase Contrast Imaging

Phase contrast imaging is a noncontrast MR angiographic technique that can extract velocity information by measuring changes in the phase of protons. Currently its primary applications are in venography, cerebrospinal fluid (CSF) flow, cardiovascular flow, and three-dimensional (3D) vascular studies. *The information from phase contrast can be used in two separate ways: (1) to produce conventional angiographic images and (2) for flow quantification.* Phase contrast is not commonly used to produce angiographic images because time-of-flight (TOF) and contrast angiography are much faster sequences. Instead, phase contrast is generally used to obtain physiologic information or to solve problems when other angiographic images provide equivocal results.[3] Specifically, *it is the most sensitive sequence for detecting slow-flowing blood, and it is the only MR sequence that can provide velocity, flow, and pressure data.[3–5]*

Two types of information are acquired when an MR echo is recorded: magnitude information and phase information. This can be conceptualized as analogous to a vector, in which the magnitude determines the length of the vector and phase information determines the direction of the vector (from 0–360 degrees). To generate most images, the phase information is disregarded, and only the magnitude information is displayed. However, the phase information is useful in some scenarios. For example, phase information is frequently used to localize signal in the phase-encoding direction. Protons along the phase-encoding gradient acquire different phases, depending on their location along the gradient. A proton at the weaker end of the gradient that experiences a 1.49-T magnetic field will precess slightly slower than a proton in the middle of the gradient that experiences a 1.5-T magnetic field. Due to these differences in precession speed, the protons develop different phase shifts, which can then be used to map the location of the proton within the body.

Phase contrast sequences use this same principle but use special gradients to eliminate the phase differences between stagnant protons while accentuating the phase differences in moving protons. *In phase contrast sequences, moving protons experience a changing magnetic field and therefore accumulate a phase that is different from stationary protons, which experience a constant magnetic field. Because faster-flowing protons travel a farther distance through the gradient than slower-moving protons, their phase differences (compared with stationary protons) will be greater than those of the slower flowing protons.* In summary, in phase contrast imaging, *phase differences are proportional to a proton's velocity, which can be calculated.[3]*

In addition to velocity, the phase shift is also proportional to the magnitude of the gradient, with *larger gradients producing more phase shift per distance traveled.* Therefore for a given velocity, the degree of phase shift can be manipulated by adjusting the size of the gradient. To illustrate, consider a proton moving through a gradient with a constant velocity of 10 cm/s. In a gradient ranging from 1.49 to 1.51 T, assume that the proton accumulates +90 degrees of phase shift. If the gradient were doubled to 1.48 to 1.52 T, the proton would accumulate twice the phase shift, or +180 degrees. The ability to adjust the gradient is important because phase shifts greater than 180 degrees result in aliasing, similar to Doppler ultrasound. As another example, consider a gradient that gives a proton with a velocity of 50 cm/s a +180-degree phase and −50 cm/s a −180-degree phase. In this scenario, what if a proton has a velocity of 75 cm/s? The proton will develop a +270-degree phase shift, which will be incorrectly labeled as a −90-degree phase shift. This is an example of aliasing because the proton is incorrectly calculated to have a −25 cm/s velocity (Fig. 14.1).

Fortunately, we do not have to calculate the ideal size of the gradient ourselves. Instead, we enter a VENC value, which the computer uses to calculate the size of the gradient. This value must be specified before executing any phase contrast sequence. *The VENC value is the maximum velocity that can be correctly measured by the sequence before aliasing occurs.* In other words, the computer sets the gradient so that the VENC value (maximum projected velocity) will result in a ±180-degree phase shift (in the previous example, the VENC value would be 50 cm/s). The closer the VENC is set to the measured velocity, the more accurate the measurement. *If the VENC value is set too low (as in the example above), aliasing will occur. If*

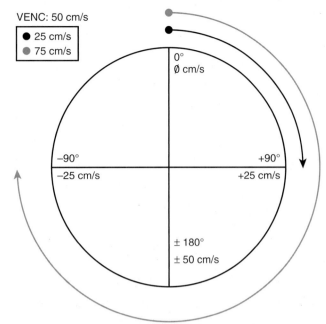

FIG. 14.1. Aliasing in phase contrast. If the VENC value is set at 50 cm/s, a proton with a velocity of 25 cm/s will develop +90 degrees of phase shift and will be calculated correctly. However, a proton with a velocity of 75 cm/s will develop +270 degrees of phase shift and will be incorrectly calculated as having a velocity of −25 cm/s.

the VENC value is set too high, slower velocities will not be measured accurately, and the signal-to-noise ratio will decrease. The ideal VENC value for evaluating the venous sinus and veins is usually around 20 to 30 cm/s.[3] For arterial blood, the VENC is usually greater than 100 cm/s and can be as high as 300 or 400 cm/s, depending on the vessel that is being evaluated and on the degree of stenosis present.[3] Adjusting the VENC value is similar to adjusting the maximum velocity of Doppler ultrasound. The ability to manipulate the VENC value is one reason that phase contrast is the most sensitive MR sequence for the detection of slowly flowing blood. In Cases 14.1 and 14.2, the VENC was set to 30 cm/s, resulting in successful detection of the slowly flowing blood in the iliac veins.

Phase contrast is a GRE sequence that uses bipolar gradients to acquire signal. The two lobes of the bipolar gradient, often called *the dephasing and rephasing lobes, are identical in magnitude and time but exactly opposite in direction. Stationary protons experience two gradients that are exactly opposite to each other, resulting in a return to a net 0-degree phase.* This occurs regardless of the position of the proton along the gradient. Moving protons, on the other hand, will change locations in between the two lobes of the bipolar gradient, which results in two different magnetic field strengths influencing the phase of the proton. This difference results in an accumulation of a net change in phase relative to the stationary proton.[6]

In practice, a single bipolar gradient is not sufficient to account for magnetic field inhomogeneities, which lead to unwanted phase changes in nonmoving protons. *To eliminate field inhomogeneities, a second mirror image bipolar gradient is applied. This gradient is identical to the first, but in the opposite order. Echoes are recorded after each bipolar gradient and are then subtracted from each other.* This results in a flow-sensitive sequence, similar to digital subtraction angiography. A stationary proton that accumulates phase during the first bipolar gradient (secondary to magnetic field inhomogeneities) will then acquire exactly the same phase during the second reversed bipolar gradient. Thus when subtracted, the stagnant spin will have a net 0-degree phase. However, the moving spin will accumulate the same magnitude but the opposite direction of phase (e.g., +15 degrees and −15 degrees) during the second bipolar gradient compared with the first. When subtracted, the opposite phase shifts will result in a net doubling of the phase shift (Fig. 14.2).

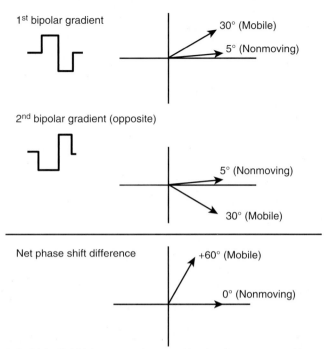

FIG. 14.2. Field inhomogeneity correction in phase contrast. Stationary spins have a phase shift as a result of field inhomogeneities. When the bipolar gradient is flipped, field inhomogeneities will still produce the same phase shift (+5 degrees in this case). However, the moving proton will have a −30-degree phase shift. By subtracting the two datasets, the phase shift of stationary protons cancel, and the phase shift of the mobile protons is doubled. (Modified from Lee VS. *Cardiovascular MRI: Physical Principles to Practical Protocols.* Philadelphia: Lippincott Williams & Wilkins; 2006:207.)

Unfortunately, obtaining echoes after each bipolar gradient makes the acquisition twice as long compared with time of flight. In addition, flow is detected only in one dimension, the dimension oriented parallel to the axis of the gradient. To obtain flow in all three dimensions, as would be required to create a traditional angiographic image, the sequence must be repeated three times, making it prohibitively long.

As noted previously, flow quantification is the most common application of phase contrast. *Flow quantification can be acquired in either one dimension (through-plane flow) or two dimensions (in-plane flow). With through-plane flow, the velocity-encoding gradient is oriented along the slice selection axis (craniocaudal for an axial scan) and information is obtained about flow that is moving through the plane of the image.* For in-plane flow, the gradients are along the frequency- and phase-encoding axes (e.g., transverse and anteroposterior dimensions for an axial slice). Information is obtained about flow that occurs in the plane of the scan. Cases 14.1 and 14.2 illustrate through-plane flow, whereas the next case (Case 14.3) illustrates in-plane flow.

Phase contrast images have a characteristic angiographic appearance similar to fluoroscopic digital subtraction angiography images. This is because two separate datasets are obtained and then subtracted from each other to create the flow quantification image.[5] *All stationary spins (0-degree phase shift) are assigned an intermediate gray signal. Mobile protons are then assigned either hypointense or hyperintense signal based on the direction of flow, with an intensity level correlating to the velocity magnitude.* Regions that contain air (and therefore are relatively devoid of signal), such as are found external to the patient, in the lungs, and in the facial sinuses, exhibit a static or snowstorm appearance, which is due to background noise and random movement of protons.

As noted, one of the major advantages of the phase contrast technique is its ability to calculate *velocity and flow data. This information is typically acquired via through-plane images with the use of cardiac gating* to obtain dynamic information throughout the cardiac cycle. With the placement of a region of interest and the use of commercially available computer software, both velocity and flow information in relation to time can be determined. These flow data can then be incorporated into the Bernoulli equation to determine intraluminal pressures, which can be used to evaluate the degree of a vessel stenosis (e.g., as in aortic coarctation). Finally, higher-order flow data such as pulsatility and jerk can be analyzed using more complex gradients. However, this application is rarely used.

Phase contrast has several disadvantages that reduce its practicality and thereby its frequency of use. First, its *long acquisition time (two to four times as long as TOF imaging)* renders it less desirable for use in MR angiographic imaging. Second, similar to digital subtraction angiography, *phase contrast is very sensitive to motion degradation*. In fact, if the patient moves during any of the acquisitions the sequence is usually nondiagnostic. Finally, regions of turbulent flow contain protons that swirl rather than move in a single direction, which results in a signal void precluding the acquisition of velocity data. Turbulent flow usually occurs immediately distal to an area of high-grade stenosis or at the bifurcation of a vessel.

Four-Dimensional Phase Contrast Imaging

Advances in phase contrast techniques have allowed for the development of time-resolved, 3D phase contrast MRI, commonly referred to as four-dimensional (4D) flow MRI. In contrast to standard phase contrast imaging, velocity-encoding data are obtained in three directions. Thus the distinct advantage of this technique is that it provides information on the temporal and spatial evolution of 3D blood flow in any particular vascular bed. However, the major disadvantage of this technique is the long scanning time required to perform velocity encoding in three directions. For example, an intracranial 4D flow examination is 50 to 100 times longer than a conventional spin echo, contrast-enhanced angiogram.[7–9] Newer techniques have shortened imaging times greatly, allowing 4D flow MRI to move from being a predominantly research sequence to providing clinically important data on vascular hemodynamics in various parts of the body, including the brain, chest, and abdomen. More clinically applicable imaging times, from 5 to 10 minutes, have been achieved by implementing a combination of strategies, including undersampling k-space, parallel imaging, and more robust reconstruction techniques.[7–9]

CASE 14.2 ANSWERS

1. **C. Stationary protons experience a static magnetic field, and moving protons experience a changing magnetic field.**
2. **A. Increase the velocity encode (VENC) value.**
3. **D. Bipolar gradients with both dephasing and rephasing lobes**

CASE 14.3

FIG. 14.C3

1. What is the most likely diagnosis?
   A. Right transverse and sigmoid sinus thrombosis
   B. Right transverse and sigmoid sinus hypoplasia
   C. Cerebellar dural arteriovenous fistula
   D. High-riding jugular bulb
2. Which of the following sequences takes the longest to acquire?
   A. 2D time of flight
   B. 3D time of flight
   C. Phase contrast
   D. Contrast MR angiography

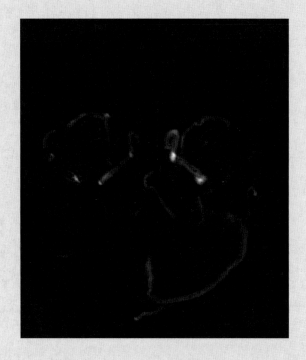

FIG. 14.C3. Axial phase contrast slab of the brain. There is absent signal in the right transverse and sigmoid sinus, signifying absence of flow.

Right Transverse and Sigmoid Sinus Thrombosis

Phase contrast can be used in MR venograms to evaluate for venous sinus thrombosis. The lack of signal in the right transverse sinus and sigmoid sinus is concerning for venous sinus thrombosis.[10] With dural venous hypoplasia, one would still expect to see flow on phase contrast venograms.

Magnetic Resonance Venogram

Phase contrast angiography is acquired and displayed differently than phase contrast for use in flow quantification. Flow is detected in all three dimensions rather than simply one or two. *In phase contrast, the net velocity* is determined by the 3D Pythagorean theorem (below) and *is thus always positive* (because the square of a negative number is positive).

$$V_{net} = \sqrt{\left(V_x^2 + V_y^2 + V_z^2\right)}$$

Signal intensity is based on net velocity of flow. The benefits of phase contrast angiography are its excellent background suppression and *the ability to detect flow in all three* dimensions. *This allows for reduced artifacts compared with TOF MR venography, which often suffers from reduced in-plane flow-related enhancement.* For this reason, assessment of the transverse sinus can occasionally be challenging on TOF MR venograms. Lengthy scanning times are phase contrast's biggest detraction because image acquisition times are at least four times longer than those in TOF, which is already much more time intensive than gadolinium-enhanced contrast angiography.

CASE 14.3 ANSWERS

1. **A. Right transverse and sigmoid sinus thrombosis**
2. **C. Phase contrast**

CASE 14.4

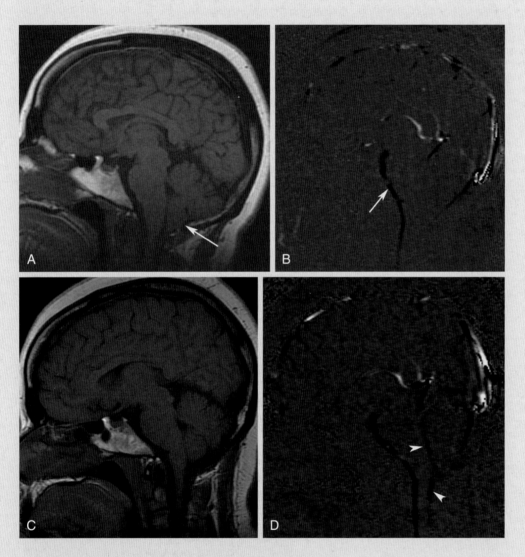

FIG. 14.C4

1. When comparing the preoperative images (Fig. 14.C4A–B) to the postoperative images (Fig. 14.C4C–D), what is the diagnosis?
   A. Intracranial hypertension with restricted CSF flow after treatment
   B. Intracranial hypotension with improved CSF flow after treatment
   C. Chiari I malformation with improved CSF flow after treatment
   D. Chiari I malformation with restricted CSF flow after treatment

2. To visualize CSF flow, the correct phase contrast imaging mode is which of the following?
   A. 2D mode
   B. 3D mode
   C. Subtraction mode
   D. Cine mode

FIG. 14.C4. (A) Sagittal T1-weighted image of the brain. There is tonsillar herniation through the foramen magnum *(arrow)*. (B) Sagittal phase contrast image of the brain. Black signal is seen anterior to the brainstem *(arrow)*. Little to no signal is seen in the region of the fourth ventricle, foramen of Magendie, or dorsal to the cerebellum. (C) Sagittal T1-weighted image of the brain. Status post–suboccipital craniectomy, resulting in resolved tonsillar herniation. (D) Sagittal phase contrast image of the brain (status post–suboccipital craniectomy). Demonstrated is a dark signal anterior to the brainstem. In addition, there is now black signal in the fourth ventricle and foramen of Magendie and dorsal to the cerebellum *(arrowheads)*.

Chiari I Malformation

In a Chiari I malformation, the cerebellar tonsils are low lying and can result in obstruction of CSF flow at the foramen magnum.[11] In the initial phase contrast image (Fig. 14.C4B), there is minimal to no flow posterior to the brainstem. However, the phase contrast image acquired post–suboccipital craniectomy for decompression demonstrates markedly improved flow in this region, which suggests resolution of the flow-limiting stenosis. Intracranial hypotension can also cause low-lying cerebellar tonsils but typically occurs secondary to a spinal CSF leak and should not be treated with suboccipital craniectomy.

Cerebrospinal Fluid Flow

In addition to flow within vessels, phase contrast can be used to evaluate CSF flow.[11] *CSF flow is even slower than venous flow, and the VENC is set quite low, usually at 5 to 7 cm/s for adults and 15 cm/s for children.* Also, CSF flow is complex, changing with the stage of the cardiac cycle.[12] Therefore these sequences are *displayed in cine mode* to characterize the flow better. Normally, there is both to-and-fro flow within the subarachnoid space corresponding to the cardiac cycle. Therefore, to confirm adequate bidirectional flow, ideally one should identify both dark and bright signals within the CSF spaces. Single static images (e.g., like those provided here) are not adequate for evaluating CSF flow dynamics in clinical practice but are sufficient for illustrating points in MRI physics texts.

CASE 14.4 ANSWERS

1. **C. Chiari I malformation with improved CSF flow after treatment**
2. **D. Cine mode**

CASE 14.5

FIG. 14.C5

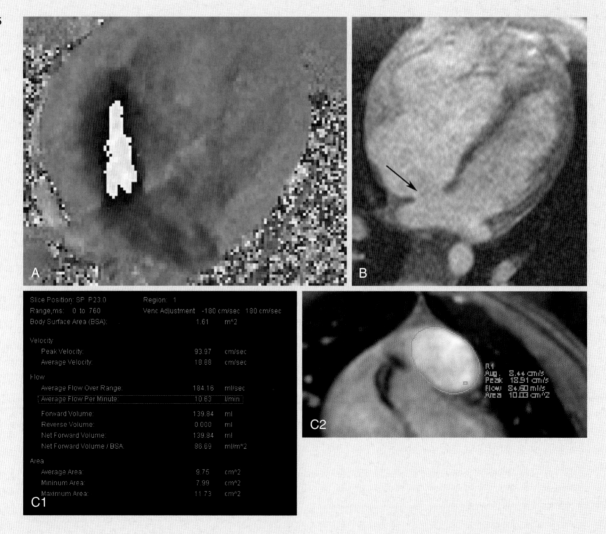

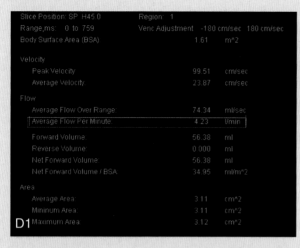

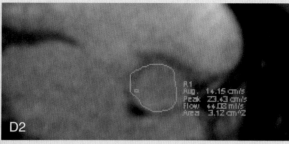

Slice Position: SP H45.0	Region: 1		
Range,ms: 0 to 759	Venc Adjustment -180 cm/sec 180 cm/sec		
Body Surface Area (BSA)	1.61	m^2	
Velocity			
Peak Velocity	99.51	cm/sec	
Average Velocity	23.87	cm/sec	
Flow			
Average Flow Over Range	74.34	ml/sec	
Average Flow Per Minute	4.23	l/min	
Forward Volume	56.38	ml	
Reverse Volume	0.000	ml	
Net Forward Volume	56.38	ml	
Net Forward Volume / BSA	34.95	ml/m^2	
Area			
Average Area	3.11	cm^2	
Mininum Area	3.11	cm^2	
Maximum Area	3.12	cm^2	

1. Which of the following may be obtained from a phase contrast sequence?
   A. Both flow direction and velocity maps and anatomic 2D imaging
   B. Only flow direction and velocity maps
   C. Only velocity maps
   D. Only velocity maps and anatomic 2D imaging
2. You are interested in measuring velocity values in a vessel with flow of 10 cm/s. Which of the following VENC values will give the most accurate measurement?
   A. 9 cm/s
   B. 15 cm/s
   C. 20 cm/s
   D. 5 cm/s
3. Anatomic images may be produced in phase contrast imaging by analyzing which of the following?
   A. Phase magnitude
   B. Signal magnitude
   C. Anatomic images cannot be produced in phase contrast imaging
   D. Time-resolved phase shifts

FIG. 14.C5. (A) Four-chamber phase contrast image of the heart. A jet of flow is noted extending from the left atrium to the right atrium (white signal). (B) Four-chamber magnitude image of the heart. There is a large defect between the right and left atrium *(black arrow).* Note the enlarged right heart from long-standing increased volume. (C1) Flow table from the region of interest (ROI) over the main pulmonary artery (C2). There is an average flow of 10.63 L/min. (D1) Flow table from ROI over the aortic root (D2). There is an average flow of 4.23 L/min.

Atrial Septal Defect

Phase contrast is an excellent method to obtain flow information in patients with cardiac shunts noninvasively.[13] In Fig. 14.C5A, the phase contrast image nicely demonstrates the jet of flow from the left atrium to the right atrium, diagnostic of an atrial septal defect. However, many alternative sequences, including the magnitude image in Fig. 14.C5B, could have provided similar information. The true benefit of the phase contrast in this case is found in the flow tables, which demonstrate the severity of the left-to-right shunt. In this case, the Qp/Qs ratio (or ratio of flow to the pulmonary circulation compared with that to the systemic circulation) is 10.63/4.23, or 2.5. Although *any value over 1 is consistent with a left-to-right shunt,[3]* this particular case reveals a severe shunt because there is more than twice as much flow to the pulmonary circulation compared with the systemic circulation.

Flow Assessment

Flow dynamics are usually calculated with cardiac gated, through-plane, phase contrast. An ROI is placed over the vessels of interest—in this case the aorta and main pulmonary artery—and the area of these vessels is traced. The computer automatically *calculates the velocity based on the phase shift and the VENC value:*

$$(\text{Phase shift [°]} \times \text{VENC [cm/sec]})/180° = \text{velocity}$$

Flow information is calculated by multiplying the average velocity by the cross-sectional area of the vessel[3]:

$$(\text{Velocity [cm/sec]} \times \text{area [cm}^2] \times 60 \text{ [sec/min]})/1000 \text{ (mL/L)} = \text{flow (L/min)}$$

Note that Fig. 14.C5B is also an image acquired from a phase contrast sequence. Remember, all echoes contain both magnitude and phase information. *The magnitude data from the phase contrast sequence can be displayed to give additional anatomical information.* In actuality, the magnitude image is a GRE sequence because the protons are realigned using bipolar gradients. In this case, the magnitude image nicely displays the large atrial septal defect.

CASE 14.5 ANSWERS

1. **A. Both flow direction and velocity maps and anatomic 2D imaging**
2. **B. 15 cm/s**
3. **B. Signal magnitude**

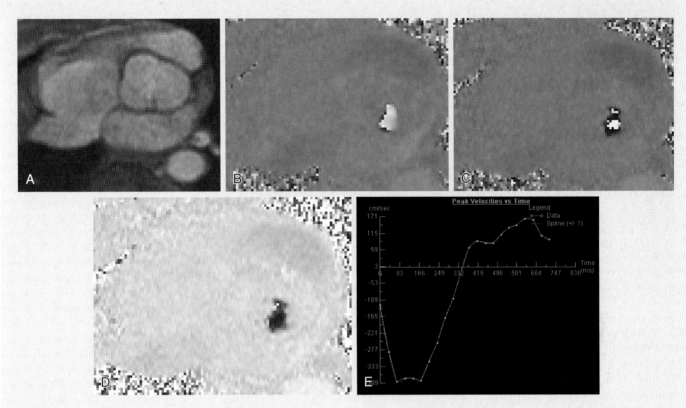

FIG. 14.C6

1. What is the diagnosis?
   A. Aortic stenosis with a component of aortic insufficiency
   B. Aortic insufficiency only
   C. Aortic stenosis only
   D. Aortic valve thrombus
2. In attempting to visualize flow within the iliac veins using phase contrast imaging, the acquisition demonstrates only flow within the iliac arteries. If the VENC input value was set to 200 cm/s, what should be done to visualize venous flow?
   A. Decrease the VENC to 30 cm/s
   B. Increase the VENC to 300 cm/s
   C. Decrease the VENC to 100 cm/s
   D. Increase the VENC to 400 cm/s
3. When using the through-plane technique in phase contrast imaging, the flow velocity is most accurately measured when it is in which direction relative to the imaging plane?
   A. 180 degrees to the imaging plane
   B. 45 degrees to the imaging plane
   C. 90 degrees to the imaging plane
   D. 60 degrees to the imaging plane

FIG. 14.C6. (A) Cross section through the aortic valve, magnitude image. Note the dilated aortic root. (B) Cross section through the aortic valve, phase contrast image (VENC = 250 cm/s). Note the mixture of both hyperintense and hypointense signal overlying the aortic valve, signifying aliasing. (C) Cross section through the aortic valve, phase contrast image (VENC = 350 cm/s). There is persistent mixed signal and aliasing. (D) Cross section through aortic valve, phase contrast image (VENC = 400 cm/s). Only black signal is present over the aortic valve, signifying no aliasing. (E) Velocity graph from the aortic jet (VENC = 400 cm/s). There is high velocity during systole and reversal of velocities during diastole.

FIG. 14.C7

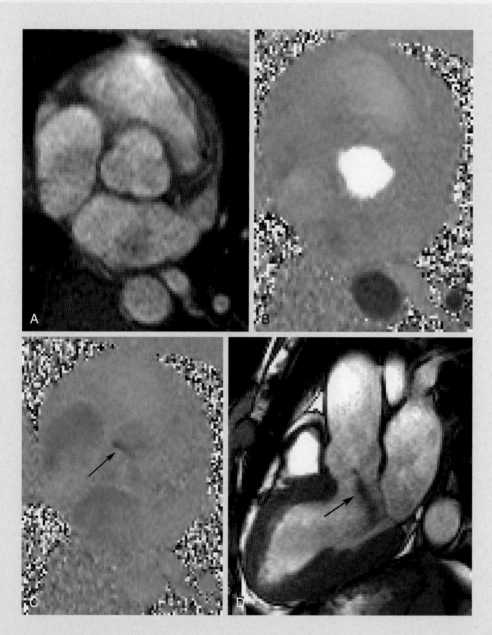

4. What is the diagnosis?
   A. Aortic stenosis
   B. Aortic insufficiency
   C. Normal aortic valve
   D. Bicuspid aortic valve

FIG. 14.C7. (A) Cross section through the aortic valve, magnitude image; normal aortic valve. (B) Cross section through the aortic valve, phase contrast image, systole. There is hyperintense signal within the aortic root and hypointense signal within the descending aorta. (C) Cross section through the aortic valve, phase contrast image, diastole. There is a slit of hypointense signal *(arrow)* over the aortic valve. (D) True fast imaging with steady-state precession of the aortic outflow tract, diastole. There is a jet of dark signal *(arrow)* extending back into the left ventricle.

Phase Contrast Assessment of Aortic Valve Pathology and Cardiac Flow Quantification

Phase contrast measurements of velocity have been validated with data from echocardiography.[14] The flow chart in Case 14.6 demonstrates *high velocities during systole consistent with aortic stenosis* (see Fig. 14.C6E). *The reversed flow during diastole means that there is also a component of aortic insufficiency.* (Note that the curve extends above the *x*-axis to the region corresponding to positive values on the *y*-axis.) Thus, the diagnosis in this case is aortic stenosis, with a component of aortic insufficiency. Determining jet velocities in aortic stenosis is important because it has both prognostic and treatment implications for the patient. Patients with jet velocities of less than 300 cm/s are unlikely to have symptoms within the next 5 years. However, if the peak velocity is more than 400 cm/s, the patient is likely to experience symptoms within the next 2 years, and there is an associated increased mortality rate.[15] The patient in Case 14.6 had a peak velocity of 382 cm/s, which was equivocal. However, he was symptomatic and therefore underwent successful elective aortic valve repair.

Complementary to the first case in this series, Case 14.7 demonstrates a jet of reversed flow during diastole on the phase contrast images (Fig. 14.C7C), confirming a diagnosis of aortic insufficiency.

Quantification of flow in Case 14.6 was accomplished using cardiac gated, through-plane, phase contrast, as previously described in this chapter. Remember that the *through-plane technique measures flow perpendicular to the imaging slice.* In contrast, the in-plane technique detects flow parallel to the imaging slice. Although flow is still detected at other angles relative to the imaging plane, *the measurement will be underestimated unless the flow jet is perpendicular to the imaging plane (90 degrees).*

Note also that the VENC needed to be adjusted during the scan in Case 14.6 to eliminate aliasing. Normal aortic velocities are less than 250 cm/s, which is usually the initial VENC setting. However, *the initial phase contrast image demonstrates both hyperintense and hypointense signal within the aortic jet, signifying aliasing artifact.* The series was repeated with an increased VENC of 350 cm/s, which reduced but did not eliminate aliasing. Finally, a series with a VENC setting of 400 cm/s was performed, which eliminated the aliasing artifact. The VENC was then set at 400 cm/s to obtain the velocity graph. Note that if one wished to visualize slower moving blood within a vein, such as the iliac vein in question 2, the VENC would need to be reduced accordingly. Remember that the ideal VENC value for evaluating veins is usually around 20 to 30 cm/s.

CASES 14.6 AND 14.7 ANSWERS

1. **A. Aortic stenosis with a component of aortic insufficiency**
2. **A. Decrease the VENC to 30 cm/s**
3. **C. 90 degrees to the imaging plane**
4. **B. Aortic insufficiency**

TAKE-HOME POINTS

Physics

1. All MR echoes contain both phase and magnitude information. Usually only the magnitude data are used to produce an image. Phase contrast makes use of the phase information.
2. Phase contrast relies on phase differences that result from protons moving through a complex magnetic field gradient.
3. The amount of phase that a proton accumulates is proportional to its velocity and to the size of the gradient—that is, the faster a proton is moving, and the larger the gradient applied, the more phase the proton will accumulate.
4. Phase shifts can be calculated from −180 degrees to +180 degrees. Protons that accumulate more phase than this result in aliasing.
5. Instead of directly calculating the appropriate size of the gradient, the physician or technologist enters a VENC value.
6. The VENC value is the maximum velocity that can be accurately measured by the sequence before aliasing occurs.
7. The closer the VENC value is to the measured velocity, the more accurate is the measurement.
8. Phase contrast uses bipolar gradients (gradients with the same magnitude and phase, but opposite direction) to return stationary protons to a 0-degree phase shift. Because moving protons change location between gradients, they do not experience the exact opposite magnetic field and thereby accumulate phase.
9. Mirror image bipolar gradients (back to back bipolar gradients with reversed order) are used to eliminate phase differences that arise from magnetic field inhomogeneities.

Clinical Considerations

1. Phase contrast is a noncontrast MR angiographic technique that is used almost exclusively for the additional physiologic information that it provides.
2. Phase contrast images have an appearance similar to those obtained with digital subtraction angiography.
3. Stationary protons result in a medium gray signal and flowing protons result in a dark or bright signal, depending on the flow direction.
4. The magnitude data from a phase contrast sequence can also be displayed to show anatomic information. It is effectively a GRE sequence.
5. Phase contrast is the most sensitive sequence for detecting flow. Thus it is often used to differentiate slow flow from thrombus.
6. Phase contrast is particularly useful in providing physiologic data during cardiac imaging.
7. Phase contrast velocity measurements are integral in making management decisions in the case of aortic stenosis.
8. Flow information from the aorta and pulmonary artery can be compared to evaluate the severity of a shunt.

References

1. Spritze CE, Norconk JJ Jr, Sostman HD, Coleman RE. Detection of deep venous thrombosis by magnetic resonance imaging. *Chest.* 1993;104(1):54–60.
2. Catalano C, Pavone P, Laghi A, et al. Role of MR venography in the evaluation of deep venous thrombosis. *Acta Radiol.* 199;38(5):907–912.
3. Lee VS. *Cardiovascular MRI: Physical Principles to Practical Protocols.* Philadelphia: Lippincott Williams & Wilkins; 2006.
4. Edelman RR, Hesselink JR, Zlatkin MB. *Clinical Magnetic Resonance Imaging.* 2nd ed. Philadelphia: Saunders; 1996.
5. Brown MA, Semelka RC. *MRI: Basic Principles and Applications.* 2nd ed. New York: Wiley-Liss; 1999.
6. Miyazaki M, Lee VS. Nonenhanced MR angiography. *Radiology.* 2008;248(1):20–43.

7. Stankovic Z, Allen BD, Garcia J, Markl M. 4D flow imaging with MRI. *Cardiovasc Diagn Ther.* 2014;4(2):173–192.

8. Roldan-Alzate A, Francois CJ, Wieben O, et al. Emerging applications of abdominal 4D flow MRI. *AJR Am J Roentgenol.* 2016;207(1):58–66.

9. Turski P, Scarano A, Hartman E, et al. Neurovascular 4Dflow MRI (phase contrast MRA): emerging clinical applications. *Neurovasc Imaging.* 2016;2(1):8.

10. Provenzale JM, Joseph GJ, Barboriak DP. Dural sinus thrombosis: findings on CT and MR imaging and diagnostic pitfalls. *AJR Am J Roentgenol.* 1998;170(3):777–783.

11. Roldan A, Wieben O, Haughton V, et al. Characterization of CSF hydrodynamics in the presence and absence of tonsillar ectopia by means of computational flow analysis. *AJNR Am J Neuroradiol.* 2009;30(5):941–946.

12. Bhadelia RA, Bogdan AR, Kaplan RF, Wolpert SM. Cerebrospinal fluid pulsation amplitude and its quantitative relationship to cerebral blood flow pulsations: a phase-contrast MR flow imaging study. *Neuroradiology.* 1997;39(4):258–264.

13. Beerbaum P, Körperich H, Barth P, et al. Noninvasive quantification of left-to-right shunt in pediatric patients: phase-contrast cine magnetic resonance imaging compared with invasive oximetry. *Circulation.* 2001;103(20):2476–2482.

14. Kilner PJ, Manzara CC, Mohiaddin RH, et al. Magnetic resonance jet velocity mapping in mitral and aortic valve stenosis. *Circulation.* 1993;87(4):1239–1248.

15. Otto CM, Burwash IG, Legget ME, et al. Prospective study of asymptomatic valvular aortic stenosis. Clinical. echocardiographic. and exercise predictors of outcome. *Circulation.* 1997;95(9):2262–2270.

CHAPTER 15

Diffusion Magnetic Resonance Imaging

Charles M. Maxfield

OPENING CASE 15.1

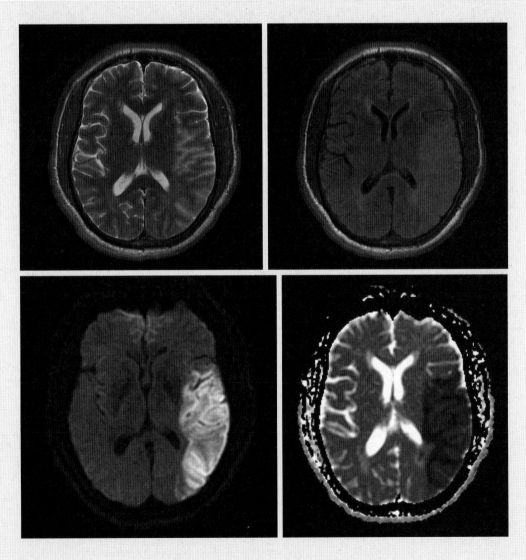

1. Which of the following is responsible for the bright signal in the left middle cerebral artery distribution on the diffusion-weighted image (part C)?
   A. Subacute hemorrhage
   B. Acute hemorrhage
   C. Vasogenic edema
   D. Cytotoxic edema

2. What is the purpose of the apparent diffusion coefficient map (part D)?
   A. Corrects for T2 blackout effect
   B. Corrects for T2 shine-through
   C. Increases sensitivity for blood products
   D. Identifies brain tissue that is ischemic but not yet infarcted

CASE ANSWERS

OPENING CASE 15.1

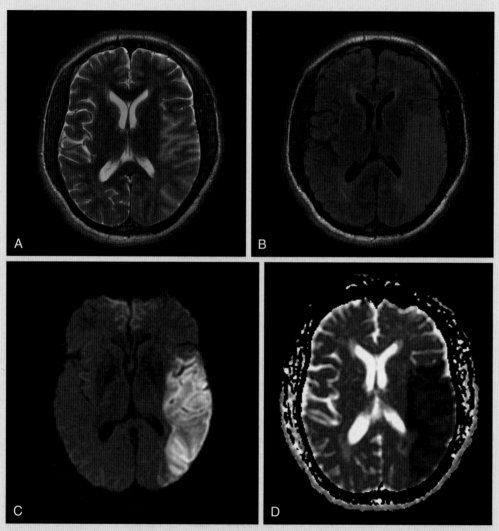

FIG. 15.C1. T2-weighted image (A) and fluid-attenuated inversion recovery image (B) demonstrate areas of increased T2 signal, with associated gyral swelling and sulcal effacement in the left middle cerebral artery (MCA) distribution. (C) Diffusion-weighted image demonstrates increased signal in the left MCA distribution with corresponding low signal in this region on the apparent diffusion coefficient map (D), consistent with restricted diffusion.

1. Which of the following is responsible for the bright signal in the left middle cerebral artery distribution on the diffusion-weighted image (part C)?
   D. Cytotoxic edema

2. What is the purpose of the apparent diffusion coefficient map (part D)?
   B. Corrects for T2 shine-through

Discussion

The random motion of water molecules, driven by thermal agitation, is highly dependent on their cellular environment. Ischemia alters that environment. When neurons become ischemic, oxidative metabolism fails, and the adenosine triphosphate–dependent ion transporters stop functioning. This results in an ion gradient across the cell membrane, which causes a shift of water molecules from the extracellular space into the intracellular space. This is cytotoxic edema. Water molecules in an excessively fluid-distended cell will have restricted mobility, which results in high signal of the tissue on diffusion-weighted imaging (DWI).[1] In contrast to cytotoxic edema, vasogenic edema is characterized by enlarged extracellular spaces. This increases molecular mobility and results in low signal at DWI.

Because T2 contrast contributes to the signal intensity on spin echo echoplanar sequences used for DWI, there is an element of T2 contrast within a DWI that can manifest as increased signal that is not attributable to restricted diffusion. This is called *T2 shine-through* and is most prevalent in tissues with long T2 relaxation times. This T2 shine-through must be distinguished from signal resulting from restricted diffusion. This can be done with an apparent diffusion coefficient (ADC) map. The ADC is generated by combining two diffusion-weighted sequences with different B values. The ratio of these two can then be used to calculate an ADC, which can be mapped by voxels to create an image. If the area of increased signal on the DWI is low in signal on the ADC map, this confirms restricted diffusion. If the corresponding area on the ADC map is high in signal, then the increased signal is due to T2 shine-through rather than restricted diffusion.

Physics

DWI generates images based not on differences in T1 recovery or T2 relaxation, but on local differences in the random (brownian) motion of molecules, particularly water molecules, in biologic tissues.

In a perfectly homogeneous and unrestricted environment, the direction of molecular motion is completely random and isotropic, meaning that it has an equal probability of moving in any direction. However, biologic tissues are not homogeneous; they present a complex environment in which water is divided among intravascular, intracellular, and extracellular compartments. Molecules in extracellular environments experience relatively free diffusion, whereas those in an intracellular environment are relatively restricted in their diffusion. Because different biologic tissues vary in their proportion of intracellular and extracellular compartments and in their cellular architecture, each has characteristic diffusion properties. Water molecules in any of these tissues must also interact with cell membranes, fibers, and macromolecules, all of which can further restrict their motion.

Pathologic processes also affect the diffusion of water molecules. Tissues with intact cellular membranes, high cellular density, or complex fluid-containing macromolecules will have restricted mobility of water molecules. This explains the appearance of highly cellular tumors, abscesses, and cytotoxic edema related to acute tissue infarction on DWI.[2]

Pulse sequences have been developed to make use of MR's ability to measure and display molecular diffusion. These diffusion-weighted sequences can differentiate fast-moving protons (e.g., unrestricted diffusion) from slow-moving protons (e.g., restricted diffusion). Diffusion within each individual voxel can be mapped and displayed in a DWI.

Spin echo echoplanar imaging is the most commonly used imaging sequence in DWI primarily because of its speed, which helps minimize macroscopic motion artifact. The distinguishing feature of a diffusion-weighted sequence is that two strong and symmetric gradients are placed on two sides of the 180-degree refocusing pulse. The first gradient pulse dephases the protons, and the second gradient pulse is intended to rephase the protons. If the protons remain static throughout the course of the pulse sequence, they will be rephased by the second gradient and will not contribute to any signal changes. However, if the protons move significantly (undergo diffusion) during the pulse sequence, they will not be completely rephased by the second gradient and, instead, the result will be the loss of phase coherence, leading to the loss of signal.[3]

The degree of diffusion weighting is determined by the b value, which reflects the strength (amplitude), duration, and temporal separation of the two motion-probing gradients.

The b value is expressed in seconds per square millimeter (sec/mm^2) and is calculated as follows:

$$b = \gamma^2 G^2 \delta^2 \left(\Delta - \delta/3\right)$$

where G is the amplitude of the applied gradient, δ is the time of the applied gradient, Δ is the duration between the two gradients, and $\gamma = 42$ Mz/T.

A baseline image, called b_0, is typically acquired in diffusion MRI, where no motion-probing gradients are applied. The result is essentially a T2-weighted image, which is used in conjunction with the DWIs to derive all diffusion-related coefficients. A higher b value is achieved by increasing the gradient amplitude and the duration of, and time between, the gradients. This increases sensitivity to diffusion and reduces signal due to T2 decay. At the highest b values, nearly all signal received is from very restricted molecules. The signal intensity from a diffusion-weighted sequence is generated according to the following equation (Stejskal-Tanner sequence):

$$S = S_0 e^{-bD}$$

where S_0 is the baseline signal in the b_0 image, b is the b value, and D is the diffusion coefficient.

T1, T2, and proton density contrast all contribute to signal intensity in DWI. Because T2 contrast tends to predominate in spin echo echoplanar sequences, significant signal seen on DWI may be due to T2 contrast, particularly in tissues with very long T2 relaxation times. This T2 shine-through must be distinguished from bright signal resulting from restricted diffusion. This is done using the ADC map, which effectively eliminates the contribution of all contrast except that resulting from diffusion.

The ADC for any voxel is generated by combining two sequences, which are performed at different b values, keeping all other parameters equal. Typically, one spin echo echoplanar sequence is performed in which the b factor is 0 and a second sequence is performed in which the b factor is greater than 0. The ADC is then calculated by taking the negative logarithm of the ratio of those two image sets according to the equation:

$$D = -\left(1/b\right) \ln\left(S/S_0\right)$$

The ADC is expressed in square millimeters per second. Each voxel is assigned an ADC and can be mapped to generate a DWI. An ADC value in any tissue can be derived by drawing a region of interest on the ADC map.

Diffusion within a voxel, then, can be quantitatively or qualitatively displayed. Tissue with restricted diffusion, such as an acute brain infarct or high-grade tumor, will appear bright on the trace image and dark on the ADC map and will have a low ADC value.[2]

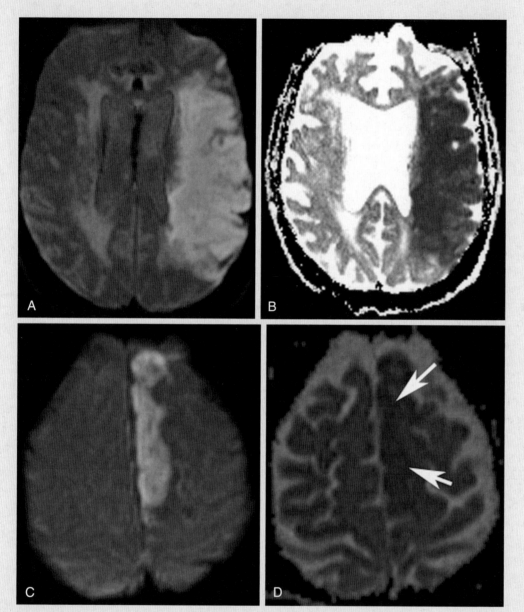

FIG. 15.C2

1. Of the following imaging tools, which is most sensitive in the diagnosis of hyperacute ischemic stroke?
   A. Noncontrast CT
   B. Perfusion CT
   C. Fluid-attenuated inversion recovery (FLAIR) MR
   D. Diffusion-weighted MRI
2. Restricted diffusion is seen in the left MCA and left anterior cerebral artery (ACA) territories. The measured ADC value in the left MCA distribution infarct is decreased by 50% and, in the left ACA infarct, it is decreased by 20%. Which of the following statements is true concerning the timing of the two infarcts?
   A. The MCA distribution infarct is acute and the ACA infarct is subacute.
   B. The MCA distribution infarct is subacute and the ACA infarct is acute.
   C. Both infarcts are acute.
   D. DWI cannot date stroke.

Diagnosis

The diagnosis is left MCA and ACA infarcts of different ages.

FIG. 15.C2. (A) Diffusion-weighted and (B) ADC images demonstrating restricted diffusion in the left MCA territory. (C) Diffusion-weighted and (D) ADC images (same patient and examination) demonstrate restricted diffusion in the left anterior cerebral artery territory *(arrows)*.

Discussion

DWI is currently the most sensitive diagnostic tool for acute ischemic stroke in patients presenting within 6 hours of symptom onset. The sensitivity of DWI to ischemia in this setting is 95%, far superior to the 50% sensitivity of CT and conventional MRI without DWI. DWI, in fact, can detect abnormalities due to ischemia within 3 to 30 minutes of onset.

FLAIR MRI is more sensitive than T2-weighted MRI in the acute stage of stroke, but even FLAIR is usually negative in the first 6 to 12 hours. Therefore in this clinical setting, a focal brain abnormality that is abnormal on DWI but negative on FLAIR suggests hyperacute stroke.

Most centers will perform noncontrast CT scanning in the hyperacute phase because the presence of hemorrhage will change management. MR protocols that include DWI sequences and susceptibility methods (e.g., gradient recalled echo) can reliably diagnose both acute ischemic stroke and acute hemorrhage in the emergency setting and have obviated the use of CT at some centers.

On conventional T2-weighted MR images, it is often difficult to distinguish among new stroke, old stroke, and new extension of a previous stroke. All appear as increased signal on T2-weighted images. Similarly, signal on DWI can remain bright for months—initially due to restriction from ischemia and, later, from T2 shine-through. The ADC map, however, is quantitative and, because its evolution is predictable over time, it can be used to age an infarct.

Within minutes of the onset of ischemia, ADC values drop, reaching a nadir at approximately 3 to 5 days, at which time the ADC value is typically 50% that of normal brain parenchyma. The ADC then gradually returns to baseline over the next week in a process termed *pseudonormalization*. ADC values can even exceed normal levels as time passes, in some cases helping to differentiate acute, subacute, and chronic injuries.

This predictable pattern can be used to determine the age of an infarct. Although visually there is no difference in signal between the MCA and ACA infarcts in this case, the question indicates that ADC values were decreased by 50% in the left MCA distribution and by 20% in the left ACA infarct; 50% is consistent with acute infarct. An ADC value of 20% suggests some normalization of diffusion and corresponds to a subacute infarct.

A chronic infarct would show increased signal on both the DWIs and the ADC map. The signal inverts from low (dark) to high (bright) signal on the ADC map after about 7 to 12 days because of T2 bright signal.[4,5]

CASE 15.2 ANSWERS

1. **D. Diffusion-weighted MRI**
2. **A. The MCA distribution infarct is acute and the ACA infarct is subacute.**

CASE 15.3

FIG. 15.C3

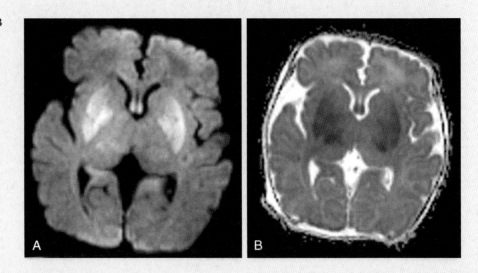

1. Of the following, which clinical scenario most likely explains the pattern of injuries to this neonatal brain?
   A. Acute profound hypoxia in a term infant
   B. Acute profound hypoxia in a premature infant
   C. Partial prolonged hypoxia in a preterm infant
   D. Partial prolonged hypoxia in a term infant
2. What is the optimal timing of MRI of the neonate suspected of suffering from hypoxic-ischemic injury?
   A. First day of life
   B. Any time after the first day of life
   C. After the first day but before the end of the first week of life
   D. Any time after the first week of life

Diagnosis

Hypoxic-ischemic injury to the newborn.

FIG. 15.C3. (A) Diffusion-weighted and (B) ADC images in a newborn demonstrate restricted diffusion in the basal ganglia and thalamus.

Discussion

The distribution of ischemic injury in neonatal hypoxic ischemic encephalopathy depends on three factors: the intensity of the hypotensive-hypoxic insult, duration of the insult, and maturity of the brain at the time of insult. Although there is considerable overlap in the mechanism of injury and imaging findings, the distribution of injuries on MRI can often characterize the insult.

With partial prolonged ischemia (sustained but incomplete loss of oxygenation, such as with a prolonged difficult labor), the brain is able to shift blood flow to the more critical areas (e.g., basal ganglia, thalamus, brainstem), which are preserved at the expense of white matter in a watershed distribution. The watershed distribution for term newborns is typically interarterial and parasagittal, as it is in older patients. Premature babies, however, have a unique watershed distribution, which is periventricular. This explains the distribution of injury in periventricular leukomalacia, a common injury seen in premature infants.

With acute profound loss of brain oxygenation (e.g., from placental abruption or umbilical cord prolapse), there is insufficient blood to shunt to critical areas. Thus it is these same critical areas—basal ganglia, thalamus, perirolandic cortex—that are injured first. They are particularly susceptible because they are the most metabolically active. If the acute profound insult lasts less than 20 minutes, they may be the only areas affected, as in Case 15.3. If the insults last beyond 20 to 30 minutes, the entire brain, including the cortex, will be involved.[6]

MRI is the most sensitive and specific imaging tool to evaluate for neonatal hypoxic-ischemic injury. DWI reveals restricted diffusion earlier than signal intensity changes appear on conventional T1- or T2-weighted sequences. DWI results can be negative in the first 24 hours after hypoxic-ischemic encephalopathy insult. DWI abnormalities generally peak 3 to 5 days after the insult and normalize by day 7. The ideal time to detect hypoxic-ischemic injury in a newborn infant is therefore between 24 hours and 7 days.

CASE 15.3 ANSWERS

1. **A. Acute profound hypoxia in a term infant**
2. **C. After the first day but before the end of the first week of life**

CASE 15.4

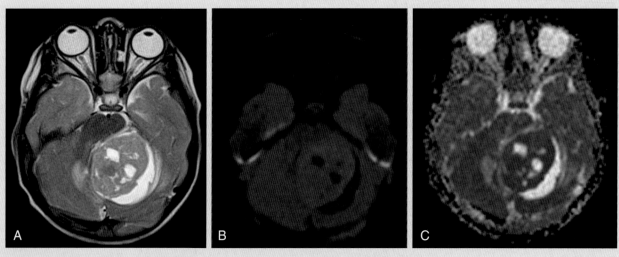

FIG. 15.C4

1. A 6-year-old presents with a posterior fossa tumor. Based on the figures, which of the following is the most likely tumor type?
   A. Ependymoma
   B. Medulloblastoma
   C. Juvenile pilocytic astrocytoma
   D. Hemangioblastoma

FIG. 15.C4. (A) T2-weighted, (B) diffusion-weighted, and (C) ADC images demonstrate restricted diffusion in a posterior fossa tumor.

Discussion

Medulloblastoma, ependymoma, and juvenile pilocytic astrocytoma are the three most common posterior fossa tumors in the pediatric age group. It can be difficult to differentiate the three tumor types on CT or conventional MRI. All may present in the midline, all may have solid and cystic components, and all may have calcifications.

DWI and ADC maps can often suggest the correct diagnosis preoperatively, based on tumor cellularity. Fig. 15.C4B, the DWI, shows that the signal in this midline posterior fossa tumor is slightly greater than that of normal brain. This indicates that the tumor restricts diffusion and is characteristic of a medulloblastoma.

It has been shown that medulloblastoma, due to its dense cellularity, tends to restrict diffusion and exhibit low ADC values. The dense cellularity and high nuclear-cytoplasmic ratio provides an increased number of membrane barriers to microscopic water diffusion.

Using ADC values to discriminate tumors is not limited to the posterior fossa in children. Lower ADC values have been reported in other highly cellular tumors, such as central nervous system lymphoma and high-grade gliomas. Low ADC values have been shown to predict higher grade tumors and poorer prognosis.

CASE 15.5

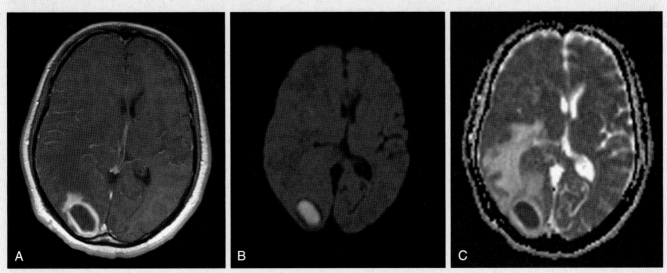

FIG. 15.C5

1. Based on the images provided, which of the following is the most likely diagnosis?
   A. Brain abscess
   B. Brain infarct
   C. Necrotic tumor
   D. Evolving hematoma

2. Of the following, which is the best explanation for the increased signal in the white matter surrounding the lesion on the ADC map?
   A. Inflammation
   B. Gliosis
   C. Cytotoxic edema
   D. Vasogenic edema

FIG. 15.C5. (A) Axial postcontrast, T1-weighted image demonstrates a rim-enhancing lesion in the right occipital lobe. (B) Diffusion-weighted and (C) ADC images demonstrate restricted diffusion within the lesion.

Discussion

Fig. 15.C5A, the postcontrast T1-weighted image, demonstrates a rim-enhancing lesion in the right occipital lobe. The differential diagnosis for a rim-enhancing lesion is extensive and includes necrotic tumor, abscess, demyelinating disease, metastatic disease, radiation necrosis, infarct, and evolving hematoma. The appearance on conventional MR sequences is rarely able to distinguish among these entities. The clinical history is most helpful in arriving at a final diagnosis, but DWI with ADC mapping can help distinguish between an abscess and a necrotic primary brain tumor or metastatic lesion.

Demonstration of restricted diffusion within the central portion of the lesion, as seen in Fig. 15.C5B and 15.C5C, strongly suggests abscess as the diagnosis. It is hypothesized that an abscess has restricted diffusion centrally because of the physical characteristics of pus. The increased viscosity and cellularity of pus limit the motion of water molecules, resulting in restricted diffusion, with increased signal on DWI and corresponding decreased signal on ADC maps.

Necrotic tumor, in contrast, will often demonstrate increased diffusion centrally and appear dark on DWI. An acute brain infarct could restrict diffusion but would not have rim enhancement.

The bright signal in the periatrial white matter on the ADC map results from vasogenic edema, related to mass effect from the lesion. In contrast to cytotoxic edema, in which fluid accumulates within cells as a result of cell injury, vasogenic edema represents extracellular edema as a result of leakage of fluid from capillaries, typically into white matter. The extracellular fluid of vasogenic edema does not restrict diffusion and appears dark on DWIs. This dark signal, however, is counterbalanced by the T2 shine-through effect, resulting in a signal that is isointense to white matter (Fig. 15.C5B).

CASE 15.5 ANSWERS

1. **A. Brain abscess**
2. **D. Vasogenic edema**

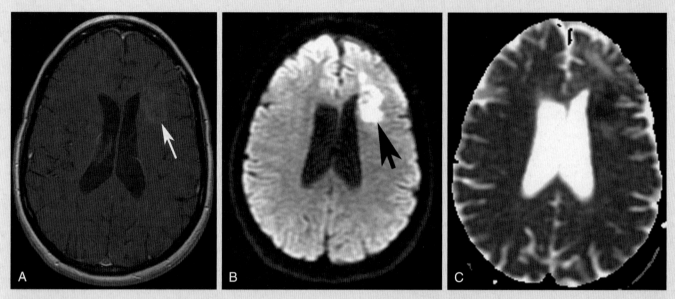

FIG. 15.C6

1. Which of the following can explain the increased contrast enhancement in the resection bed on MRI following treatment for a GBM?
   A. Tumor recurrence
   B. Postoperative ischemia
   C. Pseudoprogression
   D. Radiation necrosis
   E. All of the above

2. Which of the following is the best explanation for the new enhancement at the inferior aspect of the resection cavity in the left frontal white matter of this 55-year-old woman 6 months after resection of a glioblastoma multiforme?
   A. Tumor recurrence
   B. Postoperative ischemia
   C. Pseudoprogression
   D. Radiation necrosis

FIG. 15.C6. (A) Axial postcontrast, T1-weighted image demonstrates a subtle area of focal hyperenhancement in the left anterior corona radiata *(arrow)* along the inferior aspect of a resection cavity for a glioblastoma multiforme (GBM). Increased signal is seen on the DWI (B), *arrow*), with low signal seen in this region on the ADC map (C), consistent with restricted diffusion corresponding to the area of hyperenhancement on the postcontrast T1-weighted image.

Discussion

The current standard therapy for glioblastoma multiforme (GBM) is surgical resection, followed by radiotherapy and chemotherapy. Immediately after surgery and throughout continued treatment, MR surveillance is performed to evaluate for tumor recurrence. The development of new contrast enhancement generates concern for tumor recurrence but can also be seen with postoperative ischemia, pseudoprogression, and radiation necrosis.

In the process of surgical tumor resection, small adjacent arteries can be injured and lead to a rim of cytotoxic edema at the margins of the resection bed that restricts diffusion in the immediate postoperative period. This often leads to enhancement for weeks to a few months following surgery. DWI cannot distinguish the restricted diffusion caused by cytotoxic edema from that caused by the hypercellularity of recurrent tumor. Fortunately, however, the distinction can be made based on evolution over time. Restricted diffusion from tumor hypercellularity will persist or progress, whereas that from cytotoxic edema will resolve in 1 week and eventually evolve into encephalomalacia or a gliotic cavity.

Occasionally, a transient increase in lesion size is observed on imaging weeks to months following radiation therapy. This phenomenon, termed *pseudoprogression,* is thought to be due to endothelial damage to oligodendrocytes from the radiation. Patients are usually asymptomatic and its course is transient and resolves spontaneously. On MR images, pseudoprogression manifests as new or increasing enhancement that stabilizes with time. Pseudoprogression does not restrict diffusion and can usually be differentiated from tumor recurrence on that basis.

Radiation necrosis typically appears several months after radiation therapy. It can be harder to distinguish from tumor recurrence on MR because, unlike ischemic injury and pseudoprogression, it can have mass effect and vasogenic edema along with the contrast enhancement.

Imaging has a role in differentiating these entities, but they are best distinguished by time course and symptoms. If the new enhancement is seen within months of radiation, and the patient is asymptomatic, pseudoprogression is favored. New enhancement after 3 months, particularly with symptoms, suggests tumor recurrence or radiation necrosis. DWI can often help distinguish between those two entities.

The time frame and mass effect exclude postoperative ischemia and pseudoprogression as causes for the new enhancement and limit the differential diagnosis to radiation necrosis and tumor recurrence. Conventional MRI sequences are insufficient to distinguish between the two reliably, but diffusion-weighted MRI, along with perfusion imaging and positron emission tomography, can be helpful in differentiating tumor recurrence from radiation necrosis.

Recurrent malignant brain tumors retain their high tumor cellularity, which restricts diffusion, resulting in increased signal DWI and low ADC values on the ADC map. This allows differentiation from tumor necrosis, which usually does not restrict diffusion.

In this case, bright signal is seen on the DWI (Fig. 15.C2B), and dark signal is seen on the ADC map (Fig. 15.C2C), consistent with restricted diffusion corresponding to the area of hyperenhancement on the postcontrast T1-weighted image (Fig. 15.C2A). This strongly suggests the presence of residual or recurrent tumor.

1. E. All of the above
2. A. Tumor recurrence

CASE 15.7

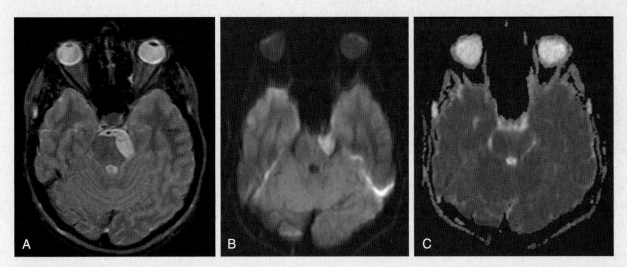

FIG. 15.C7

1. The images provided show an incidental finding from an MR scan on a 14-year-old female. Of the following, which is the most likely diagnosis?
   A. Acoustic schwannoma
   B. Meningioma
   C. Arachnoid cyst
   D. Epidermoid cyst

FIG. 15.C7. Axial (A) T2-weighted, (B) diffusion-weighted, and (C) ADC images demonstrate a focal abnormality in the left cerebellopontine angle.

Discussion

Fig. 15.C7A demonstrates a mass in the left cerebellopontine angle. The postcontrast T1-weighed image (not shown) suggested a cystic rather than a solid mass, excluding schwannoma and meningioma.

Arachnoid and epidermoid cysts both appear as cerebrospinal fluid (CSF) density lesions on CT, and both follow CSF in signal on most MR sequences. They can be distinguished by DWI.[7]

Arachnoid cysts are well-circumscribed cysts with an imperceptible wall. They characteristically displace adjacent structures and follow CSF in CT density (water density) and all MR sequences (hyperintense on T2 with FLAIR suppression).

Epidermoid cysts are T2 bright but are often more heterogeneous on FLAIR. They can be more lobulated in shape than arachnoid cysts and tend to engulf adjacent nerves and arteries rather than displacing them. They have a thin capsule and are filled with desquamated epithelial keratin and cholesterol crystals. These macromolecules restrict diffusion of water molecules, resulting in bright DWI signal that can distinguish epidermoids from arachnoid cysts.

In this case, the lesion demonstrates restricted diffusion—increased signal on the DWI (Fig. 15.C7B) and low signal on the ADC image (Fig. 15.C7C), suggesting the final diagnosis of epidermoid cyst, which was confirmed at surgery.

CASE 15.7 ANSWER

1. D. Epidermoid cyst

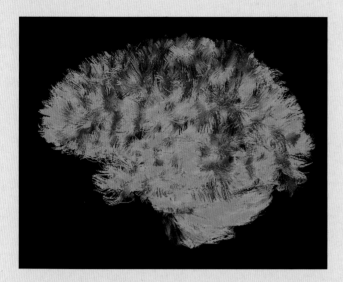

FIG. 15.C8

1. Diffusion tensor imaging is based on which of the following?
   A. Isotropic diffusion
   B. Anisotropic diffusion
   C. Changes in blood flow
   D. Changes in oxygen consumption

FIG. 15.C8. Normal appearance of nerve tract fibers within an adult brain displayed from the lateral projection.

Discussion

If only one diffusion direction is used in DWI, then the anisotropy of the water diffusion cannot be characterized. When more than six noncolinear diffusion directions are used, the anisotropy of water diffusion can be delineated based on the mathematical model of diffusion tensor. These diffusion MRI methods are known as diffusion tensor imaging (DTI).

DTI has had its greatest application in the imaging of white matter, which lends itself to anisotropic imaging because bundles of parallel-oriented axons all run along a single direction. Water molecules are more likely to diffuse along the long axis of a nerve fiber, rather than perpendicular to it (and rather than randomly). DTI exploits this principle to produce microstructural images of white matter tracts. In effect, it uses structural connectivity to generate images of white matter tracts. Clinically, it can be used to evaluate for the structural integrity of these tracts, the loss of which can indicate early pathology.

DTI images are acquired by applying gradients sensitized to the direction of diffusion, which are then compared to a reference b_0 image to derive a quantitative ADC for each voxel, as in DWI. By applying at least six different direction-sensitive gradients, a three-dimensional trajectory of diffusion (the diffusion tensor) can be generated for each voxel, which indicates the dominant direction of diffusion and the spectrum of directions of diffusion within that voxel. This can be represented conceptually by a diffusion ellipsoid. The long axis of this ellipsoid indicates the dominant direction of diffusion within that voxel, and the spectrum of directions within any one voxel is indicated by the girth of that ellipsoid, which is also expressed as fractional anisotropy (FA), a number between 0 (isotropy) and 1 (anisotropy).

A dense nerve tract will have a high FA value because diffusion will be uniform along one axis. The diffusion ellipsoid will be long and narrow, oriented in the direction of the nerve fibers. In intraventricular CSF, in contrast, motion is unrestricted in all directions. There is no dominant direction of diffusion and so movement is isotropic; the ellipsoid is spherical, and the FA value is near zero.[8]

The diffusion ellipsoid vector can be plotted for each individual voxel, allowing computer tracking algorithms to map out pathways of continuous direction of diffusion on grayscale or color-coded images as evidence of connectivity as landmarks of white matter tracts. This is diffusion tractography, as illustrated in Fig. 15.C8A.

The clinical applications of DTI are promising. Clinical studies have shown that DTI can detect microstructural changes early in various white matter diseases, including multiple sclerosis and Alzheimer disease. Tractography is being used increasingly in preoperative neurosurgical planning.

CASE 15.8 ANSWER

1. B. Anisotropic diffusion

FIG. 15.C9

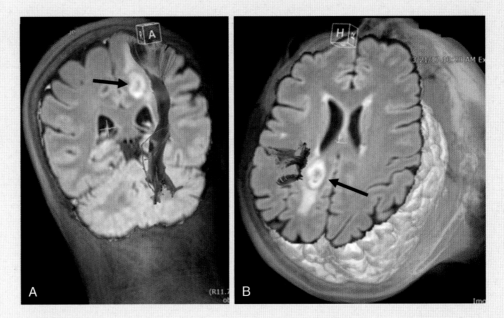

A

B

1. A preoperative MRI is obtained on a 55-year woman with a left frontal GBM. What is the significance of the blue color in the figures?
   A. Blue depicts actual nerve fibers of the corticospinal tract.
   B. Blue indicates areas of low fractional anisotropy.
   C. Blue depicts nerve conduction from superior to inferior.
   D. Blue depicts diffusion from superior to inferior.
   E. Blue depicts degenerated axons distal to the tumor.

FIG. 15.C9. Preoperative (A) coronal and (B) axial DTI tractography images in a 55-year old woman with a left parietal GBM show the relationship of the corticospinal tracts *(blue)* to the left parietal tumor *(arrows)*.

Discussion

Data obtained in DTI can be displayed in different ways. Currently at our institution, the most common clinical use of DTI uses three-dimensional (3D) fiber tractography, in which color-coded 3D images are reconstructed for use in neurosurgical planning for tumor resection. Fig. 15.C9 displays the relationship of the vital corticospinal tracts to the left frontal tumor.

The blue color does not represent structural nerve fibers, but shows virtual tracts depicting the principal direction of diffusion. A computer algorithm considers the principal direction of diffusion within each voxel in a user-defined region of interest and reconstructs fiber tracts based on the assumption that the direction of diffusion tends to be parallel to the orientation of axonal fibers; it statistically depicts likely connections from voxel to voxel. In the case of the corticospinal tracts, the direction is superior to inferior. By convention, blue is assigned for diffusion in this *z*-axis.[9]

CASE 15.9 ANSWER

1. D. Blue depicts diffusion from superior to inferior.

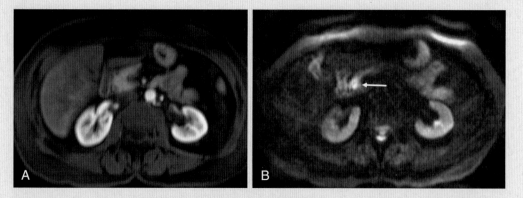

FIG. 15.C10

1. Which of the following is an established benefit of DWI
   over conventional MR sequences in body imaging?
   A. Reliable discrimination of malignant from benign liver
      masses
   B. Reliable characterization of response to chemotherapy
   C. Increased conspicuity of lesions
   D. All of the above

FIG. 15.C10. Postcontrast volumetric interpolated breath-hold examination sequence in the arterial phase (A) fails to demonstrate a primary pancreatic head tumor, which is nicely demonstrated on the DWI (B, *arrow*). Pathology confirmed a malignant neuroendocrine tumor.

Discussion

DWI is best established clinically in neuroimaging, but it has been increasingly making contributions in body imaging. Although DWI shows promise in lesion characterization and response to chemotherapy and is being investigated in other areas, its greatest utility to date has been in lesion detection.

T2 bright abdominal lesions that restrict diffusion are usually more conspicuous on DWI than on T2-weighted imaging because most other entities lose signal on DWIs. Highly cellular lymph nodes and liver lesions can be quite conspicuous. Whole-body DWI is being investigated for the detection of metastases and the evaluation of lymphoma.

Although studies have shown that malignant abdominal tumors tend to show lower ADC values (more diffusion restriction) than benign tumors, there is considerable overlap in ADC values between malignant and benign lesions, so the differentiation cannot be made reliably. Even within tumors, there can be considerable variability in diffusion restriction, probably reflecting biologic variation within tumors.

Because the dense cellularity of malignant tumors is the cause for the diffusion restriction, it was hoped that a decrease in restriction (rise in ADC) might be predictive of the response to chemotherapy, which destroys cell membranes, thereby increasing the diffusion of water molecules. Although some studies have shown an increase in ADC values of tumors being treated with chemotherapy before changes in tumor size, the findings have not been reproducible, and the technique is not relied on in cancer treatment.[10]

CASE 15.10 ANSWER

1. **C. Increased conspicuity of lesions**

FIG. 15.C11

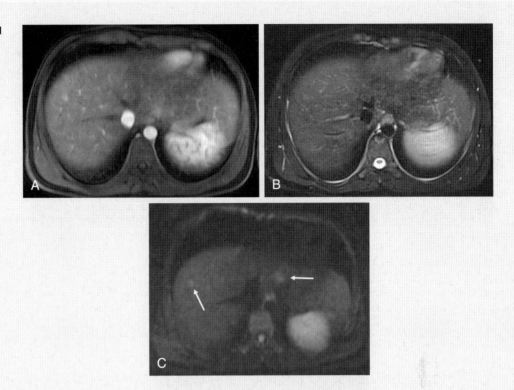

1. In body imaging, which of the following is an advantage
   of DWI over conventional spin echo sequences?
   A. Improved signal-to-noise ratio (SNR)
   B. Superior spatial resolution
   C. Motion artifact suppression
   D. Improved contrast resolution for some lesions

FIG. 15.C11. (A) Postcontrast arterial phase volumetric interpolated breath-hold examination, (B) T2-weighted, and (C) DWI through the upper liver in a 14-year-old with glycogen storage disease. New hepatic adenomas *(arrows)* are demonstrated on the DWI that were not detected on the postcontrast or T2-weighted images. Based on the detection of these additional lesions, the patient underwent liver transplantation.

Discussion

As illustrated in Cases 15.9 and 15.10, focal abdominal lesions can often be detected on DWI due to their improved contrast resolution relative to background. SNR, spatial resolution, and motion artifact are liabilities of DWI in the abdomen, rather than advantages.

Most DWI in the abdomen uses single-shot echoplanar sequences, which have low spatial resolution, poor SNR, and susceptibility to various artifacts. Breathing, cardiac pulsations, and bowel peristalsis all make motion artifact a greater problem in the abdomen than in the brain. The breath-hold technique can minimize motion artifact, but at the cost of further lowering the SNR. It also limits the minimum slice thickness and the number of b values that can be used.

The shorter inherent T2 relaxation times of abdominal organs and muscles, compared with brain tissue, result in poor signal return and a reduced SNR. Several strategies can be used to offset this low SNR, including higher field strength (3.0 vs. 1.5 T), increasing the number of signals acquired, and increasing slice thickness, but each has its costs. SNR can also be improved by using high b values for DWI in the abdomen, which are lower than those used in neuroimaging. High b values of 500 to 600 sec/mm^2 are typically used in the liver. New parallel imaging techniques permit rapid imaging and reduce motion artifacts and allows the application of b values in multiple directions. This increases the SNR.

CASE 15.11 ANSWER

1. **D. Improved contrast resolution for some lesions**

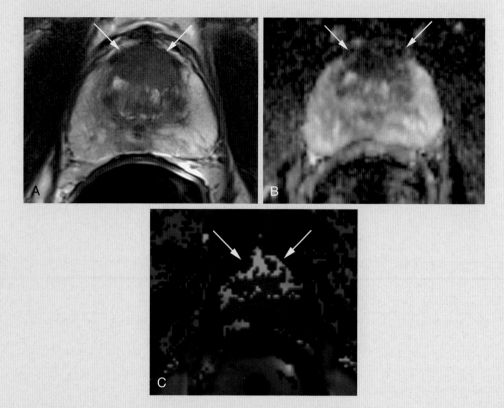

FIG. 15.C12

1. Which of the following findings are suggestive of prostate cancer on MRI?
   A. Capillary permeability demonstrated on dynamic contrast-enhanced (DCE) MRI
   B. Restricted diffusion
   C. Low T2 signal within normally high-signal peripheral zone
   D. All of the above

FIG. 15.C12. (A) Axial T2-weighted image in a 59-year-old man with rising prostate specific antigen levels and multiple prior negative biopsies demonstrates a large area of abnormal low signal along the anterior aspect of the prostate gland at the level of the midgland *(arrows)*. (B) ADC map reveals this same area *(arrows)* to have markedly restricted diffusion, most compatible with a high-grade prostate cancer. (C) Colorized perfusion map created using postprocessing software from dynamic contrast-enhanced MRI acquisition shows highly suspicious enhancement kinetics and abnormal perfusion *(arrows)*, corresponding with findings seen on the T2-weighted images and ADC map. The patient underwent confirmatory biopsy, revealing a high-grade (Gleason 4 + 3 = 7) adenocarcinoma at the site of MRI suspicion.

Discussion

Multiparametric MRI uses multiple MR parameters, both functional and anatomic, to maximize performance. In prostate MRI, DWI, with the calculation of ADC maps and DCE MRI, are the preferred functional parameters. MR spectroscopy has been studied as an additional functional parameter, but is not as widely used. When combined with high-resolution T2-weighted images, particularly when using a 3-T field strength magnet and an endorectal coil, positive predictive values of 98% can be achieved for cancer detection.[11]

Characteristically, prostate cancer will present as a mass of low T2 signal relative to the surrounding high-signal peripheral zone of the gland, restricted diffusion, and increased tissue capillary permeability using DCE MRI.

CASE 15.12 ANSWER

1. **D. All of the above**

TAKE-HOME POINTS

1. DWI is based on the principle of brownian movement of water molecules.
2. In the stroke setting, increased signal on DWI is primarily due to cytotoxic edema (cellular swelling).
3. There is an element of T2 contrast within a DWI that can manifest as increased signal, termed *T2 shine-through*. This is distinguished from restricted diffusion by means of an ADC map. If the area of increased signal on the DWI is low in signal on the ADC map, this confirms restricted diffusion. If the corresponding area on the ADC is high in signal, then the increased signal is due to T2 shine-through, which is seen in facilitated diffusion (noncytotoxic edema) associated with many types of lesions.
4. The distinguishing feature of a DWI sequence is that two strong equal and opposite gradients are applied on either side of the 180-degree refocusing pulse.
5. The ADC map is quantitative and can be helpful in aging infarcts.
6. DWI can be helpful in narrowing the differential diagnosis of a rim-enhancing lesion and in distinguishing between an arachnoid cyst and epidermoid cyst.
7. DWI is primarily helpful in abdominal imaging in lesion detection.
8. DTI is unique in that is measures anisotropic diffusion, as seen along white matter tracts.

References

1. Srinivasan A, Goyal M, Al Azri F, Lum C. State-of-the-art imaging of acute stroke. *Radiographics.* 2005;26(suppl 1):S75–S95.
2. Stadnik TM, Luypaert R, Jager T, Osteaux M. Diffusion imaging: from basic physics to practical imaging. *RSNA EJ/Radiographics.* 1999.
3. Bitar R, Leung G, Perng R, et al. MR pulse sequences: what every radiologist wants to know but is afraid to ask. *Radiographics.* 2006;26:513–537.
4. Schlaug G, Siewert B, Benfield A, et al. Time course of the apparent diffusion coefficient (ADC) abnormality in human stroke. *Neurology.* 1997;49:113–119.
5. Fiebach J, Jansen O, Schellinger P, et al. Serial analysis of the apparent diffusion coefficient time course in human stroke. *Neuroradiology.* 2002;44:294–298.
6. Momjian-Mayor I, Baron J-C. The pathophysiology of watershed infarction in internal carotid artery disease: review of cerebral perfusion studies. *Stroke.* 2005;36:567–577.
7. Stadnik TW, Demaerel P, Luypaert RR, et al. Imaging tutorial: differential diagnosis of bright lesions on diffusion-weighted MR images. *Radiographics.* 2003;23:e7.
8. Hagmann P, Jonasson L, Maeder P, et al. Understanding diffusion MR imaging techniques: from scalar diffusion-weighted imaging to diffusion tensor imaging and beyond. *Radiographics.* 2006;26(suppl 1):S205–S223.
9. Abhinav K, Yeh F-C, Pathak S, et al. Advanced diffusion MRI fiber tracking in neurosurgical and neurodegenerative disorders and neuroanatomical studies: a review. *Biochim Biophys Acta.* 2014;1842(11):2286–2297.
10. Qayyum A. Diffusion-weighted imaging of the abdomen and pelvis: concepts and applications. *Radiographics.* 2009;29:1797–1810.
11. Turkbey B, Mani H, Shah V, et al. Multiparametric 3T prostate magnetic resonance imaging to detect cancer: histopathological correlation using prostatectomy specimens processed in customized magnetic resonance imaging based molds. *J Urol.* 2011;186:1818–1824.

CHAPTER 16

Perfusion Magnetic Resonance Imaging

Neal K. Viradia, Mustafa R. Bashir, Carlos Torres, Elmar M. Merkle, Allen W. Song, and Wells I. Mangrum

OPENING CASE 16.1

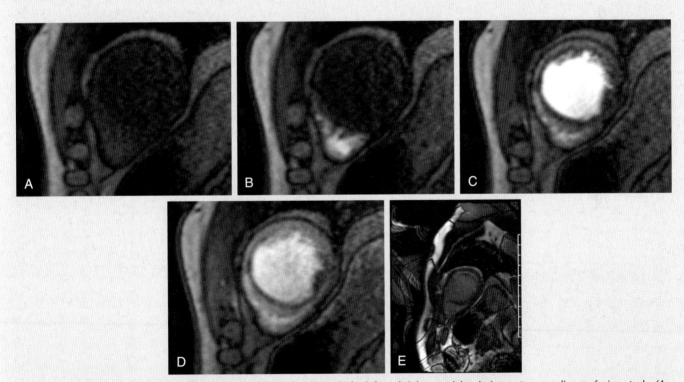

FIG. 16.C1. Short-axis fast low-angle shot images of the heart through the left and right ventricles during a stress cardiac perfusion study. (A–D) images of the same slice shown over time. Contrast progresses from the right ventricle to the left ventricle and then perfuses the myocardium, as evidenced by a blush of myocardial enhancement. There is no perfusion of the subendocardial muscle in the anterior and septal walls and a dense nonperfused area of subendocardial muscle in the inferolateral wall. (E) Delayed postcontrast TRUE fast imaging with steady-state precession short-axis view of the heart. Delayed enhancement is seen in the anterior and septal walls of the left ventricle. No delayed enhancement is seen in the inferolateral wall. Also noted is the presence of a moiré fringe artifact along the periphery of the image, which is the result of field inhomogeneity of the main magnetic field, resulting in superimposition of signals of different phasicity.

1. Given the pattern of subendocardial enhancement on the delayed imaging (Fig. 16.C1E), what coronary artery is involved in the infarct?
   A. Multicoronary artery infarct
   B. Right coronary artery
   C. Left anterior descending coronary artery
   D. Circumflex coronary artery

OPENING CASE 16.1

1. Given the pattern of subendocardial enhancement on the delayed imaging (Fig. 16.C1E), what coronary artery is involved in the infarct?
   C. Left anterior descending coronary artery

Discussion

Perfusion MRI

The perfusion of an organ is a basic physiologic process that can be altered by disease. *The main utilities of perfusion imaging include providing information about the presence or absence of ischemia (as shown in Case 16.1), assessing the metabolic activity of the tissue of interest, and evaluating the status of relevant vasculature.[1] MRI is one of many available techniques to measure perfusion.*

Cardiac Perfusion MRI

Cardiac MRI perfusion studies are primarily used to evaluate the cardiac vasculature and myocardium. They are analogous to nuclear cardiac perfusion studies. *Cardiac stress perfusion studies in MRI are generally performed with the same pharmacologic stress agents used in nuclear medicine perfusion studies.[1]* The cardiac perfusion study (Fig. 16.C1A–D) is performed during the first minute after the injection of contrast. The delayed image (Fig. 16.C1E) is obtained 10 minutes after the injection of contrast. *Ischemic and infarcted myocardium both exhibit the absence of subendocardial enhancement on stress perfusion images. However, on delayed imaging, only infarction will show subendocardial enhancement.[2] In chronic infarcts, the delayed enhancement is due to fibrotic scar, whereas in acute infarcts the enhancement is caused by edema and inflammatory cells. Chronic infarcts also generally have corresponding wall thinning.* The area of delayed enhancement in Fig. 16.C1D is in the left anterior descending artery (LAD) territory compatible with an acute infarct, given the presence of subendocardial enhancement and lack of wall thinning. *The LAD normally supplies the apical, anterior, and septal walls of the left ventricle. The circumflex coronary artery normally supplies the lateral wall of the left ventricle, and the right coronary artery (RCA) normally supplies the posterior wall of the left ventricle.* If the nonperfused myocardium in the lateral wall had shown delayed enhancement, then it would have been a multiterritory infarct involving both the LAD and circumflex territories. The lateral wall does not show delayed enhancement.

Rest perfusion images are helpful in distinguishing ischemic from hibernating myocardium. Hibernating myocardium has decreased blood flow at rest, differentiating it from exercise-induced ischemia, which appears normal at rest.[3] Hibernating myocardium can be differentiated from infarcted myocardium by the fact that hibernating myocardium will not enhance on delayed images, whereas infarcted myocardium will enhance. If we assume that the rest images (not provided) in Case 16.1 were normal, the stress perfusion defect of the inferolateral wall and the lack of delayed enhancement would be compatible with a significant area of inducible myocardial ischemia in the left circumflex arterial distribution.

Several MRI techniques are used to maximize detection of ischemia in cardiac perfusion imaging.[1] *First, a preparatory inversion recovery pulse is applied with the effective time to inversion set to null the signal from nonenhancing myocardium. Then multiple postcontrast images are obtained of the heart.* These images are electrocardiographically gated to reduce cardiac motion. *A fast gradient echo technique is used to acquire an image series of the heart during diastole rapidly.* At our institution, during first-pass perfusion stress testing, images are obtained at three or four levels from base to apex during every R-R interval. The sequence is repeated for first-pass perfusion and washout over approximately 1 minute. When viewing the acquired images in cine mode, gadolinium is seen to pass from the right heart to the left heart and then to equilibrate in the blood pool. *The normal myocardium will show rapid uptake of contrast agent followed by rapid washout.*

CASE 16.2

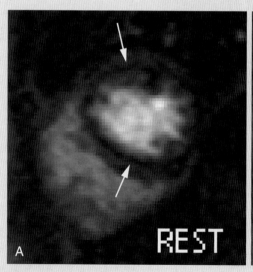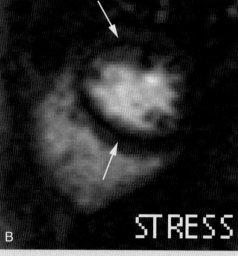

1. What artifact is seen in the rest and stress images?
   A. No artifact; circumferential infarct
   B. Ring artifact
   C. Chemical shift artifact
   D. Magic marker artifact

FIG. 16.C2

FIG. 16.C2. (A) Short-axis view from a rest cardiac MRI perfusion study. A low signal ring *(arrows)* is seen circumferentially around the subendocardium. (B) Short-axis view from a stress cardiac MRI perfusion study. Again, a low signal ring *(arrows)* is seen circumferentially around the subendocardium.

Discussion

Theoretically, a circumferential infarct could also have this appearance. However, it would be unusual for an infarct to involve the entire heart so uniformly. In addition, the clinical presentation, cardiac wall motion, and ejection fraction would all be different in these two patient populations.

Ring Artifact

Transient hypointense artifacts are frequently seen along the myocardium–blood pool interface that can mimic diffuse subendocardial hypoperfusion. This artifact is manifested as a low signal intensity ring encircling the subendocardium and is likely due to susceptibility effects from the divergent magnetic susceptibility of intravascular gadolinium and the adjacent myocardium. To differentiate this artifact from true hypoperfusion, resting perfusion images can be obtained. *On the resting studies, if the transient hypointense subendocardial signal persists, the finding is likely artifactual.* Because cardiac perfusion imaging is T1 weighted, the time to echo is shorter and the sequence is less sensitive to susceptibility effects than a T2*-weighted sequence (e.g., T2*-weighted dynamic susceptibility perfusion images in the brain).[1] However, susceptibility artifact can still be an issue in cardiac perfusion imaging, as illustrated by this case.

Chemical shift artifact occurs at an interface between water-dominant and fat-dominant tissues, not at muscle/blood interface. Ring artifact and chemical shift artifact both have an appearance of being drawn by a magic marker, but there is no artifact by this name.

CASE 16.2 ANSWER

1. **B. Ring artifact**

CASE 16.3

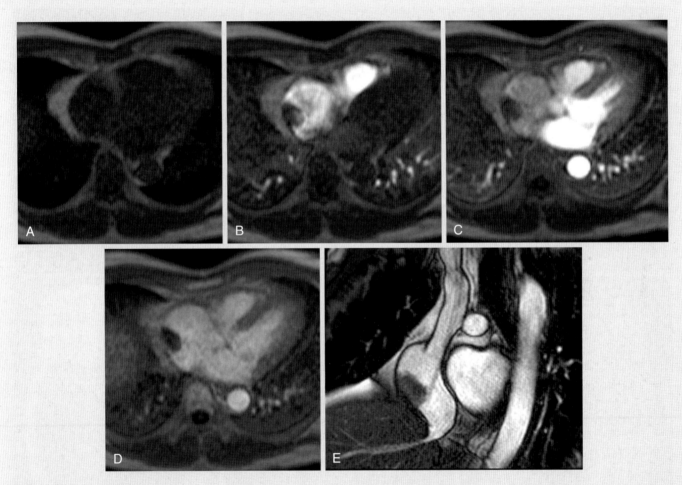

FIG. 16.C3

1. What is the most likely diagnosis?
   A. Atrial thrombus
   B. Atrial myxoma
   C. Metastatic disease
   D. Valve vegetation

FIG. 16.C3. Axial four-chamber view cardiac perfusion images centered at the level of the right atrium. (A–D) Perfusion images of the same level shown over time. There is a predominantly low signal intensity mass abutting the posterior wall of the right atrium. The mass shows no enhancement in the last perfusion image (D). (E) A coronal steady-state free precession image shows that the mass is associated with a central line entering through the superior vena cava.

Discussion

The differential diagnosis of an intraatrial mass includes both thrombus and neoplasm. In some cases, the diagnosis is difficult to make based on structural features alone. *Perfusion imaging can be helpful because enhancement of the lesion excludes bland thrombus.* This lesion shows no enhancement. In addition, the mass is clearly associated with a central line. No muscular invasion or enhancement is present. Atrial myxomas often have a pedicle attaching them to the fossa ovalis. Valve vegetations can show some level of enhancement; however, this mass is not associated with the tricuspid valve.

Cardiac Perfusion MRI: Further Considerations

Cardiac MRI perfusion analysis is generally qualitative. Qualitative analysis means that the raw perfusion data are analyzed visually, and no quantitative analysis is performed. In this example, the perfusion of the atrial mass is assessed by simply observing the signal change of the mass over time. In quantitative perfusion analysis, a single computational image is created mathematically that represents perfusion. Examples of quantitative perfusion analysis are given later in this chapter.

It is also important to note that cardiac MRI perfusion uses gadolinium-based contrast material as the perfusion agent and assesses the concentration of gadolinium with T1-weighted imaging. This is referred to as *dynamic contrast enhancement.* Alternate methods used in other organ systems to acquire MRI perfusion images are briefly explored later in this chapter.

CASE 16.3 ANSWER

1. **A. Atrial thrombus**

CASE 16.4

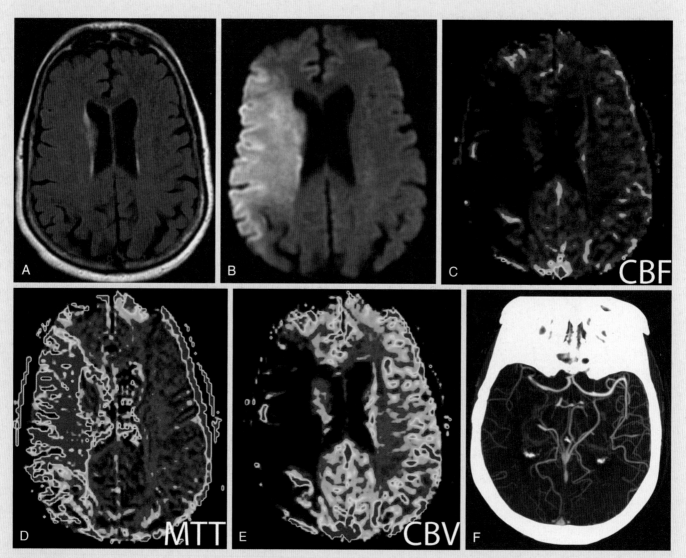

FIG. 16.C4

1. A patient is seen in the emergency department after collapsing. What is the correct diagnosis?
   A. Right MCA distribution infarct with no ischemic penumbra
   B. Right MCA distribution infarct with ischemic penumbra
   C. Gliomatosis cerebri
   D. Herpes encephalitis

FIG. 16.C4. (A) Axial fluid-attenuated inversion recovery image of the brain. There is subtle increased T2 signal in the periventricular white matter, right worse than left. (B) Axial diffusion-weighted imaging. Restricted diffusion is noted in the right frontal and parietal lobes in the distribution of the right middle cerebral artery (MCA). (C) Axial cerebral blood flow (CBF) calculation from an MRI perfusion study. Decreased blood flow in the right MCA distribution matches the diffusion abnormality. (D) Axial mean transit time (MTT) calculation from an MRI perfusion study. Increased mean transit time is noted in the right MCA distribution. This matches the CBF abnormality. (E) Axial cerebral blood volume (CBV) calculation from an MRI perfusion study. Decreased cerebral blood volume is noted in the right MCA distribution. This matches the MTT and CBF abnormalities. (F) Axial CT angiography maximal intensity projection image. There is an abrupt cutoff of the right M1 segment. Very little flow is documented in the right MCA distribution.

Brain Perfusion MRI

A brief review of stroke imaging and therapy will help explain the current role of perfusion imaging in stroke. Intravenous administration of a thrombolytic has been shown to improve clinical outcomes in patients treated within the first 3 to 4.5 hours of ischemic stroke onset, assuming patients do not meet exclusion criteria.[4,5] After 4.5 hours, the risks of giving intravenous thrombolytics may outweigh the benefits.[5]

Multiple multicenter trials (e.g., ESCAPE, SWIFT-PRIME, Extended-IA) have established intraarterial intervention, principally in the form of mechanical thrombectomy, as an accepted adjuvant treatment for acute ischemic stroke or even as a primary treatment in the setting where intravenous thrombolytics are contraindicated.[6] One as-of-yet unanswered question is whether perfusion imaging should be used to exclude patients from receiving intraarterial therapy. Two randomized controlled trials used perfusion imaging to exclude patients from receiving intraarterial therapy and found statistically significant beneficial results of therapy in their selected patient populations.[7,8] This would seem to indicate the need for perfusion imaging. However, other randomized controlled trials have found intraarterial therapy to be beneficial, even when no perfusion imaging was applied.[9–11] In summary, it is still unclear whether perfusion imaging should be used to include or exclude patients from intraarterial stroke therapy. This chapter does not weigh in on the need for perfusion imaging in ischemic stroke but does present the theory behind its potential utility.

Perfusion imaging seeks to depict the infarct core and the ischemic penumbra during an ischemic stroke accurately. The infarct core is in that portion of the brain that has already suffered irreparable damage. The ischemic penumbra refers to the ischemic brain tissue that is at risk to progress to infarction but that is potentially salvageable (Fig. 16.1). The larger the infarct core, the greater the risk for reperfusion hemorrhage and the greater the risk of treatment. The smaller the penumbra, the less potential benefit of therapy. The ideal candidate for intraarterial therapy would have a small infarct core and a large surrounding penumbra.

Vital to this management strategy is the theory that MRI (or CT) perfusion can accurately depict the infarct core and the ischemic penumbra. According to this theory, *the infarct core restricts on diffusion-weighted imaging, whereas areas of the brain with reduced perfusion and normal diffusion are thought to represent the ischemic penumbra.*[12] Identifying an area of restricted diffusion is relatively straightforward by MRI. However, characterizing perfusion defects is more complex. One way to assess perfusion is by analyzing the source image data that depict perfusion over time. This technique is termed *qualitative analysis* and is the

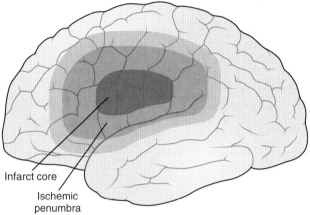

FIG. 16.1. Depiction of the concept of the ischemic penumbra. An arterial occlusion causes an area in the adjacent brain to undergo irreversible infarction. This area is known as the *infarct core*. A surrounding portion of the brain is at risk for infarction but is not yet irreversibly damaged. This separate area is termed the *ischemic penumbra*.[16] Experimental models have shown that the penumbra remains viable for hours; these studies have also shown that the infarct core gradually expands into the ischemic penumbra.[16,17] Early intervention to reperfuse the penumbra may prevent the ischemic tissue from progressing to complete infarction.

same method used in cardiac perfusion studies described earlier in this chapter. The main advantage of qualitative analysis is speed.[13] However, qualitative analysis of stroke perfusion data is challenging, not specific, and not commonly practiced. Instead, quantitative analysis is used. In quantitative analysis, mathematical models are applied to the perfusion data to calculate hemodynamic parameters that describe the physiologic character of tissue vasculature. *Common hemodynamic parameters that can be derived from perfusion imaging include CBV, MTT, and CBF. CBV is the volume of blood within the vasculature in a given volume of the brain. MTT is the time it takes for blood to traverse the capillary bed. CBF is the volume of blood flowing through a given volume of tissue per unit time.*

Applying the classic ischemic penumbra theory to Case 16.4, it can be seen that the perfusion defects in the right MCA distribution (characterized by reduced CBF, reduced CBV, and increased MTT) are similar in size to the diffusion defect. Consequently, this patient has no ischemic penumbra and theoretically would not benefit from intraarterial therapy.

CASE 16.4 ANSWER

1. A. Right MCA distribution infarct with no ischemic penumbra

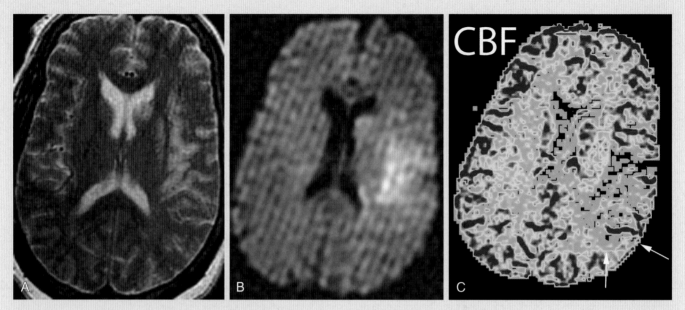

FIG. 16.C5

1. Given the imaging findings, what is the diagnosis?
   A. Normal study; increased signal on the diffusion study is artifactual and related to T2 shine-through
   B. Left perisylvian infarct in the left MCA distribution with small ischemic penumbra in the posterior left parietal lobe
   C. Left perisylvian infarct in the left MCA distribution without ischemic penumbra in the posterior left parietal lobe
   D. Transient perfusion defect in the posterior left parietal lobe

FIG. 16.C5. (A) Axial T2-weighted image of the brain. High T2 signal is present in the left caudate, the putamen, and the cortex of the left sylvian region. (B) Axial diffusion-weighted image. High signal in the region of the left perisylvian region represents restricted diffusion (confirmed by apparent diffusion coefficient map, not shown). Also note that this image has a stripe artifact (see "Other Artifacts" section in Chapter 9 for a more detailed discussion of this artifact). (C) CBF map. There is decreased flow in the left perisylvian region extending posteriorly into the posterior left parietal lobe. The CBF defect is slightly larger than the diffusion defect (mismatch shown by *arrows*), indicating the presence of a small penumbra.

MRI Perfusion Limitations

If the patient in Case 16.5 presented 8 hours after symptom onset, should he or she receive intraarterial mechanical thrombectomy? The answer is controversial, in part because there is ongoing debate regarding the utility of perfusion data in stroke patients. *Some argue that changes in CBF better represent the final infarct size (ischemic penumbra + infarct core) than changes in MTT or CBV,[14,15] MTT perfusion defects can overestimate the area of ischemic penumbra,[14,16] and CBV most closely follows restricted diffusion changes.[13]* Using these principles, one may conclude that the infarct core is represented by a marked decline in CBV with associated restricted diffusion and that the ischemic penumbra is represented by reduced CBF, with normal CBV. However, such a conclusion would sometimes be erroneous because these general principles do not always hold in the individual patient. For example, *areas of the brain with restricted diffusion and decreased CBV do not always go on to infarction.[16,17]* In addition, *changes in CBF are not 100% sensitive for areas of the brain that go on to infarction.* Another seeming contradiction to the above theory is the demonstration that *MTT can occasionally underestimate infarct expansion.[14] Thus MRI and CT cannot yet definitively characterize areas of ischemic penumbra or infarct core in the human brain during ischemic stroke.[16]*

CASE 16.5 ANSWER

1. **B. Left perisylvian infarct in the left MCA distribution with small ischemic penumbra in the posterior left parietal lobe**

CASE 16.6

FIG. 16.C6

1. Given the imaging findings, what is the most likely cause for the stroke?
   A. Left M2 MCA occlusion
   B. Left M3 MCA occlusion
   C. Hypertensive infarct of small perforators supplying the caudate
   D. Left internal carotid artery dissection

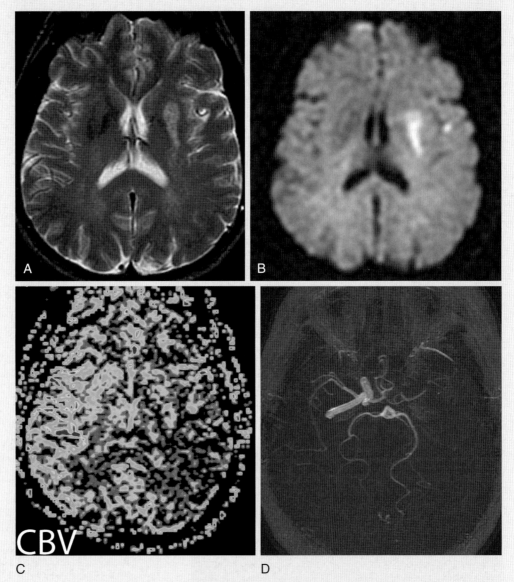

FIG. 16.C6. (A) Axial fast spin echo T2-weighted image. High T2 signal is seen in the left putamen. (B) Axial diffusion-weighted image. Restricted diffusion is noted in the left putamen and in the perisylvian left frontal lobe (confirmed on apparent diffusion coefficient (ADC) maps [not shown]). (C) Axial CBV map. There is decreased CBV in the left MCA distribution involving the left parietal more than the left frontal lobes. (D) Maximum intensity projection (MIP) image from a two-dimensional time-of-flight sequence. There is no flow in the left internal carotid artery. There is some flow in the bilateral anterior cerebral arteries and the left M1 segment, likely from collateral flow via the circle of Willis. There is an abrupt termination of the left M1 segment.

Discussion

In this case, most of the posterior distribution of the left MCA demonstrates decreased CBV, but the corresponding area of restricted diffusion is relatively small. Given the perfusion findings, left internal carotid artery dissection is the most correct answer. This is in contradistinction to the hypothesis that both the CBV and DWI maps can be used interchangeably to represent infarct core. (One example of the use of this hypothesis is the fact that many use CBV to represent infarct core in CTA perfusion cases where no DWI is available.[13]) Some have argued that the presence of a *CBV-DWI mismatch is strong evidence for the existence of an ischemic penumbra and that these patients would benefit the most from therapy.*[18] Based on the DWI, answer choice C would seem appropriate, but is incorrect given the perfusion abnormality and the lack of internal carotid artery (ICA) seen on the maximal intensity projection imaging. Answer choices A and

B are incorrect because no ICA is seen on the left. Filling of the proximal portion of the left MCA is likely through collateral flow. This patient was treated conservatively and recovered, with relatively few long-term sequelae from this left ICA dissection.

MRI Perfusion Methods

There are two general methods by which MR perfusion can be performed—bolus techniques and arterial spin labeling (ASL). Bolus perfusion techniques include dynamic susceptibility-weighted (DSC) and dynamic contrast-enhanced (DCE) MRI. These bolus techniques derive physiologic information from assessment of the concentration of gadolinium passing through the tissue microcirculation over time. This is done by repeatedly scanning the volume of interest, typically every second or so, before and after the administration of contrast agent.

DSC-MRI is based on the sequential acquisition of T2*-weighted images following contrast administration. Gadolinium's paramagnetic properties cause heterogeneity in the local magnetic field as it passes through the vasculature and/or tissues. These field heterogeneities cause dephasing of protons, resulting in a shortened T2* time and signal loss (see Chapters 2 and 8 for discussions on T2* and susceptibility artifact, respectively). Because these *susceptibility effects extend several millimeters beyond the actual gadolinium molecules (i.e., adjacent to a vessel), this method is particularly sensitive to the presence of contrast in areas of low vascular density*—for example, in capillary beds. Fig. 16.2 shows an example of the effects of gadolinium on the T2*-weighted signal of a region of interest of the brain over time.

Because the signal intensity over time reflects the concentration of gadolinium over time, a concentration-time curve (CTC) can be calculated from the signal intensity curve (Fig. 16.3).[19] *Physiologic parameters can then be calculated from the CTC as follows. The area under the CTC provides an estimate of the CBV within the voxel, MTT is estimated from the width of the contrast bolus, and regional CBF is calculated using the central volume theorem: CBF = CBV/MTT.*

The shape of the CTC is affected by various factors, including infusion rate, cardiovascular function, and vascular stenoses. These variations can invalidate direct interindividual (or even interscan) comparison of the derived parameters. One approach to this problem is to measure the concentration of arterial contrast agent over time—the arterial input function—from a large nearby artery and use this information to calculate CBF (Fig. 16.4). This process, termed *deconvolution,* estimates the CTC in each voxel that would be seen if the input were a bolus of infinitely short duration. By controlling for some of the variability in contrast delivery, deconvolution can be used as the basis for absolute measurements of CBF.[20] In Case 16.6, the provided CBV map is normalized to the reference arterial inflow. CBF and MTT can also be normalized in this way.[20]

In contrast to DSC-MRI, DCE-MRI uses T1-weighted sequences to characterize the CTC. The cardiac perfusion cases shown in the beginning of this chapter are examples of MRI perfusion using DCE-MRI. *Compared with susceptibility-related signal loss, gadolinium-induced T1 shortening is less susceptible to relatively remote alterations of the magnetic field outside of the vasculature, resulting in an extremely short radius of action. It is therefore particularly suitable to characterize the passage of contrast agent between the intravascular space and the extracellular-extravascular spaces.* There are many ways to characterize the CTC in DCE-MRI, including subjective, semiquantitative, and quantitative methods. Although more technically demanding, pharmacokinetic modeling can be used to extract quantitative physiologic information about the microcirculation. *Commonly modeled parameters include the fractional plasma volume, fractional volume of the extracellular-extravascular space, and K_{trans} (the transfer coefficient between the intravascular and extravascular spaces). The last*

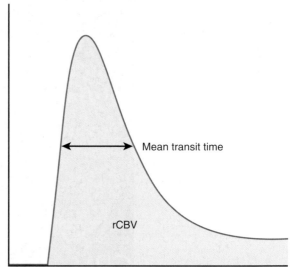

FIG. 16.3. Concentration-time curve (CTC). The *y*-axis is the concentration of contrast in a voxel; the *x*-axis is time. The CTC is mathematically derived from the signal intensity curve shown in Fig. 16.2. The cerebral blood volume (CBV) is estimated from the CTC by calculating the area underneath the curve. Mean transit time is estimated as the width of the contrast bolus. Cerebral blood flow can then be derived by dividing the CBV by the mean transit time. *rCBV,* relative CBV.

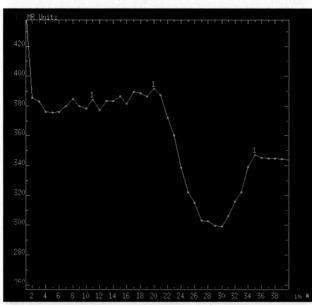

FIG. 16.2. Signal intensity curve over time of a region of interest in the brain during a dynamic susceptibility weighted perfusion study. The *y*-axis represents the net T2*-weighted signal intensity. The *x*-axis represents the image number (in this case, 40 images were obtained of the region of interest over a period of 1 minute). Note that during the first 21 images, the T2*-weighted signal in the selected region of interest is relatively unchanged. The contrast agent then enters the region of interest, and the signal begins to fall as a result of the T2*-shortening effects of gadolinium. The T2* signal hits a trough when the gadolinium concentration from the first pass reaches a maximum. Then, as the contrast agent washes out, the T2* signal begins rising again. The new baseline is lower than the precontrast images because the intravascular gadolinium has not yet been totally cleared from the intravascular pool.

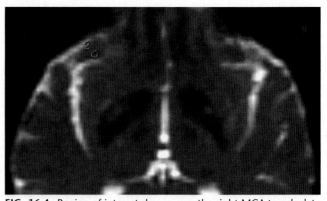

FIG. 16.4. Region of interest drawn over the right MCA to calculate an arterial input. The changes in signal over time in the artery reflect the changes from various parameters that are otherwise difficult to quantify, such as cardiovascular function and contrast bolus technique. This measurement is then used to calculate a more accurate CBF, CBV, and MTT (see text for more detailed discussion).[21]

parameter, which provides a measure of vessel permeability, is of particular interest in characterizing the effects of antiangiogenesis treatment in patients with high-grade primary brain tumors.

Compared to bolus techniques, *ASL perfusion imaging does not require an exogenous contrast agent, but uses a radiofrequency pulse to invert the spins of protons in flowing blood proximal to the areas of interest* (e.g., while blood is in the neck before cerebral perfusion imaging). *Inflow of these protons into a given voxel therefore results in a reduction in its signal intensity. The labeled image volume can then be subtracted from the dataset obtained using* *an identical MR sequence performed without the labeling pulse. The result is an image with contrast that is based primarily on tissue perfusion.* This technique is completely noninvasive, avoids the use of contrast agent, and is inherently quantitative, advantages that make it particularly well suited for certain populations. ASL perfusion techniques are thus under active development to be translated to routine clinical use.

CASE 16.6 ANSWER

1. **D. Left internal carotid artery dissection**

CASE 16.7

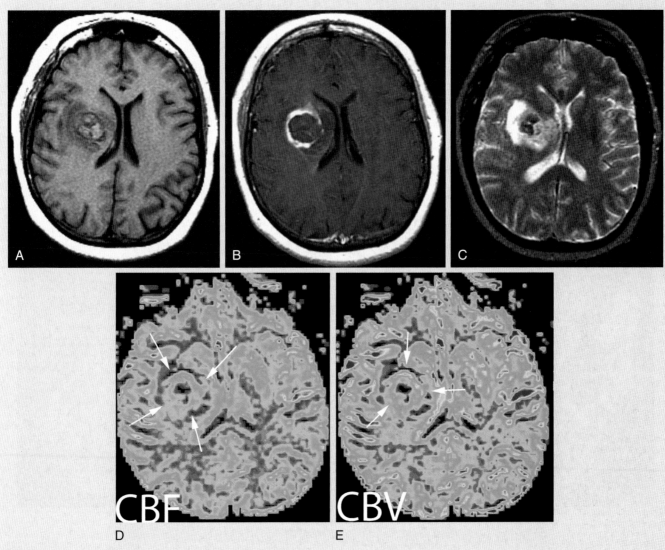

FIG. 16.C7

1. What is the most likely diagnosis given the imaging findings?
   A. Hypertensive parenchymal hemorrhage
   B. Hemorrhagic glioblastoma (glioblastoma multiforme)
   C. Meningioma
   D. Tumefactive multiple sclerosis

FIG. 16.C7. (A) Axial T1-weighted precontrast image. A heterogeneous lesion with areas that are intrinsically bright on T1-weighted imaging is centered in the right basal ganglia. (B) Axial T1-weighted postcontrast image. The lesion demonstrates thick and irregular rim enhancement. (C) Axial T2-weighted image. The lesion is heterogeneous on T2 with areas of low and high T2- weighted signal. (D) CBF and (E) CBV perfusion images. There is increased CBF and increased CBV along the rim of the lesion *(arrows)*.

Discussion

Hypertensive hemorrhage is the most common cause of spontaneous (nontraumatic) intraparenchymal hemorrhage in the adult brain. The diagnosis of hypertensive hemorrhage is often suggested by its location and a clinical history of hypertension. In Case 16.7, imaging demonstrates a heterogeneous lesion centered in the right basal ganglia, with signal characteristics consistent with blood products. There is a smooth rim of peripheral enhancement, a finding commonly seen as a parenchymal hematoma resolves. *The adjacent increased CBV is the only indicator that this bleed may not be hypertensive in cause. Hypertensive hemorrhage would be expected to have decreased perfusion in the area of the bleed.[21]* The patient in this case was ultimately diagnosed with glioblastoma multiforme. Tumefactive multiple sclerosis frequently has an incomplete rim of enhancement on MRI and does not have the complete thickened rim of enhancement shown in this case.

Other Uses of MRI Perfusion

Although perfusion imaging is useful to evaluate for ischemia, it also has a role in nonischemic disease, such as the characterization of neoplasms.[22] For example, perfusion imaging can help differentiate a highly vascular, high-grade tumor (relatively high CBV) from a low-grade tumor (low CBV),[23] although this does not always hold true—some low-grade tumors can have high CBV values, and some clinically benign intracranial tumors are highly vascular, such as meningiomas and choroid plexus tumors.[23] *Perfusion imaging can also help differentiate tumor recurrence (high CBV) from radiation necrosis (low CBV).[24]* This indication is particularly useful because tumor recurrence and radiation necrosis can have a similar appearance with conventional MRI techniques, manifesting as a mass with variable degrees of surrounding edema and ring enhancement on serial MRI evaluation.[24]

Less commonly, *perfusion imaging is used to evaluate the status of the intracranial vasculature.* For example, it can be used to evaluate overall brain perfusion before and after an extraintracranial bypass procedure.[25] *Perfusion imaging can also be used to characterize the vasculature of the brain adjacent to a mass before functional MRI.* In this situation, perfusion imaging can warn of possible false-negative results on functional MRI caused by tumor-induced failure of autoregulation (see Chapter 17 for a more thorough explanation).[26]

CASE 16.7 ANSWER

1. **B. Hemorrhagic glioblastoma (glioblastoma multiforme)**

CASE 16.8

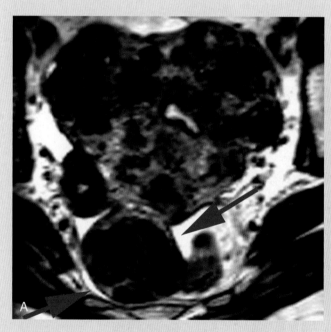
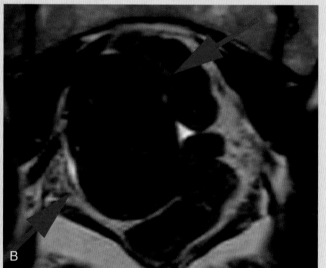

FIG. 16.C8

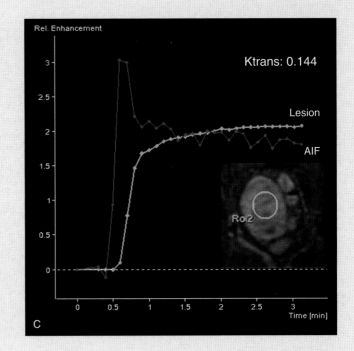

1. What is the most likely diagnosis for the posterior pelvic mass?
   A. Subserosal pedunculated leiomyoma
   B. Normal rectum filled with fecal material
   C. Ovarian fibroma
   D. Sacrococcygeal teratoma

FIG. 16.C8. (A) Axial T2-weighted image of the pelvis showing multiple uterine fibroids. There is also a low signal mass posterior to the uterus and adjacent to the uterus and rectum *(arrows)*. (B) Coronal T2-weighted image centered over the low signal mass in the posterior pelvis. The low T2-weighted signal mass is ovoid in shape and surrounded by multiple loops of bowel *(arrows)*. (C) Graph depicting relative enhancement of the lesion *(green curve)* following contrast administration. The *red curve* measures the enhancement in the aorta and thereby depicts the arterial input function (AIF; note that the region of interest for the aorta is not included in the field of view on these images). The inset coronal T1 DCE image in the right lower quadrant shows the region of interest drawn to acquire the perfusion data. The calculated K_{trans} for the region of interest was 0.144.

Discussion

Subserosal pedunculated uterine fibroids and ovarian fibromas can be difficult to differentiate with conventional MRI because they can be low in signal on T1- and T2-weighted images. Dynamic contrast enhancement can potentially be used to distinguish these masses. Uterine leiomyomas have greater maximal enhancement and higher rates of enhancement than ovarian fibromas.[27] In Case 16.8, a subserosal leiomyoma was favored, given the lesion's brisk homogeneous enhancement, similar to the patient's other intramural leiomyomas (not shown) and its apparent connection with the uterus on the axial image (Fig. 16.C8A). The normal rectum is adjacent to this mass.

Other Uses of MRI Perfusion

In addition to cardiac and neurologic evaluations, perfusion imaging is also being used to study genitourinary and gastrointestinal diseases. Perfusion imaging in these organ systems is frequently performed using T1-weighted dynamic contrast enhancement, the same technique used in the cardiac cases shown in the beginning of this chapter. Intravenous gadolinium is administered and multiple image volumes are acquired over time. A graph can then be generated describing the relative enhancement of the area of interest (see Fig. 16.C8C). Using the arterial input as a control, the concentration of gadolinium over time can then be computed.

Quantitative perfusion analysis is also frequently performed in body imaging. K_{trans} is one quantitative parameter often measured. K_{trans} measures the rate of diffusion of contrast between the intravascular space and the extravascular-extracellular space. K_{trans} is proportional to both the rate of flow in the vessels and their permeability.[28] As flow increases, there is more contrast to diffuse into the extravascular space; similarly, if the vessels are leaky (as in tumor vascularity), a higher percentage of contrast will leak into the extravascular space. *K_{trans} can be a useful quantitative parameter in oncology. As a malignant tumor grows, it promotes the growth of additional small vessels through angiogenesis. In general, the vessels recruited by tumor angiogenesis are abnormal in that they are especially fragile and leaky. Measuring this property, as expressed by K_{trans} can yield useful diagnostic information about the physiology of the lesion of interest.[28]*

CASE 16.8 ANSWER

1. **A. Subserosal pedunculated leiomyoma**

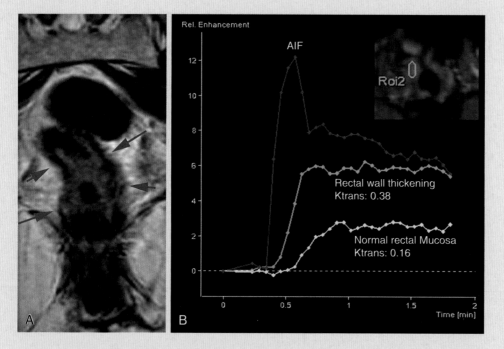

FIG. 16.C9

1. What is the most likely cause of the rectal wall thickening
   seen on this T2-weighted MRI image of the pelvis?
   A. Stercoral colitis
   B. Diverticulitis
   C. *Clostridium difficile* colitis
   D. Rectal carcinoma

FIG. 16.C9. (A) Coronal T2-weighted image of pelvis. There is masslike circumferential rectal wall thickening that is intermediate in T2-weighted signal intensity *(arrows)*. (B) Graph depicting relative enhancement over time. The *red curve* represents the arterial input function (AIF). The *green curve* is the enhancement of the masslike area of rectal wall thickening. The *yellow curve* is derived from a region of interest selected over normal rectal mucosa (not shown). Inset in the right upper corner is a coronal T1-weighted, DCE image showing the region of interest drawn over the rectal wall thickening. Qualitatively, the masslike area enhances much more quickly and reaches a higher peak than the normal rectal mucosa. Quantitatively, the perfusion is also increased in the area of rectal wall thickening. The measured K_{trans} of the area of wall thickening was 0.38, whereas the normal rectal mucosa K_{trans} measured 0.16.

Discussion

Inflammatory conditions, such as diverticulitis and various forms of colitis, can cause colorectal wall thickening. However, perfusion is not typically as elevated in these conditions.[29] Rectal carcinoma requires angiogenesis to ensure continued growth. Dynamic contrast enhancement has been shown to predict the degree of rectal carcinoma angiogenesis,[30] which can be used for diagnostic purposes. For example, one study has shown that *colon cancer and diverticulitis can be accurately distinguished using perfusion imaging; this differentiation can be difficult using anatomic criteria alone. Colorectal cancer has significantly higher levels of blood flow, blood volume, and vascular permeability.*[29] Given the increased perfusion, answer choice D is the correct answer. The level of perfusion would not be as elevated in diverticulitis and colitis; in addition, no diverticula are seen.

CASE 16.9 ANSWER

1. **D. Rectal carcinoma**

CASE 16.10

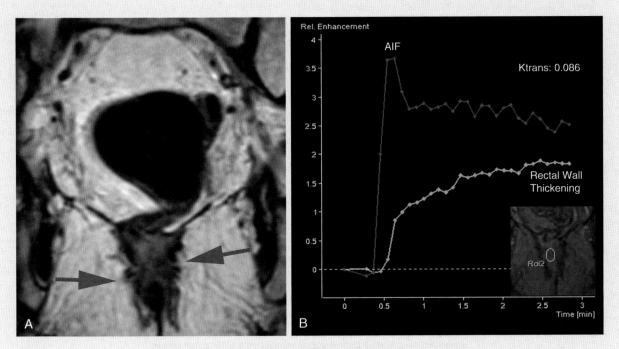

FIG. 16.C10

1. What is the most likely cause for the rectal wall thickening in this patient status post–low anterior resection for rectal carcinoma?
   A. Postsurgical scar
   B. Tumor recurrence
   C. Normal study; no wall thickening seen

FIG. 16.C10. (A) Coronal T2-weighted image through the pelvis in a patient with a history of low anterior resection for rectal carcinoma and coloanal anastomosis. Colonic wall thickening is noted at the anastomosis *(arrows).* (B) Graph depicting relative enhancement over time. The *red curve* is the arterial input function (AIF). The *green curve* is the enhancement of the area of rectal wall thickening. The inset coronal T1-weighted, DCE image in the right lower quadrant shows the region of interest used to calculate the curve. Qualitatively, the perfusion of the area of wall thickening appears low. This is supported by quantitative data that calculated K_{trans} for the area of abnormality at 0.086 (for perspective, this is <25% of the K_{trans} measured in the rectal carcinoma shown in Case 16.9).

Discussion

The primary imaging dilemma is whether the rectal wall thickening seen in Fig. 16.C10A represents postoperative scar or recurrent tumor. On conventional imaging, this can be a difficult distinction because both entities enhance and can be morphologically identical. *Perfusion imaging can help by characterizing the enhancement pattern in further detail. One study has shown that recurrent tumor demonstrates increased perfusion compared with scar.[31] That study specifically found that the relative* *enhancement of the wall thickening with respect to the arterial input was less in scar than in tumor.[31] Another as-yet unproven but possible distinction is that the enhancement curve for fibrosis continues to increase over time (**Fig. 16.C10B**), whereas tumor enhancement plateaus and then washes out.*

CASE 16.10 ANSWER

1. **A. Postsurgical scar**

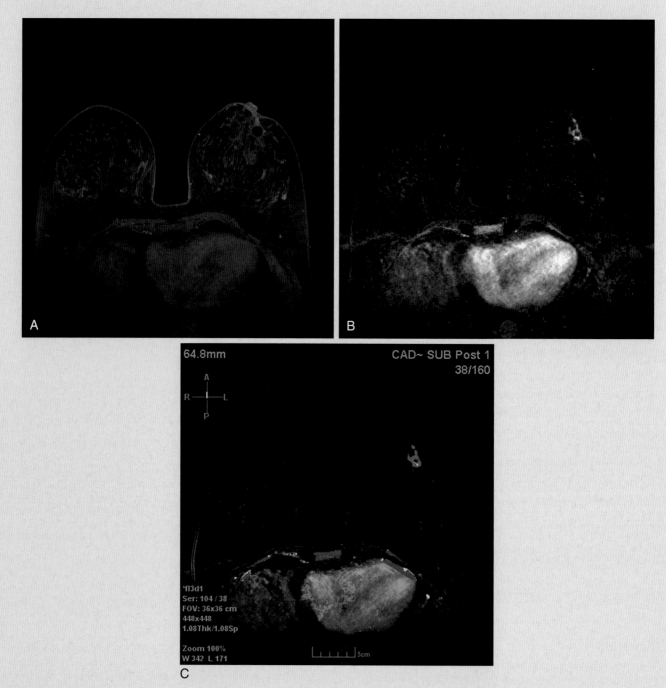

FIG. 16.C11

1. What postcontrast perfusion and kinetic characteristics
   would best describe this area of enhancement surrounding
   the susceptibility from a prior biopsy clip?
   A. Persistent
   B. Plateau
   C. Washout

FIG. 16.C11. (A) T1-weighted postcontrast, fat-suppressed axial image from breast MRI. Note the susceptibility artifact in the left anterior breast. There is enhancement surrounding the area of susceptibility with associated nipple retraction. (B) T1-weighted postcontrast subtraction MRI image better shows the degree of abnormal enhancement in the left breast (C). Computer-assisted diagnosis. This postsubtraction T1-weighted perfusion color-coded image shows the perfusion and kinetic characteristics in the area of abnormal enhancement. *Red* = washout; *yellow* = plateau; *blue* = persistent.

Discussion

Contrast-enhanced breast MRI is often performed after the diagnosis of breast cancer or ductal carcinoma in situ to evaluate the extent of disease or as a highly sensitive screening modality in women with a strong family history, history of mantle radiation, or increased genetic susceptibility to breast cancer. The addition of perfusion-based, DCE breast MRI and the resulting qualitative assessment of the type of contrast enhancement curve can result in higher diagnostic performance for establishing or excluding malignancy.[32] *Assessment of the type of time-signal intensity curve, more often called the kinetic curve, is performed by categorizing the washout pattern of a gadolinium contrast agent. There are three patterns of kinetic curves— type I, persistently enhancing (progressive), which is suggestive of benignity and by convention is color-coded as blue; type II, plateau type, which has an intermediate probability for malignancy and is color-coded as yellow; and type III, washout type, which is highly indicative of malignancy and is color-coded as red.[32] The washout patterns are typically assessed qualitatively and assigned on the most suspicious type of kinetics present.*

In Case 16.11, there is an area of abnormal enhancement surrounding the susceptibility artifact from the previous biopsy clip as seen on the T1 contrast-enhanced and subtracted images. The subtracted image is formed by subtracting the T1 precontrast series from the T1 postcontrast series, which serves to highlight the areas of abnormal enhancement. The kinetic curve and color overlay is generated using computer-assisted diagnosis software. The abnormal enhancement primarily shows persistent kinetics. However, there is an area of plateau and washout kinetics along the posterior aspect of the enhancement. Because the overall kinetics is based on the most suspicious characteristic, this area of abnormal enhancement has washout kinetics and is indicative of residual malignancy as opposed to postbiopsy changes.

CASE 16.11 ANSWER

1. **C. Washout**

TAKE-HOME POINTS

Defining Perfusion

1. The perfusion of an organ is an inherent physiologic parameter that can be altered in disease states. Perfusion can be measured with many different techniques, including MRI.
2. MRI perfusion can be assessed by two main types of techniques—bolus techniques that use a gadolinium-based contrast agent and ASL.
3. DCE is a T1-weighted bolus technique used frequently in cardiac perfusion imaging and body perfusion imaging.
4. DSC is a T2*-weighted bolus technique used frequently in brain perfusion imaging.
5. ASL does not use any contrast. Flowing intravascular protons are instead labeled using radiofrequency pulses applied upstream to the images.

Cardiac Perfusion Imaging

1. Cardiac perfusion imaging is a useful tool to evaluate for stress-induced myocardial ischemia.
2. Electrocardiographically gated T1-weighted images are obtained postcontrast. Cardiac perfusion analysis is usually qualitative; the raw images are analyzed visually.
3. Occasionally, cardiac perfusion imaging can also be helpful to distinguish between tumor and thrombus.

Brain Perfusion Imaging

1. The penumbra is the area of the brain that is ischemic but not yet infarcted. This is the area of the brain that is potentially salvageable with intervention.

2. MRI seeks to define the penumbra. In theory, a diffusion defect represents the infarcted core, and the perfusion defect is the entire ischemic area. The difference between the diffusion and perfusion images is the penumbra.
3. Brain perfusion analysis uses quantitative techniques. Perfusion parameters such as CBF, CBV, and MTT are mathematically computed and displayed in a series of color-coded images.
4. The CBV is the volume of blood within the small vessels and capillary bed in a given area of the brain.
5. The MTT is the time it takes for blood to traverse the capillary bed: CBF = CBV/MTT.
6. Brain perfusion imaging can also be used to characterize the grade of tumors, to distinguish between radiation necrosis and tumors, and to characterize blood flow.

Body Perfusion Imaging

1. Dynamic contrast enhancement can be used in the genitourinary and gastrointestinal systems to characterize lesions.
2. Malignant tumors rely on angiogenesis to grow. This angiogenesis creates fragile and leaky vessels. The leakiness of these vessels can be measured using K_{trans}, a quantitative parameter derived from perfusion imaging.
3. Qualitative assessment of contrast enhancement perfusion kinetics can result in higher diagnostic performance for establishing or excluding malignancy with breast MRI.

References

1. Lee VS. *Cardiovascular MRI: Physical Principles to Practical Protocols*. Philadelphia: Lippincott Williams & Wilkins; 2006.
2. Kim RJ, Fieno DS, Parrish TB, et al. Relationship of MRI delayed contrast enhancement to irreversible injury, infarct age, and contractile function. *Circulation.* 1999;100:1992–2002.
3. Tadamura E, Yamamuro M, Kubo S, et al. Hibernating myocardium identified by cardiovascular magnetic resonance and positron emission tomography. *Circulation.* 2006;113:e158–e159.
4. The National Institute of Neurological Disorders and Stroke rt-PA Stroke Study Group. Tissue plasminogen activator for acute ischemic stroke. *N Engl J Med.* 1995;333:1581–1588.
5. Lees KR, Bluhmki E, von Kummer R, et al. ECASS, ATLANTIS, NINDS and EPITHET rt-PA Study Group Investigators. Time to treatment with intravenous alteplase and outcome in stroke: an updated pooled analysis of ECASS, ATLANTIS, NINDS, and EPITHET trials. *Lancet.* 2010;375:1695–1703.
6. Powers WJ, Derdeyn CP, Biller J, et al. American Heart Association Stroke Council.
7. Campbell BC, Mitchell PJ, Kleinig TJ, et al. Endovascular therapy for ischemic stroke with perfusion-imaging selection. *N Engl J Med.* 2015;372:1009–1018.
8. Saver JL, Goyal M, Bonafe A, et al. Stent-retriever thrombectomy after intravenous

2015 AHA/ASA focused update of the 2013 guidelines for the early management of patients with acute ischemic stroke regarding endovascular treatment: a guideline for healthcare professionals from the American Heart Association/American Stroke Association. *Stroke.* 2015;46(10):3020–3035.

t-PA vs. t-PA alone in stroke. *N Engl J Med.* 2015;372:2285–2295.

9. Fransen PS, Beumer D, Berkhemer OA, et al. MR CLEAN, a multicenter randomized clinical trial of endovascular treatment for acute ischemic stroke in the Netherlands: study protocol for a randomized controlled trial. *Trials.* 2014;15:343.

10. Goyal M, Demchuk AM, Menon BK, et al. Randomized assessment of rapid endovascular treatment of ischemic stroke. *N Engl J Med.* 2015;372:1019–1030.

11. Jovin TG, Chamorro A, Cobo E, et al. Thrombectomy within 8 hours after symptom onset in ischemic stroke. *N Engl J Med.* 2015;372:2296–2306.

12. Srinivasan A, Goyal M, Al Azri F, Lum C. State-of-the-art imaging of acute stroke. *Radiographics.* 2006;26(suppl 1):S75–S95.

13. de Lucas ME, Sánchez E, Gutiérrez A, et al. CT protocol for acute stroke: tips and tricks for general radiologists. *Radiographics.* 2008;28:1673–1687.

14. Parsons M, Yang Q, Barber A, et al. Perfusion magnetic resonance imaging maps in hyperacute stroke. *Stroke.* 2000;32:1581–1587.

15. Rohl L, Ostergaard L, Simonsen C, et al. Viability thresholds of ischemic penumbra of hyperacute stroke defined by perfusion-weighted MRI and apparent diffusion coefficient. *Stroke.* 2001;32:1524–1628.

16. Kidwell C, Alger J, Saver J. Evolving paradigms in neuroimaging of the ischemic penumbra. *Stroke.* 2004;35:2662–2665.

17. Kranz PG, Eastwood JD. Does diffusion-weighted imaging represent the ischemic core? An evidence-based systematic review. *AJNR Am J Neuroradiol.* 2009;30(6):1206–1212.

18. Schaefer P, Hunter G, He J, et al. Predicting cerebral ischemic infarct volume with diffusion and perfusion MR imaging. *ANJR Am J Neuroradiol.* 2002;23:1785–1794.

19. Atlas SW. *Magnetic Resonance Imaging of the Brain and Spine.* 4th ed. Philadelphia: Lippincott Williams & Wilkins; 2009.

20. Rempp KA, Brix G, Wenz F, et al. Quantification of regional cerebral blood flow and volume with dynamic susceptibility contrast-enhanced MR imaging. *Radiology.* 1994;193:637–641.

21. Kidwell CS, Saver JL, Mattiello J, et al. Diffusion-perfusion MR evaluation of perihematomal injury in hyperacute intracerebral hemorrhage. *Neurology.* 2001;57:1611–1617.

22. Wintermark M, Sesay M, Barbier E, et al. Comparative overview of brain perfusion imaging techniques. *Stroke.* 2005;36:e83–e99.

23. Cha S, Knopp EA, Johnson G, et al. Intracranial mass lesions: dynamic contrast-enhanced susceptibility-weighted echo-planar perfusion MR imaging. *Radiology.* 2002;223:11–29.

24. Barajas RF, Chang JS, Segal MR, et al. Differentiation of recurrent glioblastoma multiforme from radiation necrosis after external beam radiation therapy with dynamic susceptibility-weighted contrast-enhanced perfusion MR imaging. *Radiology.* 2009;253:486–496.

25. Caramia F, Santoro A, Pantano P, et al. Cerebral hemodynamics on MR perfusion images before and after bypass surgery in patients with giant intracranial aneurysms. *AJNR Am J Neuroradiol.* 2001;22:1704–1710.

26. Hou BL, Bradbury M, Peck KK, et al. Effect of brain tumor neovasculature defined by rCBV on BOLD fMRI activation volume in the primary motor cortex. *Neuroimage.* 2006;32:489–497.

27. Thomassin-Naggara I, Daraï E, Nassar-Slaba J, et al. Value of dynamic enhanced magnetic resonance imaging for distinguishing between ovarian fibroma and subserous uterine leiomyoma. *J Comput Assist Tomogr.* 2007;1:236–242.

28. Yankeelov TE, Gore JC. Dynamic contrast-enhanced magnetic resonance imaging in oncology: theory, data acquisition, analysis, and examples. *Curr Med Imaging Rev.* 2009;3(2):91–107.

29. Goh V, Halligan S, Taylor SA, et al. Differentiation between diverticulitis and colorectal cancer: quantitative CT perfusion measurements versus morphologic criteria—initial experience. *Radiology.* 2007;242:456–462. 2007.

30. Zhang XM, Yu D, Zhang HL, et al. 3D dynamic contrast-enhanced MRI of rectal carcinoma at 3T: correlation with microvascular density and vascular endothelial growth factor markers of tumor angiogenesis. *J Magn Reson Imaging.* 27:1309–1316.

31. Dicle O, Obuz F, Cakmakci H. Differentiation of recurrent rectal cancer and scarring with dynamic MR imaging. *Br J Radiol.* 1999;72:1155–1159.

32. El Khouli RH, Macura KJ, Jacobs MA, et al. Dynamic contrast-enhanced MRI of the breast: quantitative method for kinetic curve type assessment. *AJR Am J Roentgenol.* 2009;193(4):W295–W300.

CHAPTER 17

Magnetic Resonance Spectroscopy

Wells I. Mangrum, Allen W. Song, and Jeffrey R. Petrella

OPENING CASE 17.1

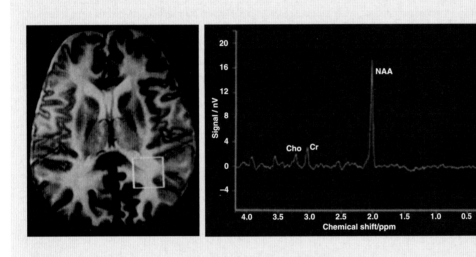

1. What is the diagnosis?
   A. Metachromatic leukodys-
      trophy
   B. HIV encephalopathy
   C. Postradiation therapy
   D. Canavan disease

CASE ANSWER

OPENING CASE 17.1

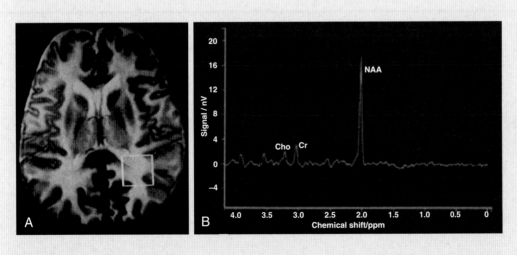

FIG. 17.C1. (A) Axial T2-weighted MR image. There is diffusely increased T2 signal in the white matter, including the subcortical white matter. The *square* overlying the left parietal white matter marks the voxel analyzed by spectroscopy. (B) Point-resolved, single-voxel spectroscopy waveform (echo time = 30 ms). *N*-acetyl aspartate (NAA), choline (Cho), and creatine (Cr) peaks are labeled. The NAA peak is markedly elevated with respect to the choline and creatine peaks.

1. What is the diagnosis?
   D. Canavan disease

Discussion

Canavan disease is an autosomal recessive dysmyelinating disease that is thought to result from a deficiency of aspartoacylase. This deficiency leads to elevated *N*-acetyl aspartate (NAA) levels in the brain, serum, and urine. Patients present in the first year of life with macrocephaly and spasticity. Death usually occurs within the first few years of life. Imaging findings include diffuse and symmetric increased T2 signal in the cerebral subcortical and deep white matter. The elevated NAA peak on spectroscopy is a characteristic finding of Canavan disease.[1] Metachromatic leukodystrophy, HIV encephalopathy, and radiation changes could all have a similar appearance on the T2-weighted sequence. However, they would not have the markedly elevated NAA peak that is more characteristic of Canavan disease.

Magnetic Resonance Spectroscopy

MR spectroscopy (MRS) creates a waveform on a graph (often referred to as a spectrum) and does not produce an image. *The spectrum reflects the concentration of molecules in a voxel of interest.* Knowing the chemical environment can be useful to help make the diagnosis.

Proton spectroscopy, the technique most often used clinically, identifies the molecules in a voxel by measuring the effect that these molecules have on a proton's precession frequency. A proton in pure free water precesses at a frequency defined by the Larmor equation (at 1.5 T, the precession frequency of a proton in water is ~64 MHz). If that proton is not free in water but instead is free in a chemically different molecule, such as NAA, then the precession frequency of that proton is slightly altered. This alteration of frequency is measured in Hertz and is therefore expressed in parts per million with respect to the precession frequency of water (measured in MHz). For example, *the chemical shift for NAA is 2.02 ppm. This means that a proton in NAA in a 1.5-T magnet has a precession frequency that is shifted from that of water by 128 Hz* (64 million × [2/million] = 128).

Each molecule, because of the unique environment of its protons, has a specific chemical shift—for example, the chemical shift of NAA is 2.02 ppm, lactate is 1.33 ppm, and choline is 3.22 ppm. Because parts per million is a normalized quantity, the chemical shift does not change with field strength. NAA has a chemical shift of 2.0 ppm at 1.5 and 3 T. Similarly, choline is always 3.2 ppm and lactate is always 1.33 ppm. *By measuring the precession frequency of a proton and calculating the chemical shift, the relative quantity and type of molecules in a given voxel can be determined.* This molecular environment is represented graphically by the spectroscopy waveform. *The x-axis of the waveform represents the chemical shift in ppm. The y-axis is proportional to the relative number of protons with that chemical shift. The area under the curve of each peak represents the relative concentration of the molecule of interest.*

To interpret the results of MRS, one needs to understand the function of the different molecules being measured (Table 17.1).[2,3] NAA is synthesized in the mitochondria of neurons, and its function is unknown. Clinically, NAA serves as a marker for the presence of neurons, including neuronal axons in white matter. Creatine (Cr) is used clinically as a marker for energy metabolism. Low levels of creatine suggest that the area of interest is highly metabolically active. Creatine is also often assumed to be stable and is used for calculating metabolite ratios (e.g., Cho:Cr, NAA:Cr). Choline (Cho) is found in the cell membrane. It serves as a marker for the cellular turnover of a lesion. Choline is elevated in the setting of increased cellular production, such as in a tumor, and in the setting of cellular breakdown, such as in leukodystrophy and multiple sclerosis. Lactate is a marker for anaerobic metabolism. Normally, lactate levels in the brain are so low that they cannot be measured by spectroscopy. Increased anaerobic metabolism, such as with ischemia or tumor necrosis, results in lactate peaks. Myoinositol (Myo) is a sugar. It is absent from neurons but present in glial cells. It is used as a marker for glial proliferation or an increase in glial size. Lipids are markers for fat, as seen in the subcutaneous tissues or in the diploic space of the calvarium.

It is important to know a few of the limitations of spectroscopy. *First, the molecular levels are often not specific.* For example, a novice may see a lactate peak in a lesion and use that information to conclude that the lesion is due to an infarct. Although it is true that lactate peaks can be seen in infarcts, many other conditions can cause lactate peaks, including tumors, seizures, metabolic conditions, and inflammatory conditions.[4] Similarly, an increase in the choline level may cause one to conclude that the lesion in question is a tumor. However, increased choline levels are also noted in infarctions, inflammation, and multiple sclerosis.[4] One must therefore always interpret the MRS finding in the context of conventional MRI findings.

A second limitation to spectroscopy is a low signal-to-noise ratio (SNR) due to the extremely low concentrations of the chemical moieties being measured. To overcome the low SNR, *voxel size needs to be large (i.e., on the order of centimeters), resulting in low spatial resolution.* At times, this can be a limiting factor clinically, where we are often concerned about lesions smaller than 1 cm³.

Table 17.1 COMMON SPECTROSCOPY MOLECULES: CHEMICAL SHIFTS, MAIN FUNCTIONS, AND CLASSIC ASSOCIATIONS

Molecule	Chemical Shift (ppm)	Function	Examples of Classic Association
Lipids	0.8–1.5	Fat	↑ Dipolic space and subcutaneous fat
Lactate	1.33	Anaerobic activity	↑ Ischemia, infarction, seizures, mitochondrial disorders, necrotic tumors
N-acetyl aspartate (NAA)	2.02	Neuronal, axonal marker	↓ Leukodystrophy, malignant neoplasm, multiple sclerosis, infarction ↑ Elevated in Canavan disease
Creatine (Cr)	3.02	Marker of metabolic activity	Assumed to be unchanged and used to calculate ratios (Cho:Cr and NAA:Cr)
Choline (Cho)	3.22	Cellular turnover	↑ Increased in tumors, inflammation, infection, multiple sclerosis
Myoinositol (Myo)	3.56	Glial marker	↑ Gliosis, astrocytosis, Alzheimer disease

↑, Increased; ↓, decreased.

FIG. 17.C2

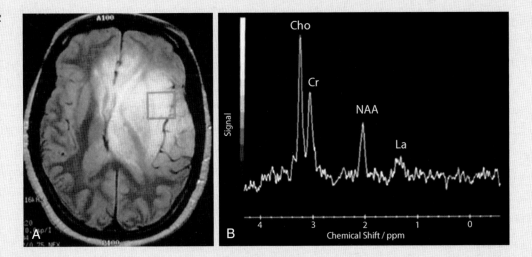

1. What abnormalities are seen in the spectrum?
   A. Elevated NAA:Cr ratio
   B. Decreased Cho:Cr ratio
   C. Lactate peak
   D. Increased chemical shift of NAA

2. What is the diagnosis?
   A. Acute infarct
   B. Gliomatosis cerebri
   C. Metastatic disease
   D. Multiple sclerosis

FIG. 17.C2. (A) Axial FLAIR image of brain. Increased T2 signal is centered in the left frontal lobe but is seen to extend into the left basal ganglia and, via the corpus callosum, into the right frontal lobe and basal ganglia. There is relative preservation of the normal brain architecture. A small amount of mass effect with a left to right midline shift is noted. The square overlying the left perisylvian region demarcates the single voxel measured in the corresponding spectroscopy waveform. (B) Point-resolved, single-voxel spectroscopy spectrum (echo time = 30 ms) demonstrates elevation of the Cho:Cr ratio and decrease of the NAA:Cr ratio. A small, poorly defined peak at 1.2 to 1.4 ppm is consistent with a lactate (La) peak. The NAA peak is at the 2.02 level; this peak does not change with pathology.

Discussion

Gliomatosis cerebri is a diffusely infiltrating neoplasm associated with a poor prognosis that occurs predominantly in middle-aged adults (40s–50s). MRI usually reveals diffuse and contiguous infiltration of the white matter of at least two lobes that is isointense on T1-weighted images and hyperintense on T2-weighted images. The overlying brain structure is preserved. Frequently, there is bihemispheric extension through the corpus callosum into the basal ganglia.[5,6]

Gliomatosis cerebri usually has a decrease in the NAA peak on spectroscopy.[5] The choline peak can be variable. There is some evidence that elevation of the choline peak, as seen in this case, is inversely related to patient prognosis.[5,7] Elevation of the lactate peak is another concerning finding.[5]

Normal Spectrum

To know whether a peak is abnormally elevated or decreased, one must first know the appearance of a normal spectrum. The spectrum of the normal human brain is predominantly made up of NAA, creatine, choline, and myo-inositol peaks. *In the normal brain, a line can usually be drawn connecting the peaks of these four molecules. This line makes a 45-degree angle with the x-axis, an angle referred to as Hunter's angle.* An alteration in the angle or a peak outside the line is a cause for concern (Fig. 17.1).

Hunter's angle can help interpret the changes in the molecular peaks of a spectrum. In Case 17.2, the choline peak at 3.2 ppm is higher than the creatine peak at 3.0 ppm. Assuming that creatine is unchanged, and recalling that in the normal situation choline is less than creatine (think of Hunter's angle), we can conclude that choline is elevated in this case. Similarly,

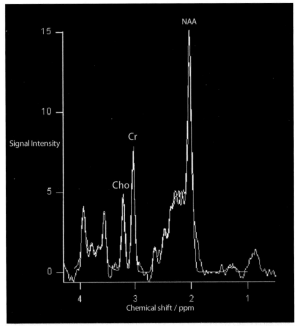

FIG. 17.1. Spectroscopy waveform in normal brain (TE = 135 ms). A peak of the waveform at 2.02 ppm means that NAA is abundant in the area of interest; conversely, a trough of the waveform at 1.33 ppm means that there are relatively few molecules of lactate in the area of interest. Note that a line forming a 45-degree angle to the x-axis can be drawn connecting the peaks of Myo, Cho, Cr, and NAA. The angle that this line forms is known as *Hunter's angle.*

NAA is less than creatine, a reversal of the normal relationship, indicating a decrease in NAA levels. A lactate peak, which presents as a doublet peak above baseline at a short echo time (TE) (~30 ms) and inverts at a long TE (~135 ms), is always abnormal.

Hunter's angle is a useful visual aid for beginners as they introduce themselves to spectroscopy but, like many rules, it has many exceptions and should be used with caution. Hunter's angle generally applies to images obtained of the cortex with a stimulated echo acquisition mode (STEAM) sequence and a short TE. (The STEAM sequence is an alternative to the point-resolved, single-voxel spectroscopy [PRESS] sequence and is further discussed in Case 17.3.) Changing any of these technical factors, even in the normal brain, can cause a disruption of Hunter's angle.[8]

Another factor complicating the understanding of the normal spectrum is its variability in healthy subjects. The normal spectrum changes from infancy to adulthood. At birth, NAA levels are low, and choline and myoinositol levels are high. By 4 years of age, the spectra have a more adult appearance.[3,9]

The normal spectrum also differs within specific regions of the brain. Above the level of the ventricles, choline is higher in the frontal than parietal lobes and higher in the white matter than the cortical gray matter. Below the level of the third ventricle, choline levels are elevated in the insular cortex, thalamus, and hypothalamus.[3,10]

Because the normal spectrum changes with age, regional location within the brain, and imaging technique, it is often difficult to predict what it should look like. For this reason, it is often helpful to obtain a spectrum of the contralateral normal hemisphere for purposes of comparison in cases of localized pathology. Fortunately, metabolites are highly symmetric between the left and right hemispheres in normal patients.[11]

CASE 17.2 ANSWERS

1. **C. Lactate peak**
2. **B. Gliomatosis cerebri**

CASE 17.3

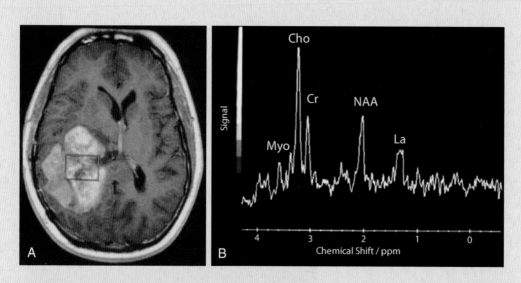

FIG. 17.C3

1. What metabolite changes in an astrocytoma predict a higher grade?
   A. Lower Cho:NAA ratio
   B. Lower Cho:Cr ratio
   C. Lower myoinositol level
   D. Lower lactate level

FIG. 17.C3. (A) Axial T1-weighted postcontrast MR image. A heterogeneously enhancing mass is centered in the right parietal periventricular white matter. There is associated mass effect with mild right to left midline shift. The square within the mass in the right parietal lobe marks the area characterized by spectroscopy. (B) PRESS spectrum (TE = 30 ms). There is a small but abnormal lactate peak. NAA levels are decreased, and choline levels are markedly increased. Myoinositol levels are also decreased.

Astrocytoma Grading

In general, the higher the grade of the primary brain tumor, the greater the Cho:NAA and Cho:Cr ratios and the lower the myoinositol level.[12,13] This case of a glioblastoma multiforme (GBM) with markedly elevated choline and decreased myoinositol levels supports the spectroscopy grading hypothesis.

However, it should be noted that some low-grade tumors have elevated choline levels, and some high-grade tumors can have low choline levels, so it is difficult to assign a grade to an individual tumor based on spectroscopy alone.[3] However, MRS combined with conventional imaging is quite effective at distinguishing high- and low-grade tumors.[4]

Single-Voxel Versus Multivoxel Spectroscopy

Spectroscopy techniques can be divided into single-voxel and multivoxel techniques. In the single-voxel technique—the technique used to produce the waveform in the preceding cases—the spectrum is generated from a single region of the brain. Three 90-degree, slice-selective pulses are used to select the voxel of interest (Fig. 17.2). This technique is termed **point-resolved, single-voxel spectroscopy (PRESS).** The selected voxel size is usually on the order of 8 cm³ (2 × 2 × 2 cm). Even though the voxel of interest is specifically selected, signal from outside the voxel can still manifest. To minimize this outside noise, so-called crusher gradients and outer-volume suppression pulses are also used. An alternative to the PRESS technique is the STEAM technique. The STEAM sequence uses three 90-degree pulses to generate a stimulated echo (which only captures half of the available signal) and the corresponding three slice-selective gradients along three different axes to localize the voxel of interest. STEAM is seldom used today in clinical practice, in part because PRESS has a higher SNR.[3]

The advantages of a single-voxel technique include short scan times and the relative ease with which short TE studies can be performed. The main disadvantage of the single-voxel technique is that only one voxel is measured, limiting the ability to determine changes in metabolite concentration over different areas in the brain. The single-voxel technique can be performed multiple times to get different samples over space, but such a strategy often exceeds the time constraints of a normal clinical MRI.[3] The other disadvantage of the single-voxel technique is its large voxel size. A large voxel size makes it difficult to obtain an accurate spectrum from smaller regions, such as the enhancing rim of a centrally necrotic tumor, because of partial volume averaging with adjacent areas.

POINT-RESOLVED SPECTROSCOPY

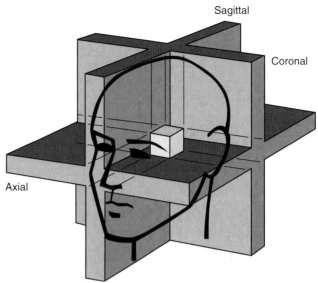

FIG. 17.2. Image representing voxel selection in PRESS. The voxel of interest is defined by the cube created by the intersection of the three 90-degree slice selection pulses. (Courtesy Cecil Charles, PhD.)

CASE 17.3 ANSWER

1. **C. Lower myoinositol level**

CASE 17.4

FIG. 17.C4

1. What chemical levels in an astrocytoma predict a low grade?
   A. Elevated Myo:Cr ratio
   B. High NAA:Cr ratio
   C. High Cho:Cr ratio
   D. Lactate peak

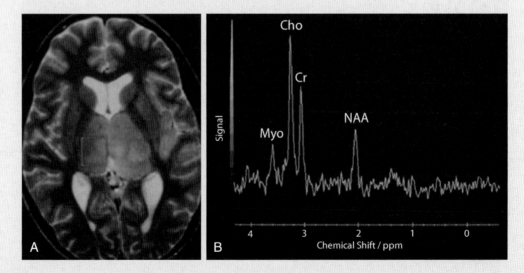

FIG. 17.C4. (A) Axial fast spin echo (FSE) T2-weighted MR image. There is high T2 signal and masslike expansion involving the bilateral thalami. The lesion is well defined, and there is relatively little vasogenic edema in the surrounding white matter. A square demarcates the voxel of interest for the spectroscopy waveform. (B) PRESS spectrum (TE = 30 ms). The NAA:Cr ratio is low, and the Cho:Cr ratio is high. A myoinositol peak at 3.6 ppm is noted. The Myo:Cr ratio is not elevated.

Low-Grade Astrocytoma

The diagnosis of a tumor is supported by the spectroscopy waveform, but the spectroscopy results are equivocal with respect to tumor grade. Elevated NAA:Cr and Cho:Cr ratios in this case support a higher-grade tumor. Furthermore, the Myo:Cr ratio is not elevated in this case. In a well-differentiated astrocytoma, we would expect to see an elevated Myo:Cr ratio. One study found the Myo:Cr ratio to average 0.8 in low-grade astrocytomas, 0.5 in normal control patients, 0.3 in anaplastic astrocytomas, and 0.15 in GBM.[13] At the same time, the lack of a lactate peak argues against a high-grade tumor such as GBM. The equivocal spectroscopy findings in this case demonstrate that it is difficult to discern the grade of an astrocytoma based on the spectroscopy waveform alone and that such findings need to be interpreted in the context of conventional MRI findings.[14]

Spectroscopy Changes With Field Strength and Time to Echo

Although the general positions of the chemical peaks in a spectrum do not change with the field strength, the MRS spectrum does improve with the field strength and the TE used. With higher field strength, the SNR increases, and the spectral resolution improves. The spectral resolution improvement is visually manifested as a narrowing of the molecule peak width. This allows for improved resolution of molecules with similar chemical shifts. For these reasons, spectroscopy is often preferred in magnets with higher field strength.[3]

The MRS spectrum changes with TE because of the different T2 times of each compound measured. *At long TEs (140–280 ms), only choline, creatine, and NAA are detected in normal patients. Lactate, alanine, or other molecules may be detectable if their concentrations are abnormally elevated.* Compounds with short T2 relaxation times, such as myoinositol and lipids, are not visible with long TEs. This is because the short T2 relaxation time of these molecules causes these molecules to lose all of their signal with long TEs. At a short TE (≤35 ms), all the aforementioned molecules can be visualized.[3] MRS protocols need to be created with these TE effects in mind. If the myoinositol level is important for the diagnosis, a short TE is required. If one is only interested in the NAA, choline, and creatine peaks, then a long TE should be used because there will be less noise caused by the molecules with a short T2 relaxation time.

CASE 17.4 ANSWER

1. **A. Elevated Myo:Cr ratio**

CASE 17.5

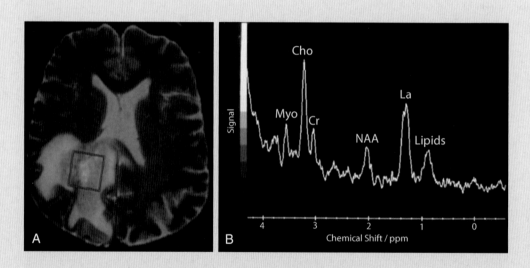

FIG. 17.C5

1. If a diseased area of the brain has an elevated lactate level, then the presence of the lactate level decreases the likelihood of which disease?
   A. Infarct
   B. Chronic multiple sclerosis plaque
   C. GBM
   D. Mitochondrial disease

FIG. 17.C5. (A) Axial fast spin echo T2-weighted MR image of the brain. A mass is centered in the right periventricular white matter. T2 prolongation is seen in the surrounding white matter. The square demarcates the area of interest for spectroscopy. (B) PRESS spectrum (TE = 30 ms). Lactate levels are markedly elevated, NAA levels are reduced, choline levels are elevated, and myoinositol levels are neither elevated nor decreased.

Lactate Peaks

This patient has a GBM. The elevated lactate levels are presumably secondary to the central ischemia and necrosis. Under normal conditions, the lactate levels in the brain are so low that they are not detectable. However, local hypoxia or ischemia can result in anaerobic metabolism in the brain and the production of lactate. Elevated lactate levels can be seen in brain tumors (e.g., in this case), mitochondrial disease, infarcts, and other diseases. Acute demyelinating plaques of multiple sclerosis can contain elevated lactate levels, but these lactate levels typically resolve on follow-up imaging.[15]

The lactate peak has a characteristic double peak at 1.33 ppm. This double peak is a useful marker to remember because sometimes lipid peaks, which range from 0.8 to 1.55 ppm, can overlap in appearance with lactate peaks. However, it would be unusual for a lipid to have a similar double peak at 1.33 ppm. Another way to distinguish between lactate and lipid peaks is to lengthen the TE. Lipids have a short T2 relaxation time and are only seen on short TEs. If a long TE is used, the lipid signal will be eliminated, and only the lactate peak will remain. It is interesting to note that if an intermediate TE is used (144 ms), the lactate peak will invert along the y-axis and result in a negative double peak! The reason for this inversion of the lactate peak is scalar coupling between methyl groups in the lactate molecule.[16]

CASE 17.5 ANSWER

1. **B. Chronic multiple sclerosis plaque**

CASE 17.6

FIG. 17.C6

1. What metabolite changes would be expected in an acute infarct?
   A. No lactate peak
   B. Decreased NAA:Cr ratio
   C. Elevated Cho:Cr ratio
   D. Elevation of the creatine peak

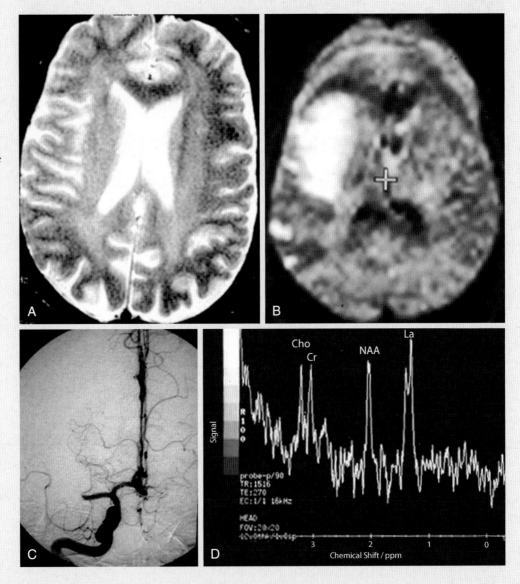

FIG. 17.C6. (A) Axial fast spin echo T2-weighted MR image. There is poorly defined increased T2 signal in the right perisylvian cortex in the right middle cerebral artery (MCA) distribution. (B) Axial diffusion-weighted MRI. Restricted diffusion is seen in the right basal ganglia and right frontal and parietal lobes in the right MCA distribution. (C) Right internal carotid arteriogram. An abrupt cutoff of flow is seen in the M1 segment of the right MCA. (D) PRESS spectrum (TE = 270 ms). The lactate doublet peak is the dominant peak. There is also a slight increase in the Cho:Cr ratio and a decrease in the NAA:Cr ratio. The creatine peak is used as a reference peak for the other chemical constituents.

Acute Infarct

The MRI and angiographic images are diagnostic of an acute stroke. The MRS spectrum demonstrates the changes of an acute stroke. NAA levels are decreased as a result of neuronal loss, and lactate levels are elevated as a result of increased anaerobic metabolism. (Note that at a TE of 270 ms, the lactate doublet peak is now again positive. See discussion of Case 17.5 regarding inversion of the lactate peak at intermediate TE values.) Choline levels in ischemic stroke are less

predictable.[17] Although elevated lactate peaks can also be seen in high-grade tumors (as shown in previous cases), the lactate peaks in infarctions tend to be more pronounced.[2] Note that in this case the lactate peak is the dominant peak of the spectrum.

CASE 17.6 ANSWER

1. **B. Decreased NAA:Cr ratio**

CASE 17.7

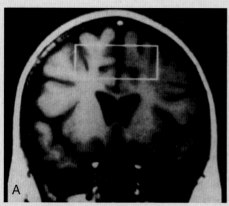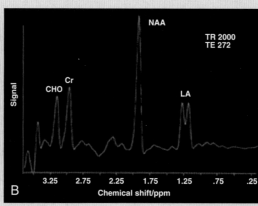

FIG. 17.C7

1. What is abnormal about this spectrum?
   A. Elevated NAA:Cr ratio
   B. Decreased Cho:Cr ratio
   C. Elevated lactate peak
   D. Double peak (doublet) in lactate

FIG. 17.C7. (A) Normal coronal T1-weighted MRI used for localization of spectroscopy volume. A rectangle demonstrates the voxel of interest. (B) PRESS spectrum (TE = 272 ms). A prominent lactate peak is identified. The peak doublet is characteristic of a lactate peak. NAA:Cr and Cho:Cr ratios are normal.

Kearns-Sayre Syndrome

This patient has a rare mitochondrial disorder, Kearns-Sayre syndrome. The typical MRI appearance of this disorder is high T2 signal in the subcortical cerebral white matter, brainstem, globus pallidus, and thalamus.[18] The abnormal elevation of the lactate peak is likely secondary to the dysfunctional mitochondria, resulting in impaired oxidative metabolism. Serial

studies have empirically demonstrated that the lactate peak in this condition precedes T2 signal abnormalities, suggesting that metabolic dysfunction precedes parenchymal damage.[19]

CASE 17.7 ANSWER

1. **C. Elevated lactate peak**

FIG. 17.C8

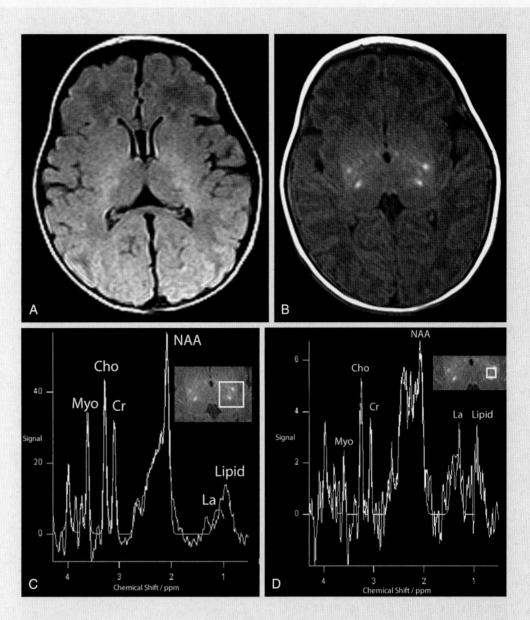

1. In neonates with hypoxic ischemic encephalopathy, which metabolite changes portend a poor prognosis?
   A. No lactate peak
   B. Low NAA:Cho ratio
   C. Elevated NAA:Cr ratio

FIG. 17.C8. (A) Axial FLAIR image, normal brain. (B) Axial T1-weighted MR image without contrast. Increased T1 signal is seen in the bilateral thalami and putamen. (C) PRESS spectrum (TE = 30 ms). The axial T1-weighted MR image in right upper corner with a large white square over the left basal ganglia demarcates the voxel of interest for the waveform. The NAA:Cho ratio is decreased. A small lactate peak is suggested, although it is overlapping with lipid. (D) PRESS repeated but now with smaller voxel of interest (note the small white box overlying the left basal ganglia); TE = 30 ms. Again, the NAA:Cho peak is decreased. A peak at 1.3 ppm likely represents a lactate peak. Note that there is increased fluctuation in the waveform as a whole compared with that in the prior spectroscopy study.

Hypoxic-Ischemic Encephalopathy

Neonatal hypoxic-ischemic encephalopathy (HIE) is an acquired condition caused by reduced cerebral perfusion and oxygenation in preterm and term infants. One classic sign of HIE with conventional imaging is foci of increased T1 signal in the basal ganglia, thalami, and posterior limb of the internal capsule. Diffusion-weighted imaging (DWI) with apparent diffusion coefficient maps is the most sensitive sequence to detect cytotoxic edema between the ages of 24 hours and 8 days, although the appearance can be less conspicuous in infants compared with adults, and the DWI images can underestimate the extent of disease.[20] Fluid-attenuated inversion recovery (FLAIR) sequences and postcontrast sequences are less sensitive sequences for HIE.[21] Spectroscopy is occasionally used in an attempt to characterize the severity of the HIE.[22] Lower NAA:Cr and lower NAA:Cho ratios are thought to indicate a poor prognosis.[23] Additionally, elevated lactate levels are thought to portend a poor prognosis.[24]

Voxel Size in Spectroscopy

This case also demonstrates the effect of voxel size on the spectroscopy waveform. A larger voxel size allows for a higher SNR and results in a smoother spectrum. However, the downside of this large voxel size is low spatial resolution. In this case, the MRI technician repeated the PRESS sequence with a smaller voxel size, trying to capture the molecular changes better in the small T1 bright foci in the left putamen and thalamus. The smaller voxel size did show a lactate peak more clearly, possibly because of decreased partial volume averaging. However, the smaller voxel size also resulted in significantly increased noise in the waveform, as manifested by the irregular appearance of the waveform.

CASE 17.8 ANSWER

1. **B. Low NAA:Cho ratio**

CASE 17.9

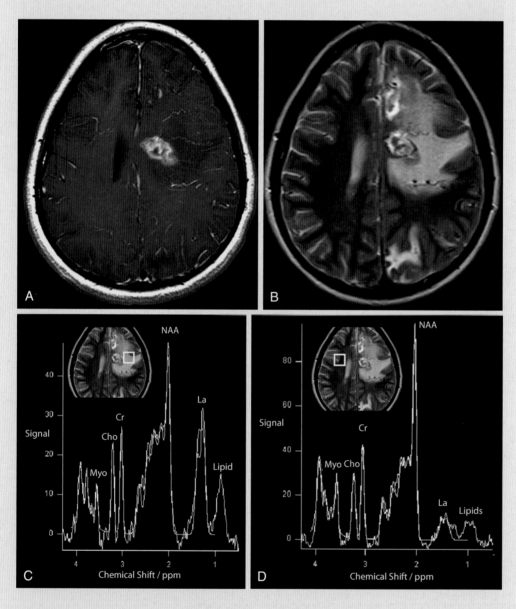

FIG. 17.C9

1. The findings in the spectroscopy waveform makes which diagnosis most likely?
   A. Gliomatosis cerebri
   B. Metastatic disease
   C. Primary angiitis of the central nervous system
   D. GBM

FIG. 17.C9. (A) Axial T1 postcontrast MRI. A rim-enhancing mass is identified in the left frontal lobe. Surrounding low T1 signal is identified. A separate site of low T1 signal is seen in the medial left parietal lobe. (B) Axial T2-weighted MR image. The rim-enhancing mass is heterogeneous on T2 weighting, with areas of high and low signal. There is surrounding T2 prolongation in the left frontal lobe white matter. A separate T2 bright area is seen posteriorly in the left parietal lobe. (C) PRESS spectrum (TE = 30 ms). The voxel of interest is shown in the white square on the inset axial T2-weighted MR image (*inset*). The voxel is in the T2 bright white matter surrounding the left frontal lobe lesion. There is an elevated lactate peak. The other levels are within normal limits. (D) PRESS waveform of contralateral hemisphere (TE = 30 ms). There may be trace elevation of lactate levels. Otherwise, the spectrum is within normal limits.

Primary Angiitis of the Central Nervous System

Primary angiitis of the central nervous system (PACNS) is a vasculitis of unknown cause that affects cerebral arteries and veins. Although PACNS can have a multitude of appearances on conventional MRI, it usually presents as multiple enhancing masses, with surrounding edema.[25] On spectroscopy, the enhancing lesions and edema may have an elevation in lactate levels. However, the real value diagnostic value of

spectroscopy is the absence of an abnormally elevated choline peak. Most neoplasms will have an elevated choline level, so a normal choline level (as shown in this case) should at least raise the possibility that the enhancing lesion is not a neoplasm.[25]

CASE 17.9 ANSWER

1. C. Primary angiitis of the central nervous system

CASE 17.10

FIG. 17.C10

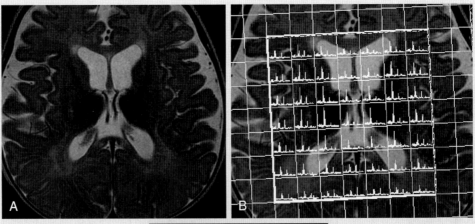

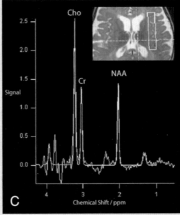

1. What is the diagnosis?
   A. Normal child brain
   B. Normal adult brain
   C. Krabbe disease
   D. HIE

2. What are advantages of single-voxel technique over a multivoxel technique?
   A. Multivoxel acquisition time is longer than a single-voxel acquisition
   B. It allows multiple voxels to be acquired simultaneously
   C. Easier for technician to localize a small voxel of interest
   D. Greater partial volume averaging

FIG. 17.C10. (A) Axial T2-weighted image of the brain reveals diffuse increased signal in the periventricular and deep white matter consistent with a metabolic or dysmyelinating process.(B) Axial T2-weighted image of the brain with an overlying grid from a multivoxel technique. (C) Spectroscopy data combining multiple voxels in the left frontal lobe. The Cho:Cr ratio is elevated, and the NAA:Cr ratio is decreased. Myoinositol is slightly increased.

Krabbe Disease

Krabbe disease is a leukodystrophy caused by a deficiency in the lysosomal enzyme galactocerebrosidase. Conventional MRI classically demonstrates extensive bilateral symmetrical abnormal T2 signal in the white matter of the bilateral cerebral hemispheres. Spectroscopy shows elevation in choline and myoinositol and a decrease in NAA. These spectroscopy findings are thought to be due to gliosis and loss of axons in the areas of demyelination.[26] The distribution of the T2 changes in the brain and the lack of a lactate peak make HIE unlikely.

Multivoxel Spectroscopy

Spectroscopic data can also be acquired using a multivoxel technique (also called *chemical shift imaging*). In this technique, data from multiple voxels are acquired simultaneously. This is achieved by using phase-encoding gradients to resolve spatial information (two phase-encoding gradients for two-dimensional spectroscopic imaging and three phase-encoding gradients for three-dimensional spectroscopic imaging). Even in the case of multivoxel spectroscopy, the volume of interest is usually still selected using the PRESS sequence. The PRESS sequence selects a large area, and the phase-encoding gradients allow data collection from multiple voxels within the area of interest. (In Case 17.10, the PRESS selection is identified as the large white square in Fig. 17.C10B while each voxel of interest is shown by the small squares in Fig. 17.C10B. Note that each small square has its own spectrum.) *The main advantage of the multivoxel technique is that it allows multiple samples to be acquired simultaneously,* with better spatial resolution.[3,27] This often alleviates the need to accurately localize a single voxel to the area of pathology before the spectroscopy acquisition. In addition, the multivoxel spectroscopic imaging technique allows for a smaller voxel size, which reduces partial volume averaging (see physics discussion of Case 17.8). One disadvantage of the multivoxel technique is that acquisition time can be much longer, although techniques such as those using echo-planar k-space trajectory can greatly reduce the imaging time.[28]

CASE 17.10 ANSWERS

1. **C. Krabbe disease**
2. **A. Multivoxel acquisition time is longer than a single-voxel acquisition**

CASE 17.11

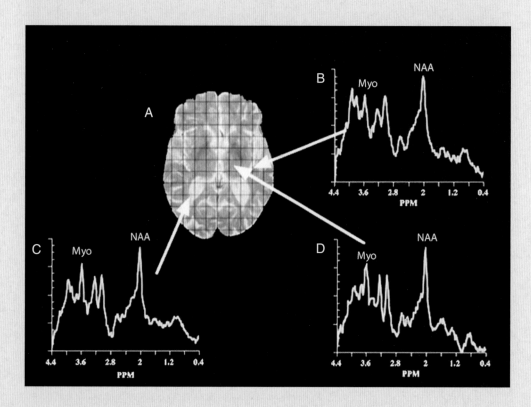

FIG. 17.C11

1. What metabolite abnormalities are present in the spectroscopy waveforms of this patient with Alzheimer disease?
   A. NAA:Cr ratio
   B. Elevated lactate peak
   C. Increased myoinositol levels
   D. Increased creatine levels

FIG. 17.C11. (A) Axial fast spin echo T2-weighted MR image. The overlying grid demonstrates the voxels captured by multivoxel spectroscopy. (B) MRS spectrum of a voxel in the left perisylvian cortex. Myoinositol levels are elevated. (C) Spectrum of a voxel in right periatrial white matter. Myoinositol levels are elevated. (D) Spectrum of a voxel in the left thalamus. Myoinositol levels are elevated. (Courtesy Cecil Charles, PhD.)

Alzheimer Disease

This patient has Alzheimer disease. Conventional MRI of Alzheimer disease reveals global or focal atrophy involving the temporal and parietal lobes, particularly the medial temporal lobes. Volumetric studies of the hippocampus and entorhinal cortex can add predictive value as to whether a patient with mild cognitive impairment will progress to Alzheimer disease.[29,30] Spectroscopy in Alzheimer disease shows a decrease in the NAA levels and an increase in myoinositol levels.[3] These changes are most pronounced in the mesial temporal lobe, hippocampus, parietotemporal region, frontal lobe, and occipital lobe. Presumably these spectroscopy changes correspond to the known pathologic changes of neuronal loss (decreased NAA levels) and increased gliosis (increased myoinositol levels). Despite the advances of spectroscopy and volumetric MRI in clinical practice, Alzheimer disease remains a clinical diagnosis. However, new criteria have been proposed in which volumetric and molecular imaging techniques will likely play a central role in early diagnostic and therapeutic assessment.[31]

CASE 17.11 ANSWER

1. **C. Increased myoinositol levels**

TAKE-HOME POINTS

1. Magnetic resonance spectroscopy measures the relative concentration of metabolites in a given voxel.
2. The molecular environment of a proton can alter its precession frequency. This frequency change, measured in parts per million relative to the precession frequency of water protons, is known as the *chemical shift*. Each molecule has a specific chemical shift.
3. On the MRS spectrum, the *x*-axis represents the chemical shift measured in parts per million. The *y*-axis measures the relative concentration of molecules at each chemical shift.
4. A line can be drawn on the spectroscopy waveform of the normal brain that connects the prominent molecular peaks. This line creates a positively sloped 45-degree angle, known as Hunter's angle, with the *x*-axis.
5. Common molecular species depicted in the spectroscopy waveform are as follows:
   - NAA: neuronal function
   - Choline: cellular turnover
   - Creatine: energy metabolism; reference marker
   - Myoinositol: gliosis
   - Lactate: anaerobic metabolism
6. Clinical pitfalls of MRS are its low specificity and low spatial resolution.
7. TE affects the spectroscopic findings. Lipids, myoinositol, and some amino acids have a short T2 relaxation time and will consequently lose signal and not be visualized on studies with a long TE. The lactate doublet peak inverts at intermediate TEs (140 ms).
8. In regard to single-voxel spectroscopy, three 90-degree, slice-selective pulses select a single voxel of interest. Advantages include a shorter scan time and the relative ease with which short TE scans can be acquired.
9. Multivoxel spectroscopy (spectroscopic imaging, or chemical shift imaging) involves multiple voxels in a plane (2D) or volume (3D) of interest that are obtained simultaneously using multiple phase-encoding gradients. This technique is useful in disorders for which multiple areas of the brain need to be sampled at a greater spatial resolution.

ACKNOWLEDGMENT

We thank Dr. David Enterline and Dr. Cecil Charles for their contributions of figures to the case material.

References

1. Michel SJ, Given CA. Case 99: canavan disease. *Radiology.* 2006;241:310–324.
2. Soares DP, Law M. Magnetic resonance spectroscopy of the brain: review of metabolites and clinical applications. *Clin Radiol.* 2009;64:12–21.
3. Barker P, Bizzi A, Stefano N, et al. *Clinical MR Spectroscopy.* New York: Cambridge University Press; 2010.
4. Hollingworth W, Medina LS, Lenkinski RE, et al. A systematic literature review of magnetic resonance spectroscopy for the characterization of brain tumors. *AJNR Am J Neuroradiol.* 2006;27:1404–1411.
5. Guzman-de-Villoria JA, Sanchez-Gonzalez J, Munoz L, et al. 1H MR spectroscopy in the assessment of gliomatosis cerebri. *AJR Am J Roentgenol.* 2007;188:710–714.
6. del Carpio-O'Donovan R, Korah I, Salazar A, Melancon D. Gliomatosis cerebri. *Radiology.* 1996;198:831–835.
7. Bendszus M, Warmuth-Metz M, Klein R, et al. MR spectroscopy in gliomatosis cerebri. *AJNR Am J Neuroradiol.* 2000;21:375–380.
8. Lin A, Ross BD, Harris K, Wong W. Efficacy of proton magnetic resonance spectroscopy in neurological diagnosis and neurotherapeutic decision making. *Neuroradiology.* 2005;2:197–214.
9. Kreis R, Ernst T, Ross BD. Development of the human brain: in vivo quantification of metabolite and water content with proton magnetic resonance spectroscopy. *Magn Reson Med.* 1993;30:424–437.
10. Pouwels PJW, Frahm J. Regional metabolite concentrations in human brain as determined by quantitative localized proton MRS. *Magn Reson Med.* 1998;39:53–60.
11. Nagae-Poetscher LM, Bonekamp D, Barker PB, et al. Asymmetry and gender effect in functionally lateralized cortical regions: a proton MRS imaging study. *J Magn Reson Imaging.* 2004;19:27–33.
12. Law M, Yang S, Wang H, et al. Glioma grading: sensitivity, specificity, and predictive values of perfusion MR imaging and proton MR spectroscopic imaging compared with conventional MR imaging. *AJNR Am J Neuroradiol.* 2003;24:1989–1998.
13. Castillo M, Smith JK, Kwock L. Correlation of myo-inositol levels and grading of cerebral astrocytomas. *AJNR Am J Neuroradiol.* 2000;21:1645–1649.
14. Panigrahy A, Krieger MD, Gonzalez-Gomez I, et al. Quantitative short echo time 1H-MR spectroscopy of untreated pediatric brain tumors: preoperative diagnosis and characterization. *AJNR Am J Neuroradiol.* 2006;27:560–572.
15. Butteriss DJA, Ismail A, Ellison DW, Birchall D. Use of serial proton magnetic resonance spectroscopy to differentiate low-grade glioma from tumefactive plaque in a patient with multiple sclerosis. *Br J Radiology.* 2003;76:662–665.
16. Lange T, Dydak U, Roberts TPL, et al. Pitfalls in lactate measurements at 3T. *AJNR Am J Neuroradiol.* 2006;27:895–901.
17. Saunders DE. MR spectroscopy in stroke. *Br Med Bull.* 2000;56:334–345.
18. Chu BC, Terae S, Takahashi C, et al. MRI of the brain in the Kearns-Sayre syndrome: report of four cases and a review. *Neuroradiology.* 1999;41:759–764.
19. Kapeller P, Offenbacher H, Stollberger R, et al. Magnetic resonance imaging and spectroscopy of progressive cerebral involvement in Kearns-Sayre syndrome. *J Neurol Sci.* 1996;135:126–130.

20. Chao CP, Zaleski CG, Patton AC. Neonatal hypoxic-ischemic encephalopathy: multi-modality imaging findings 1. *Radiographics.* 2006;26:S159–S172.

21. Liauw L, van der Grond J, van den Berg-Huysmans AA, et al. Hypoxic-ischemic encephalopathy: diagnostic value of conventional MR imaging pulse sequences in term-born neonates. *Radiology.* 2008; 247:204–212.

22. Barkovich AJ, Westmark KD, Bedi HS, et al. Proton spectroscopy and diffusion imaging on the first day of life after perinatal asphyxia: preliminary report. *Am J Neuroradiol.* 2001;22:1786–1794.

23. Graham SH, Meyerhoff DJ, Bayne L, et al. Magnetic resonance spectroscopy of N-acetylaspartate in hypoxic-ischemic encephalopathy. *Ann Neurol.* 1994;35: 490–494.

24. Malik GK, Pandey M, Kumar R, et al. MR imaging and in vivo proton spectroscopy of the brain in neonates with hypoxic ischemic encephalopathy. *Eur J Radiol.* 2002;43:6–13.

25. Panchal NJ, Niku S, Imbesi SG. Lymphocytic vasculitis mimicking aggressive multifocal cerebral neoplasm: MR imaging and MR spectroscopic appearance. *AJNR Am J Neuroradiol.* 2005;26:642–645.

26. Zarifi MK, Tzika AA, Astrakas LG, et al. Magnetic resonance spectroscopy and magnetic resonance imaging findings in Krabbe disease. *J Child Neurol.* 2001;16:522–526.

27. Atlas SW. *Magnetic Resonance Imaging of the Brain and Spine.* 4th ed. Philadelphia: Lippincott Williams & Wilkins; 2009.

28. Posse S, Dager SR, Richards TL, et al. In vivo measurement of regional brain metabolic response to hyperventilation using magnetic resonance: proton echo planar spectroscopic imaging (PEPSI). *Magn Reson Med.* 1997;37:858–865.

29. Gomar JJ, Bobes-Bascaran MT, Conejero-Goldberg C, et al. Utility of combinations of biomarkers, cognitive markers, and risk factors to predict conversion from mild cognitive impairment to Alzheimer disease in patients in the Alzheimer's disease neuroimaging initiative. *Arch Gen Psychiatry.* 2011;68:961–969.

30. Fleisher AS, Sun S, Taylor C, et al. Volumetric MRI vs clinical predictors of Alzheimer disease in mild cognitive impairment. *Neurology.* 2008;70:191–199.

31. Dubois B, Feldman HH, Jacova C, et al. Research criteria for the diagnosis of Alzheimer disease: revising the NINCDS-ADRDA criteria. *Lancet Neurol.* 2007;6:734–746.

CHAPTER 18

Functional Magnetic Resonance Imaging

Spencer J. Hood, Wells I. Mangrum, Christopher J. Roth, Allen W. Song,
James T. Voyvodic, and Jeffrey R. Petrella

OPENING CASE 18.1

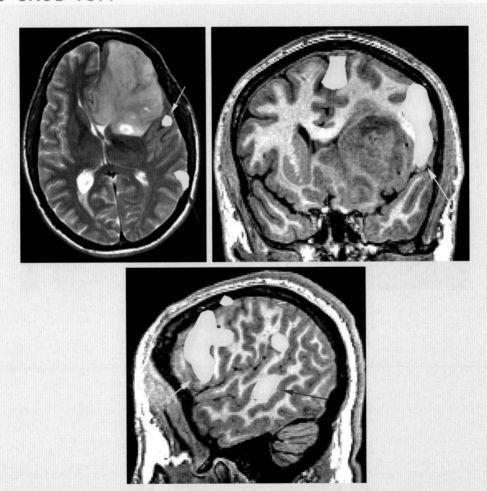

1. The functional MRI (fMRI) sequence measures the concentration of what moiety? During the functional task, is the relative concentration of this moiety increased or decreased in the yellow regions above *(yellow* and *red arrows)?*
   A. Deoxyhemoglobin, increased
   B. Deoxyhemoglobin, decreased
   C. Oxyhemoglobin, increased
   D. Oxyhemoglobin, decreased

2. How do oxyhemoglobin and deoxyhemoglobin affect the signal intensity of a T2* sequence?
   A. Deoxyhemoglobin disrupts the magnetic field uniformity of its vicinity, leads to a faster decay of transverse magnetization, and results in darker T2* signal.
   B. Elevated oxyhemoglobin appears brighter on a T2* sequence due to the blood oxygenation level–dependent (BOLD) effect.

C. Deoxyhemoglobin disrupts the magnetic field uniformity of its vicinity, leads to a faster decay of transverse magnetization, and results in brighter T2* signal.

D. Elevated oxyhemoglobin appears darker on a T2* sequence due to the BOLD effect.

3. How does increased neuronal activity in the brain affect the local relative concentrations of oxyhemoglobin and deoxyhemoglobin?

A. There is no net effect. The body's hemodynamic response maintains the oxyhemoglobin and deoxyhemoglobin concentrations at constant levels.

B. There is a decrease in the local oxyhemoglobin/deoxyhemoglobin ratio due to consumption of oxygen.

C. There is an increase in the local oxyhemoglobin/deoxyhemoglobin ratio due to a robust hemodynamic response.

D. There is a decrease in the local oxyhemoglobin/deoxyhemoglobin ratio due to the hemodynamic response.

4. Why is the spatial resolution of fMRI poor?

A. The high temporal demand of fMRI causes a decrease in spatial resolution.

B. The area of the brain affected by the hemodynamic response can often be larger than the neuronally active area of the brain.

C. All of the above.

CASE ANSWERS

OPENING CASE 18.1

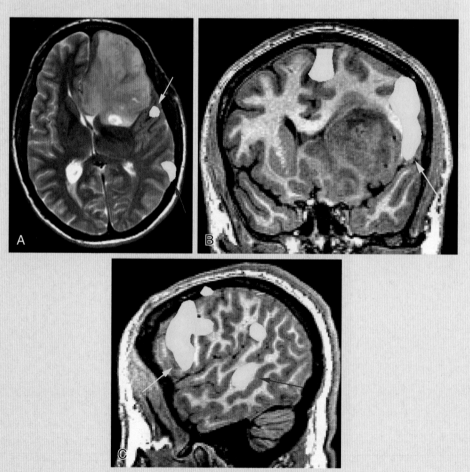

FIG. 18.C1. fMRI data obtained during language mapping. Color-coded statistical data from the fMRI has been coregistered to (A) T2 axial, (B) T1 coronal, and (C) T1 sagittal images for anatomic localization. A large mass (biopsy-proven glioblastoma multiforme) is identified in the left frontal lobe. The left inferior frontal gyral activation *(yellow arrows)* is consistent with the dominant expressive speech area. This lies within 1 cm of the posterolateral border of the left frontal mass, in the left frontal operculum, and appears separated from the insular component of the mass by the circular sulcus. The left posterior middle temporal gyrus activation *(red arrows)* is consistent with the dominant receptive speech area and lies posterolaterally, remote from the mass.

1. The functional MRI (fMRI) sequence measures the concentration of what moiety? During the functional task, is the relative concentration of this moiety increased or decreased in the yellow regions above (*yellow* and *red arrows*)?
   B. Deoxyhemoglobin, decreased
2. How do oxyhemoglobin and deoxyhemoglobin affect the signal intensity of a T2* sequence?
   A. Deoxyhemoglobin disrupts the magnetic field uniformity of its vicinity, leads to a faster decay of transverse magnetization, and results in darker T2* signal.
3. How does increased neuronal activity in the brain affect the local relative concentrations of oxyhemoglobin and deoxyhemoglobin?
   C. There is an increase in the local oxyhemoglobin/deoxyhemoglobin ratio due to a robust hemodynamic response.
4. Why is the spatial resolution of fMRI poor?
   C. All of the above.

Diagnosis

There is left-dominant expressive and receptive speech. The expressive speech cortex is within 1 cm of the left frontal glioblastoma multiforme (GBM).

Discussion

Intraoperative cortical mapping confirmed the finding of an expressive speech area in the upper part of the inferior frontal gyrus, immediately adjacent to the mass. A limited resection of the anterior and medial aspect of the tumor was performed. The patient had no postsurgical neurologic deficit.

Functional MRI

fMRI is used to identify the regions of the brain that are active during the performance of a particular sensory, motor, or cognitive task. In the clinical setting, fMRI is often used to localize the eloquent cortex anatomically. The eloquent cortex includes the sensory and motor cortices, language areas (Wernicke's and Broca's areas), and visual and auditory cortices (Fig. 18.1). Precise localization of the eloquent cortex is often needed in the preoperative management of patients with tumors near the eloquent cortex to minimize postoperative neurologic deficits; fMRI has been documented to change neurosurgical treatment planning in this regard.[1,2]

Wada Test and Intraoperative Cortical Stimulation

Alternatives to fMRI include the Wada test and intraoperative cortical stimulation. In the Wada test, a barbiturate is administered into one of the internal carotid arteries,

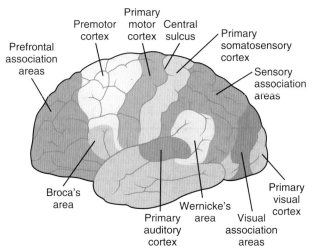

FIG. 18.1. Classic anatomic sites for functional cortical areas. The expressive speech area (Broca's area) is typically located in the inferior frontal gyrus (pars opercularis and pars triangularis). The receptive speech area (Wernicke's area) is typically located in the posterior aspect of the superior temporal gyrus. In most patients, the expressive and receptive speech areas are in the left cerebral hemisphere, but this is not always the case. The primary motor and sensory cortical areas lie anterior and posterior to the central sulcus. The visual areas in the occipital lobes are additional cortical areas that are frequently activated in fMRI scans.

resulting in temporary anesthetization and functional loss of a large portion of the cerebral hemisphere supplied by that artery. The patient is then asked to perform simple tasks that require language or memory. The Wada test is helpful to lateralize the side of dominant memory and language function. fMRI is generally preferred to the Wada test because it is less invasive and because it gives additional spatial information about the lesion and the language and memory areas.[3,4]

Intraoperative cortical stimulation is performed by the neurosurgeon during an awake craniotomy with local anesthesia. The patient is asked to perform a simple task repeatedly, such as raising and lowering the leg. Then the neurosurgeon uses a probe to stimulate the cortex electrically. The neurosurgeon marches down the cortex with a neurostimulator until the patient can no longer lift her leg and/or twitches the leg. At this point, the neurosurgeon knows that the portion of the brain just stimulated is the leg motor portion of the motor cortex. The electrical stimulation overloads the local neurons, causing them to be unable to function temporarily. *Among tests to localize the functional cortex, intraoperative cortical stimulation is the gold standard.* fMRI is not yet accurate enough spatially to replace intraoperative cortical mapping, and may never replace it, given that the techniques assess two different physiologic phenomena—the cessation of neuronal function verses changes in the deoxyhemoglobin concentration. However, fMRI is often complementary to the cortical mapping studies, enabling the use of a negative mapping technique, which reduces operative duration and allows for smaller, more tailored craniotomies.[2,3,5]

BOLD Effect and the Hemodynamic Response

fMRI works by taking advantage of the differences in the magnetic properties of oxyhemoglobin and deoxyhemoglobin. Oxyhemoglobin has no unpaired electrons and thus has essentially no magnetic moment. Conversely, *deoxyhemoglobin has unpaired electrons, resulting in paramagnetism and a significant magnetic moment. This paramagnetism disrupts the magnetic field uniformity and leads to a faster decay of transverse magnetization due to destructive addition. As the level of deoxyhemoglobin increases in the blood, the immediately adjacent regions will, as a result, appear darker on T2*-weighted imaging.*

When brain areas become active, the relative level of deoxyhemoglobin to oxyhemoglobin actually goes down, and such areas manifest brighter signal on T2*-weighted images. *This effect of increasing oxygen levels on MRI scans in* *the region of neuronal activation is known as the blood oxygenation level–dependent (BOLD) effect.*[6]

Intuitively, one may think that functionally active areas of the brain will consume oxygen, increase the local concentration of deoxyhemoglobin, and appear dark on T2*-weighted sequences. However, this is not the case. This seeming paradox can be explained by understanding how the brain responds to increased functional demands. Increased neuronal functional activity results in an increased demand for oxygen. *The body responds to this increased demand for oxygen by causing arteriolar dilation, which increases the supply of oxyhemoglobin. The vasodilation response, known as the hemodynamic response, leads to an excessive increase of arterial blood flow and results in a net increase of oxyhemoglobin concentration and a decrease of deoxyhemoglobin concentration in the activated brain regions.* As a result, functionally active areas of the brain actually increase in overall signal on fMRI images.

Creating fMRI Images

Color-coded fMRI images are statistical representations of the fMRI data. fMRI images are frequently obtained with gradient-recalled, echo-based, echo-planar imaging (EPI), a fast sequence allowing a series of more than 100 images of the entire brain volume to be acquired over a few minutes. This sequence is particularly sensitive to the T2* effects of deoxyhemoglobin. A statistical model is then applied to the EPI image series to determine which voxels have

an increase in signal during the task, compared with the rest period, beyond a chosen statistically significant noise threshold. Typically, the BOLD effect results in a signal change from baseline that is up to 3% at 1.5 T and up to 6% at 3 T for voxel volumes of about $3 \times 3 \times 3$ mm during a motor or visual task.[7] This signal change can be detected using various statistical methods. *These voxels are then color coded according to the degree of statistical significance of the increased signal. Finally, the color-coded statistical maps are overlaid on higher resolution anatomic images acquired with typical structural imaging techniques, such as a fast spin echo T2-weighted sequence or a spoiled gradient echo T1-weighted sequence.*

This last step, requiring coregistration of the fMRI images with higher resolution anatomic MRI reference images, is necessary because of the low spatial resolution of fMRI. The spatial resolution of fMRI is coarse to compensate for the low signal-to-noise ratio (SNR) associated with the BOLD effect and to meet the high temporal resolution demands of fMRI. In general, larger voxels have higher SNR and are quicker to acquire. Moreover, spatial accuracy to neuronal activation may ultimately be limited by the BOLD effect itself, which is a vascular rather than neuronal phenomenon. The area of the brain with increased perfusion due to the hemodynamic response can often be larger and may be slightly removed from the neuronally active area of the brain, particularly in the case of large draining veins.[8]

CASE 18.2

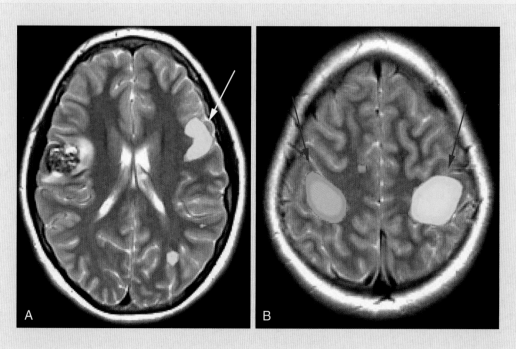

FIG. 18.C2

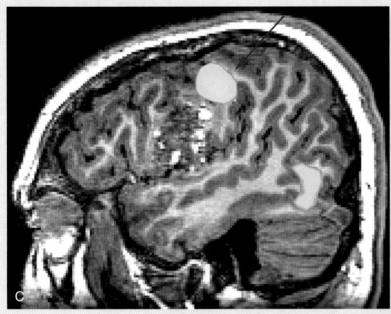
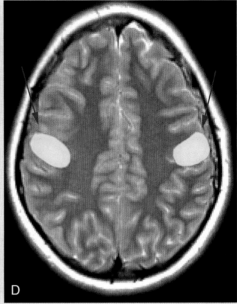

1. List in order the functional tasks that elicited the fMRI responses shown by the red, white, and purple arrows.
   A. Hand motor mapping, language mapping, mouth motor mapping
   B. Language mapping, hand motor mapping, mouth motor mapping
   C. Mouth motor mapping, hand motor mapping, mouth motor mapping
   D. Mouth motor mapping, language mapping, hand motor mapping

2. What sensitive cortical area is immediately adjacent to the cavernoma?
   A. Wernicke's receptive speech area
   B. Broca's expressive speech area
   C. The mouth-face motor cortex
   D. The hand motor cortex area

FIG. 18.C2. (A) Language mapping fMRI overlaid on axial T2-weighted image. The active area in the inferior left frontal lobe *(white arrow)* represents Broca's expressive speech area. A cavernoma is centered in the inferior right frontal gyrus, on the contralateral side of the expressive speech area. (B) Hand motor mapping fMRI overlaid on an axial T2-weighted image. The active areas *(red arrows)* correspond to the hand motor and sensory cortex. Mouth motor mapping fMRI overlaid on (C) sagittal T1-weighted and (D) axial T2-weighted images. The mouth sensorimotor areas *(purple arrows)* are lateral and inferior to the hand motor strips. The mouth motor strip in the right frontal lobe is therefore within 1 cm of the cavernoma.

Diagnosis

There is left-dominant speech; the mouth motor cortex is immediately adjacent to the cavernoma.

Discussion

The cavernoma was resected shortly after the fMRI because of recurrent and progressive seizures. Intraoperative cortical stimulation confirmed the face motor cortex to lie just posterior to the cavernoma. The cavernoma was then completely resected, with careful attention paid not to dissect into the face cortex area. At 2-year follow-up, the patient was seizure free and had no motor deficits.

fMRI Tasks

Language mapping, which is a common fMRI task for presurgical planning, can be done with multiple paradigms.[3] As mentioned previously, *one common method involves asking patients to read an incomplete sentence and mentally complete the sentence. Reading and comprehending the sentence activates the receptive speech areas, whereas mentally completing the sentence activates expressive speech areas.*

Multiple alternative tasks exist to activate nonlanguage cortices for fMRI. *In motor hand tasks, one paradigm involves having the patient alternately squeeze each hand. Note that squeezing the hand will activate both sensory and motor cortices because the hand is sensing the act of squeezing (as shown in Case 18.2). To elicit motor mouth function, as in this example, the patient is asked to pucker the mouth repetitively.* One functional paradigm often performed on patients unable to cooperate (e.g., paralyzed or comatose patients) involves rubbing a feather over a hand to determine the sensory cortices. In general, the sensory cortices are homologously aligned with the motor areas across the central sulcus. Functional paradigms also exist for many other areas of the eloquent cortex, including memory and visual cortices, with varying degrees of clinical applicability.[7] Practice parameters and guidelines for the appropriate clinical use of fMRI have been published by the American College of Radiology[9] and the American Academy of Neurology.[10]

CASE 18.2 ANSWERS

1. **B. Language mapping, hand motor mapping, mouth motor mapping**
2. **C. The mouth-face motor cortex**

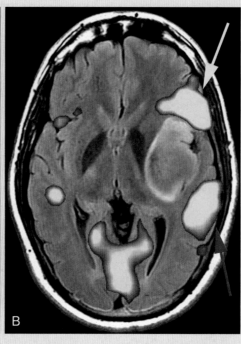

FIG. 18.C3

1. During an awake craniotomy, what cortical function should be monitored as the posterior margin of the tumor is resected?
   A. Hand sensory impairment
   B. Broca's expressive speech
   C. Wernicke's receptive speech
   D. Face motor impairment

2. What is an advantage of increasing the statistical threshold of the fMRI maps?
   A. Increased sensitivity for the cortical areas involved in the task
   B. Increased specificity for the cortical areas involved in the task
   C. Decrease in the positive predictive value of the areas selected by the fMRI
   D. Increase in the negative predictive value of the areas selected by the fMRI

FIG. 18.C3. (A) fMRI data obtained with a threshold t-value greater than 6.0. The fMRI data are then color coded and overlaid on an anatomic fluid-attenuated inversion recovery (FLAIR) image. A mass is centered in the left putamen. The dominant expressive speech area *(yellow arrow)* and receptive speech area *(red arrow)* are marked. (B) fMRI color overlay redisplayed with a lower threshold t-value (>3.0) and overlaid on the same anatomic FLAIR image. Even though the threshold value has been changed, the data in both images are statistically significant beyond a threshold of $P = .005$. With the lower threshold value (>3.0), the dominant expressive *(yellow arrow)* and receptive *(red arrow)* speech areas are larger and appear to have closer approximation with the mass.

Diagnosis

There is left-dominant speech in a patient with a well-differentiated astrocytoma (grade II). The dominant motor speech area borders the anterior margin of the tumor; the receptive speech area lies on the posterior margin of the tumor.

Discussion

The patient was taken for an awake craniotomy and the tumor was resected. When the posterior aspect of the tumor was resected, the patient did develop slow speech. In particular, the patient had difficulty understanding questions. The resection was then discontinued. At clinical follow-up, the patient had no speech difficulties.

Statistical Analysis of fMRI Data

The statistical analysis of the fMRI data is critical in the production of the fMRI image. *The activation maps are generated by calculating the* t-value *statistic of how different the BOLD signal is during the active language condition compared to the rest condition at each voxel.* The activation map threshold is set only to show voxels that exceed the statistical significance level. In Fig. 18.C3, the t-value thresholds were chosen to be 6.0 and 3.0, respectively. Both these levels are statistically significant beyond a 0.5% chance of having a false-positive result. At the higher threshold, the specificity and positive predictive value will increase due to a decrease in the number of false-positive results. However, the problem with setting the threshold too high is that there will be a higher number of false-negative results, leading to a decreased sensitivity and negative predictive value. In other words, by setting the higher threshold, one can be more confident that a positive area is truly part of the cortical function, but this comes at the cost of potentially missing some active neurons. The problem with setting the threshold too low is that the map will then include some less active voxels, which show a BOLD signal but may not be directly involved in language function. There is no a priori way to determine the optimal cutoff threshold because the activation statistical signal is dependent on task duration, patient attention levels, BOLD signal amplitude, and physiologic noise levels, all of which can be highly variable. In practice, thresholds are typically adjusted by an experienced user based on the relative overall strength of the fMRI signal, plus knowledge of the task properties and relevant functional brain anatomy.

CASE 18.3 ANSWERS

1. **C. Wernicke's receptive speech**
2. **B. Increased specificity for the cortical areas involved in the task**

CASE 18.4

FIG. 18.C4

1. What is the area marked by the blue arrow in this hand motor fMRI study?
   A. The hand motor cortex
   B. The hand sensory cortex
   C. The frontal eye fields
   D. A supplementary motor area
2. What are potential advantages of performing an fMRI before neurosurgery?
   A. fMRI results are precise enough to render intraoperative cortical mapping obsolete.
   B. The functional tasks performed by a patient during an fMRI examination prepare the patient for performing the tasks during the stressful time of surgery.
   C. The spatial resolution of fMRI is greater than that provided by intraoperative cortical mapping.
   D. fMRI can reveal a supplementary motor area, which can at times be difficult to isolate during intraoperative cortical stimulation.

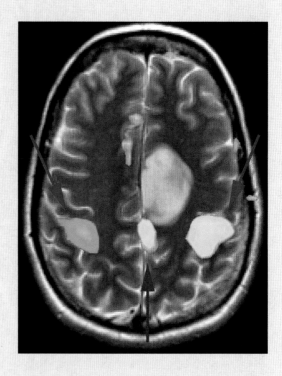

FIG. 18.C4. MRI data obtained during hand motor mapping overlaid on an axial T2-weighted image. A mass (biopsy-proven anaplastic astrocytoma) is seen along the medial aspect of the left frontal lobe. The hand motor and sensory cortices are marked by the *red arrows*. In addition, a focus of activity is noted in the cortex along the superior and medial aspect of the mass in the left hemisphere *(blue arrow)*, which is likely due to a hand supplementary motor area.

Diagnosis

The anaplastic astrocytoma is in close proximity to the left hemisphere motor cortex. The mass immediately abuts a left hemispheric hand supplementary motor area.

Discussion

The patient was taken for an awake craniotomy. Intraoperative cortical mapping demonstrated the cortical strip along the posterior aspect of the exposed brain. The tumor was then removed until the patient began to "get slow with naming." At this point, it became clear to the surgeons that they were in or immediately adjacent to the supplementary motor area. The surgical resection was then discontinued.

Supplementary Cortical Activation

This case demonstrates the complexity of cortical function. The primary motor strip has a critical role in motor function. However, other areas of the brain are also used during motor function, and loss of these other areas may or may not also result in loss of motor function. In this example, an area of cortex separate from the precentral gyrus is activated during the fMRI. Because this area is active during the motor task, the implication is that this area is used in the execution of motor function. In this example, this additional area of activation represents the supplementary motor area. The supplementary motor area is used for higher motor function, such as the planning and preparation for motor function.

fMRI is of particular value in demonstrating the supplementary motor area[11] because intraoperative cortical stimulation is often not successful in eliciting responses from the supplementary motor area.[12] As a result, if only intraoperative cortical stimulation is used, the supplementary motor area may be inadvertently excised, resulting in at least temporary paralysis after the procedure.

In this particular case, the intraoperative cortical mapping did not reveal the site of the supplementary motor area. However, the existence of the area on the fMRI scan was confirmed by the onset of symptoms when the supplementary motor area was approached during dissection.

This case shows a potential advantage of fMRI over intraoperative cortical mapping, but this does not mean that intraoperative cortical stimulation is obsolete. Intraoperative cortical mapping is still considered to be the gold standard to isolate the eloquent cortex precisely during surgery.

CASE 18.4 ANSWERS

1. **D. A supplementary motor area**
2. **D. fMRI can reveal a supplementary motor area, which can at times be difficult to isolate during intraoperative cortical stimulation.**

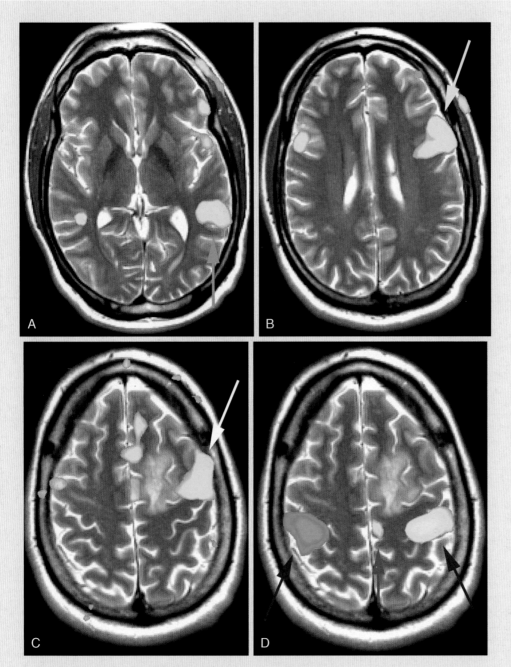

FIG. 18.C5

1. List in order the functional areas depicted by the green, yellow, white, blue, and red arrows.
   A. Expressive speech, receptive speech, frontal eye fields, hand sensorimotor cortex, supplementary motor cortex
   B. Receptive speech, expressive speech, supplementary motor cortex, hand sensorimotor cortex, frontal eye fields
   C. Receptive speech, expressive speech, frontal eye fields, hand sensorimotor cortex, supplementary motor cortex
   D. Receptive speech, expressive speech, frontal eye fields, supplementary motor cortex, hand sensorimotor cortex

FIG. 18.C5. (A–C) fMRI data from a language mapping study overlaid on axial T2-weighted images. A T2 bright mass (biopsy-proven oligo-dendroglioma) is identified in the apex of the medial aspect of the left frontal lobe. (A) The receptive speech area *(green arrow)* and expressive speech area *(yellow arrow,* B) are identified in the posterior aspect of the left superior temporal gyrus and inferior frontal gyrus, respectively. Activity is also noted more superiorly in the left frontal lobe *(white arrow,* C) that is consistent with activity in the frontal eye fields. This activity is immediately adjacent to the mass in the left frontal lobe. (D) fMRI data from a hand motor mapping study overlaid on an axial T2-weighted image. The left hemisphere hand motor and sensory cortices *(blue arrows)* are within 1 cm of the posterior-lateral aspect of the mass. In addition, a hand supplementary motor area *(red arrow)* is seen medial and posterior to the left frontal lobe mass.

Diagnosis

The oligodendroglioma is immediately adjacent to the left frontal eye fields and within close proximity to the left hemisphere hand motor cortex and supplementary motor area.

Discussion

The patient underwent an awake craniotomy. Cortical stimulation revealed the location of the primary motor strip. No language center was identified in the operative field by cortical stimulation. The tumor was then surgically removed, starting anteriorly, away from the motor area. At follow-up, the patient did not have any motor or neurologic deficits and the seizures had resolved.

Participatory Cortical Areas

This case also demonstrates the complexity of cortical mapping using fMRI. Interpreting fMRI requires a correlation between the expected location of a cortical function and the actual fMRI data. *Idealized maps of cortical function should be known to the interpreting radiologist* (Fig. 18.1). In Case 18.5, the expressive speech area is seen in the expected location of the inferior frontal gyrus. This activity is contiguous with the activity more superiorly and posteriorly in the left frontal lobe. However, this posterosuperior area is not the expected area of expressive speech function. Instead, this is the expected location of the frontal eye fields, areas of the brain that are also active when the patient is reading a sentence. *Such areas can be considered participatory in the language task, but not the eloquent (i.e., essential) language cortex.* Intraoperative cortical mapping is more specific than fMRI for identifying the eloquent cortex, defined as a brain area that if resected or injured results in cessation of a particular function. Areas of activation on fMRI include brain areas that participate in a sensorimotor or cognitive function but may not necessarily be essential to that function. Often, the role of the radiologist is to increase the specificity of fMRI by identifying which areas of activity on an fMRI might result in a deficit if injured or resected. *Only by combining the information from the fMRI data with the idealized maps of cortical function can the radiologist correctly interpret what is represented by task-related, locally decreased levels of deoxyhemoglobin,* thereby making fMRI a more clinically useful tool.

CASE 18.5 ANSWER

1. **C. Receptive speech, expressive speech, frontal eye fields, hand sensorimotor cortex, supplementary motor cortex**

CASE 18.6

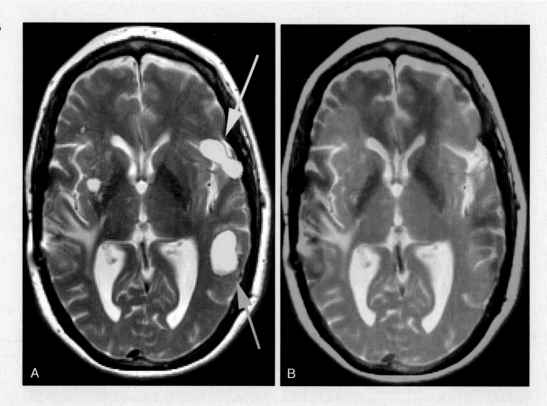

FIG. 18.C6

1. A susceptibility artifact from metal or other sources causes what effect on fMRI?
   A. No significant effect. fMRI data are not sensitive to susceptibility artifacts.
   B. Susceptibility artifact increases fMRI signal, resulting in false-positive areas of activity.
   C. Susceptibility artifact causes a loss of fMRI signal, which could potentially lead to a false-negative result.
   D. Susceptibility artifact causes blooming of the fMRI signal, resulting in an artificially increased size of the eloquent areas.

FIG. 18.C6. (A) fMRI language mapping data overlaid on an axial T2-weighted image. A poorly defined T2 bright mass is partially visualized in the right temporal and parietal lobes. Dominant expressive *(yellow arrow)* and receptive *(green arrow)* speech areas are identified in the left hemisphere. (B) Source fMRI EPI in an orange overlay superimposed on an anatomic axial T2-weighted image. On the source data, there is loss of signal from the cortex in the right frontal and temporal lobes adjacent to the patient's right pterional craniotomy site. There is also signal loss at the skull base, near the floor of the anterior and middle cranial fossa bilaterally, due to air-bone interfaces.

Diagnosis

There is left-sided dominant speech. A susceptibility artifact from a right pterional craniotomy limits evaluation of the right superior temporal gyrus.

Discussion

The clinical history in this patient is highly relevant. The patient is left handed, which increases the concern that the patient has right language dominance or that the patient is codominant. In addition, the patient's original presenting concern was speech difficulty. At the time of the fMRI, the patient was already status post–partial resection of the right parietal GBM and was returning for a repeat resection. The fMRI was ordered to help localize language function before a surgical resection.

After the fMRI, an awake craniotomy was performed with intraoperative cortical stimulation. The surgeons stimulated the area adjacent to the tumor in the right temporal lobe and could not find an area that caused the patient to be unable to say her name. The tumor was then surgically resected. The patient did not have any postoperative language deficits.

Susceptibility Artifact

This case demonstrates how susceptibility artifact can be problematic in fMRI. fMRI sequences need to be particularly sensitive to the T2* effects of deoxyhemoglobin and oxyhemoglobin. One such susceptibility-sensitive sequence is gradient-refocused EPI. This is useful in distinguishing between oxyhemoglobin and deoxyhemoglobin, but has a side effect of resulting in increased sensitivity to artifact caused by susceptibility effects.[13] This susceptibility is commonly present in the frontal lobes adjacent to

the air-filled frontal sinuses and in the temporal lobes adjacent to the mastoid air cells and petrous ridge. Patients with an intracranial hemorrhage or with metal from prior surgery will also have pronounced susceptibility effects.

In this case, the metal and blood products from the right pterional craniotomy resulted in susceptibility-induced loss of signal in the right temporal lobe. This is most evident when viewing the source EPI. This loss of signal masks any underlying activity. As a result, the interpreting radiologist could not rule out the possibility that receptive speech was also located in the right temporal lobe, even though none was detected—that is, the radiologist could not rule out a false-negative result. *When interpreting fMRI, the interpreting radiologist should be aware of any susceptibility effects that may distort the fMRI data or instruct the technologists to apply appropriate magnetic field compensation strategies (e.g., z-shimming) to recover these signal losses in the source echo-planar images.*[14] Routine quality control for fMRI needs to incorporate a method, such as the color overlay shown in Fig. 18.C6B, to help identify possible blind spots in the fMRI signal profile across the brain. In cases in which there are blind spots, the clinical history, such as the handedness of the patient and presence or absence of a speech deficit, is essential to help guide interpretation.

CASE 18.6 ANSWER

1. **C. Susceptibility artifact causes a loss of fMRI signal, which could potentially lead to a false-negative result.**

CASE 18.7

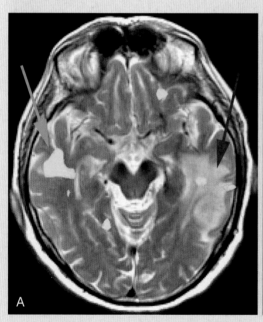 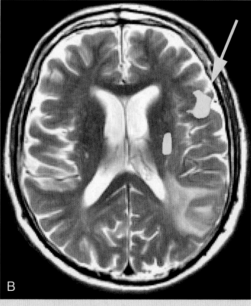

FIG. 18.C7

1. How do brain tumors affect the precision of fMRI?
   A. Tumor-induced vascular stealing can disrupt the hemodynamic response and result in false-negative findings.
   B. Mass effect from tumors can inhibit venous return, disrupt the hemodynamic response, and result in false-negative findings.
   C. Susceptibility artifact from hemorrhage or calcification in tumors can cause a drop in T2* signal, resulting in false-negative findings.
   D. All of the above.

FIG. 18.C7. Color-coded language mapping fMRI data overlaid on axial T2-weighted images. A T2 bright mass (biopsy-proven GBM) is centered in the left temporal lobe. Activation in the inferior left inferior frontal gyrus (*yellow arrow,* B) is consistent with the expressive speech area. Activation in the right superior temporal gyrus (*green arrow,* A) is most consistent with the right-sided receptive speech area. Tiny foci of activation in the superior left temporal lobe (*blue arrow,* A) are seen in the mass in the left temporal lobe.

Diagnosis

fMRI reveals left-dominant expressive speech and right-dominant receptive speech.

Discussion

The patient presented with word finding difficulty. An fMRI was ordered for preoperative management. An awake craniotomy was performed with intraoperative cortical stimulation, which demonstrated the speech area in the superior aspect of the left middle temporal lobe gyrus. The GBM was then removed by working through the inferior temporal gyrus (and avoiding the speech area).

Pathology Results in Alterations to the Hemodynamic Response

Intraoperative mapping at the time of surgery demonstrated that receptive speech was located in the superior aspect of the left middle temporal gyrus. In retrospect, there is faint activity in this location (blue arrow in Fig. 18.C7A) on the fMRI images. However, this level of activity was not called prospectively, and it is still unclear whether these tiny foci of activation on the fMRI scans correspond to the site of the receptive speech area defined by intraoperative cortical mapping.

To understand the source of this possible negative result, one first needs to recall the earlier discussion about the hemodynamic response. Functionally active cortical tissue normally recruits additional blood flow through autoregulatory arteriolar dilation. The increased blood flow results in a decrease in the level of deoxyhemoglobin and consequently an increase in signal on fMRI. *Tumors can locally disrupt normal blood flow autoregulation. As a result, functionally active areas of the brain near a tumor may not be able to recruit additional blood flow and thus may not be bright on fMRI. Highly vascular tumors are particularly adept at causing dysautoregulation.*

It is thought that these tumors are so aggressive at recruiting blood flow that they cause maximal vasodilation of the neighboring arterioles, even when at rest. When the cortex next to the tumor does become active, the hemodynamic response fails because the arterioles are already maximally dilated. False-negative fMRI results are more commonly seen with higher-grade tumors,[15] presumably because these tumors are associated more with dysautoregulation.[16] An alternative or possibly an additional reason why tumors decrease the sensitivity of fMRI is related to the mass effect of tumors. This mass effect may disrupt or displace venous return and, as a result, affect the hemodynamic response.[16]

Cerebrovascular disease and vascular malformations are additional causes for false-negative fMRI studies. These vascular diseases can also disrupt the brain's ability to autoregulate, limiting the hemodynamic response and decreasing or eliminating the BOLD effect during neuronal activation.[7] One strategy to assess for this source of a false-negative study in older patients with cerebrovascular disease or patients with arteriovenous malformations is to use MRI perfusion imaging. If there is decreased cerebral perfusion to an area, then the sensitivity of fMRI to cortical activity in that area will be decreased, and the interpretation should reflect this limitation.[7] Other approaches include assessment of cerebrovascular reserve capacity via an fMRI sequence with a breath-hold challenge to assess the vasodilatory response across the entire brain.[17]

CASE 18.7 ANSWER

1. **D. All of the above.**

CASE 18.8

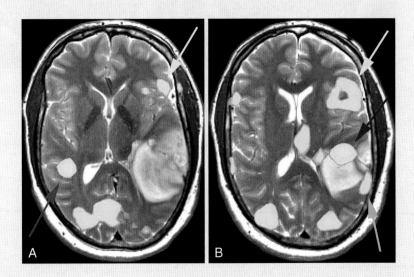

FIG. 18.C8

1. List in order the eloquent cortices depicted by the *yellow, blue, green,* and *red arrows.*
   A. Expressive speech, artifact caused by tumor, artifact caused by tumor, receptive speech
   B. Expressive speech, receptive speech, artifact caused by tumor, accessory receptive speech
   C. Expressive speech, artifact caused by tumor, receptive speech, accessory receptive speech
   D. Expressive speech, receptive speech, receptive speech (second site), accessory receptive speech

FIG. 18.C8. Color-coded fMRI data from a language mapping study overlaid on an anatomic fast spin echo T2-weighted sequence. A large T2 bright mass (biopsy-proven anaplastic astrocytoma) is centered in the left temporal lobe. Activation in the inferior left inferior frontal gyrus *(yellow arrows)* is consistent with a dominant expressive speech area. Left posterior superior temporal gyrus activation *(blue* and *green arrows,* B) is seen wrapping around the anterior, superior, and lateral margins of the tumor. This is consistent with dominant receptive speech areas being distorted by the mass. Activation in the right superior temporal gyrus *(red arrow,* A) is most consistent with an accessory receptive speech activation center.

Diagnosis

The receptive speech area is seen wrapping around the anterior, superior, and lateral margins of the tumor.

Discussion

An awake craniotomy with intraoperative cortical stimulation was performed. Intraoperative cortical stimulation revealed a speech area superior and posterior to the mass (likely the area demarcated by the green arrow in Fig. 18.C8B). Surgical dissection was then performed with care to avoid this area. The tumor was resected to the level of the ventricle. As the surgeons worked close to the anterior aspect of the tumor (near the lateral ventricle), the patient began making errors in speech (possibly the area demarcated by the blue arrow in Fig. 18.C8B). The dissection was then discontinued in this area.

Tumors Effect on Autoregulation

Tumors can disrupt autoregulation and result in false-negative findings, but that is not always the case. This is more commonly seen with higher-grade tumors, such as GBM.[15] In this example, even though the tumor is intimately involved with the dominant receptive speech area, the cortex has maintained its hemodynamic response and continues to be bright on fMRI.

CASE 18.8 ANSWER

1. **D. Expressive speech, receptive speech, receptive speech (second site), accessory receptive speech**

CASE 18.9

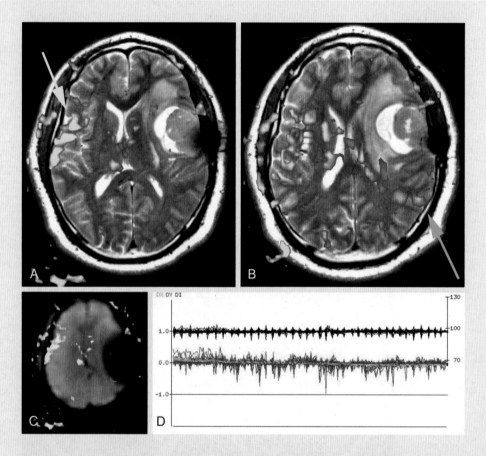

FIG. 18.C9

1. What artifacts limit this fMRI?
   A. Motion artifact from patient's intractable hiccups
   B. Susceptibility artifact from the left frontal temporal craniotomy
   C. Cerebrospinal fluid flow artifact from the ventricular compression
   D. All of the above
   E. A and B

FIG. 18.C9. (A, B) Color-coded language mapping fMRI data overlaid on anatomic axial T2-weighted images. A partially cystic and partially solid mass (biopsy-proven pleomorphic xanthoastrocytoma) is identified in the left frontal lobe. Activity is noted outside the brain and field of view of the brain, consistent with significant motion artifact. This artifact limits the ability to characterize the expressive and receptive speech areas confidently. Activity in the right inferior frontal lobe (*yellow arrow*, A) may represent an expressive speech area. Activity in the left superior temporal gyrus (*green arrow*, B) may represent a receptive speech area. (C) Color-coded language mapping fMRI overlaid on an axial echo-planar image. A large signal void is noted in the left frontal and temporal lobes from susceptibility artifact related to a prior craniotomy. This susceptibility artifact could mask activation in the left frontal and temporal lobes. (D) Graph demonstrating the motion of the head in three planes after motion correction. The *y*-axis represents how far the head has moved (measured in centimeters). The green and orange plots measure motion in the *x* and *y* planes, respectively. The black plot measures the signal intensity over time. Note the rhythmicity of the motion caused by this patient's hiccups, with excursions of up to 1 mm.

Diagnosis

Motion artifact and susceptibility artifact severely limit the study. There is possible right-dominant expressive speech and left-dominant receptive speech.

Discussion

The patient underwent an awake craniotomy and intraoperative cortical stimulation. Electrical stimulation revealed that the patient's expressive speech area was just anterior to the site of the tumor. The tumor was then resected, with careful attention paid not to dissect into the speech area. The patient had no postsurgical speech problems.

Motion and Susceptibility Artifact Limitations

This case demonstrates more limitations of fMRI. Motion can often be a significant limitation to an fMRI study. Retrospective motion correction algorithms are used to try to minimize these effects, but these algorithms have their own limitations.[18] In this case, misregistered activity is seen outside the head, even after motion correction. Prospective motion correction algorithms are increasingly becoming available and may overcome some of these limitations in the future.[19]

This is also another example of how susceptibility artifact can limit a study. The left frontal susceptibility artifact eliminated signal over the left frontal lobe, causing another false-negative result. Intraoperative cortical mapping at the time of surgery revealed the dominant expressive speech area to be just anterior to the mass in the left frontal lobe. Thus two major quality control items that should be addressed in every fMRI scan prior to interpretation are assessment of motion and susceptibility artifact.

CASE 18.9 ANSWER

1. **E. A and B**

TAKE-HOME POINTS

1. fMRI is a family of MRI techniques used to detect functionally active cortical areas of the brain.
2. Alternatives to fMRI include the following:
   - *Wada test:* Phenobarbital is administered via an internal carotid artery to numb the brain perfused by that artery. Loss of function implies that the artery supplies the cortical area in question.
   - *Intraoperative cortical stimulation:* The neurosurgeon uses electrical stimulation directly on the brain during an awake craniotomy. Loss of function implies that stimulated neurons are required for that function. Intraoperative cortical mapping is the gold standard.
3. fMRI works as follows:
   - *Hemodynamic response:* Neuronal activation results in local arteriolar dilation and local decrease of the deoxyhemoglobin level.
   - *BOLD effect:* Deoxyhemoglobin is paramagnetic and dark on T2* sequences. Consequently, reduction of the deoxyhemoglobin level (as a result of the hemodynamic response) results in increased signal on T2*-weighted images.
   - *Statistical analysis:* The color images are statistical representations of the fMRI data. Brighter areas are more functionally active. The color images are overlaid on an anatomic sequence to improve anatomic localization because fMRI usually has low spatial resolution.
4. Popular clinical techniques to activate the cortex include (1) having the patient squeeze his or her hand or pucker the mouth to assess motor function and (2) reading or listening (to assess language reception) or speaking or thinking of words (to assess language expression).
5. Limitations of fMRI include the following:
   - *Motion*
   - *Susceptibility artifact:* Although T2*-weighted imaging is sensitive to the BOLD effect, it is also greatly affected by susceptibility artifacts.
   - *Proximity to tumor:* Adjacent tumors (especially high-grade tumors) can disrupt vascular autoregulation, null the hemodynamic response, and result in false-negative fMRI results.
   - *Cerebrovascular disease* can disrupt vascular autoregulation and cause a false-negative fMRI result.

References

1. Medina LS, Bernal B, Dunoyer C, et al. Seizure disorders: functional MR imaging for diagnostic evaluation and surgical treatment—prospective study. *Radiology.* 2005;236:247–253.
2. Petrella JR, Shah LM, Harris KM, et al. Preoperative functional MR imaging localization of language and motor areas: effect on therapeutic decision making in patients with potentially resectable brain tumors. *Radiology.* 2006;240:793–802.
3. Smits M, Visch-Brink E, Schraa-Tam CK, et al. Functional MR imaging of language processing: an overview of easy-to-implement paradigms for patient care and clinical research. *Radiographics.* 2006;26(suppl 1):S145–S158.
4. Klöppel S, Büchel C. Alternatives to the Wada test: a critical view of functional magnetic resonance imaging in preoperative use. *Curr Opin Neurol.* 2005;18:418–423.
5. Sanai N, Mirzadeh Z, Berger MS. Functional outcome after language mapping for glioma resection. *N Engl J Med.* 2008;358:18–27.
6. Ogawa S, Lee TM, Kay AR, et al. Brain magnetic resonance imaging with contrast dependent on blood oxygenation. *Proc Natl Acad Sci U S A.* 1990;87:9868–9872.
7. Atlas SW. *Magnetic Resonance Imaging of the Brain and Spine.* 4th ed. Philadelphia: Lippincott Williams & Wilkins; 2009.
8. Huettel SA, Song AW, McCarthy G. *Functional Magnetic Resonance Imaging.* 2nd ed. Sunderland, MA: Sinauer; 2009.
9. American College of Radiology. Diagnostic radiology: magnetic resonance imaging (MRI) practice parameters and technical standards. https://www.acr.org/Quality-Safety/Standards-Guidelines/Practice-Guidelines-by-Modality/MRI.
10. Szaflarski JP, Gloss D, Binder JR, et al. Practice guideline summary: use of fMRI in the presurgical evaluation of patients with epilepsy: Report of the Guideline Development, Dissemination, and Implementation Subcommittee of the American Academy of Neurology. *Neurology.* 2017;88:395–402.
11. Wilkinson ID, Romanowski CAJ, Jellinek DA, et al. Motor functional MRI for pre-operative and intraoperative neurosurgical guidance. *Br J Radiol.* 2003;76:98–103.
12. Fandino J, Kollias SS, Wieser HG, et al. Intraoperative validation of functional magnetic resonance imaging and cortical reorganization patterns in patients with brain tumors involving the primary motor cortex. *J Neurosurg.* 1999;91:238–250.
13. Ojemann JG, Akbudak E, Snyder AZ, et al. Anatomic localization and quantitative analysis of gradient refocused echo-planar fMRI susceptibility artifacts. *Neuroimage.* 1997;6:156–167.
14. Song AW. Single-shot EPI with signal recovery from the susceptibility-induced losses. *Magn Reson Med.* 2001;46:407–411.
15. Bizzi A, Blasi V, Falini A, et al. Presurgical functional MR imaging of language and motor functions: validation with intraoperative electrocortical mapping. *Radiology.* 2008;248:579–589.
16. Holodny AI, Schulder M, Liu W-C, et al. The effect of brain tumors on BOLD functional MR imaging activation in the adjacent motor cortex: implications for image-guided neurosurgery. *AJNR Am J Neuroradiol.* 2000;21:1415–1422.
17. Kastrup A, Li T-Q, Takahashi A, et al. Functional magnetic resonance imaging of regional cerebral blood oxygenation changes during breath holding. *Stroke.* 1998;29:2641–2645.
18. Steger TR, Jackson EF. Real-time motion detection of functional MRI data. *J Appl Clin Med Physics.* 2004;5.
19. Maclaren J, Herbst M, Speck O, et al. Prospective motion correction in brain imaging: a review. *Magn Reson Med.* 2013;69:621–636.

CHAPTER 19

Basics of Magnetic Resonance Imaging Safety

Francesco Santini and Timothy J. Amrhein

OPENING CASE 19.1

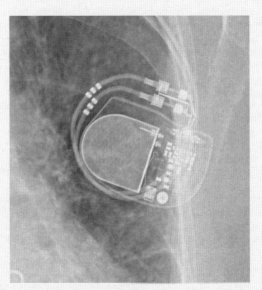

FIG. 19.C1. Magnified view of a chest radiograph from a patient with an implanted St. Jude Accent pacemaker. (Courtesy J. Bremerich.)

1. A patient with a St. Jude Accent pacemaker needs to undergo MRI of the chest wall. The generator and leads are visible on the chest radiograph. How can this scan be performed safely?

   A. This patient cannot be scanned because the chest region cannot be placed in the scanner.

   B. This patient can be scanned, with no particular precautions at any field strength.

   C. This patient can be only scanned at 1.5 T and in normal operating mode for a maximum duration of 30 minutes.

   D. This patient can be scanned at 1.5 T up to the first-level specific energy absorption rate (SAR).

OPENING CASE 19.1

1. A patient with a St. Jude Accent pacemaker needs to undergo MRI of the chest wall. The generator and leads are visible on the chest radiograph. How can this scan be performed safely?

   D. This patient can be scanned at 1.5 T up to the first-level specific energy absorption rate (SAR).

Discussion

This particular pacemaker is MR conditional; the instructions for safe scanning can be found on the manufacturer's website (https://manuals.sjm.com/~/media/manuals/product-manual-pdfs/3/7/37b11dde-7f18-491d-9348-bf99e0933952.pdf). All the instructions must be followed. In this specific case, the conditions depend on the leads used. The leads are Tendril MRI leads (note the presence of radiopaque markers); therefore no scanning region restriction is needed, and first-level SAR is allowed. The device needs to be programmed to MRI mode before the scan.

MR Safety

MRI is universally considered a safe imaging modality. This safety is primarily due to the absence of ionizing radiation, which eliminates concerns about the harmful biologic effects associated with other imaging modalities.

However, an MRI scan is still a medical procedure and carries risks and benefits that should be well understood by medical personnel and patients. Establishing this understanding can be difficult because most people never experience the effects associated with a strong magnetic field, such as that typical of a clinical MRI scanner. Although many are familiar with the direct and indirect effects of electrical potentials and currents—for example, a simple electrostatic discharge produced by touching a car door on a dry day—most people's experience with magnetic fields is usually limited to refrigerator magnets or bag latches, whose action rarely extends further than few millimeters.

In an MRI scanner, image formation is controlled by the simultaneous action of three different types of magnetic fields, each operating at different orders of magnitude in intensity and frequency: (1) the static magnetic field B_0; (2) the gradient fields $G_{x,y,z}$; and (3) the radiofrequency (RF) excitation field B_1. Each field induces different direct and indirect biologic effects and yields different associated risks. *The static magnetic field is always present,* whereas the gradient and the B_1 fields are only active during acquisition.

All these fields may have direct biologic effects (i.e., they interact directly with the body of the subject in the scanner) and indirect biologic effects (i.e., they might have a secondary interaction with the patient because they interact with objects or the environment in the vicinity of the subject).

Static Magnetic Field

The bulkiest component of an MRI scanner is the magnet creating the main magnetic field (usually called B_0). In most modern clinical scanners, this magnetic field is created by solenoids of superconducting wire in which an electrical current flows continuously. The field strength of these magnets is usually 1.5 or 3 T, and they are always active, meaning that *the magnetic field is also present when the scanner is not acquiring images.* As discussed later, this characteristic is associated with the highest safety risk in MRI. This kind of magnet can be shut off (quenched) in case of necessity; however, this procedure carries its own safety concerns and results in high costs because it requires dissipation of the large amount of liquid helium used as a coolant for the superconducting wire.

Another common configuration, only possible in lower-field systems—field strengths from 0.1 to 0.4 T—is the use of a permanent magnet. This magnet poses the same type of safety concerns as superconducting magnets, but to a lesser degree because of the lower field strengths involved. However, as a drawback, quenching is not a possibility for this class of magnets.

The purpose of the MRI magnet is to generate a strong and homogeneous magnetic field across the field of view, typically a region of approximately 50 cm in diameter. However, it is not possible to realize a field exclusively contained inside that region; instead, *around the magnet, a fringe field is present, with an intensity that decreases with the distance from the isocenter.*

Active or passive magnetic shielding, realized by additional magnets or iron cages, aims to contain the fringe fields. However, despite this shielding measurable fields are normally still present, even outside the scanner room (Fig. 19.1).

The use of active shielding helps reduce the extent of the fringe fields, which is necessary to avoid interference with sensitive electronic devices (e.g., pacemakers) that may be located outside the scanner room. *In areas open to the general public, a magnetic field intensity lower than 5 gauss (G), or 0.5 mT, is considered safe.* However, this shielding has the drawback of creating larger magnetic field variations in a smaller space. This rate at which the magnetic field intensity changes in space is termed the *spatial magnetic field gradient.* For example, Fig. 19.2 shows the approximate values of the magnetic field of a 1.5-T clinical scanner as a function of the longitudinal distance from the isocenter. *Across the edge of the magnet, in the space of approximately 1 m, the field intensity decreases 10-fold. This is an important safety concern because the spatial gradient is responsible for the most important direct and indirect effects* of the main magnetic field on the people and objects in the scanner room.

1. What is *not* a possible direct effect of the static magnetic field?
   A. Nausea
   B. Temporary loss of hearing
   C. Metallic taste
   D. Vertigo

2. Where is the attraction force on ferromagnetic objects strongest?
   A. At the entrance of the room
   B. In the middle of the bore (isocenter)
   C. At the edge of the magnet
   D. It is constant everywhere

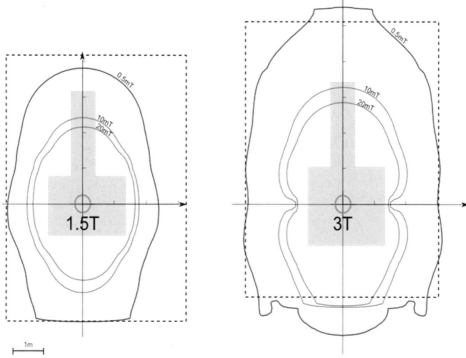

FIG. 19.1. Footprints of two commercial MRI scanners of 1.5-T (*left*) and 3-T (*right*) field strengths. The *dotted line* represents the inner walls of the room (the walls contain magnetic shielding), and the *green circle* represents the maximum field of view for imaging.

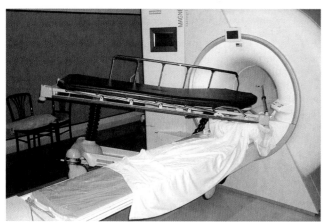

FIG. 19.2. A stretcher made of ferromagnetic material was accidentally brought into an MR scanner room. The strong resultant attraction force pulled the stretcher toward the isocenter of the magnetic field, an event that could not be prevented by staff. If a patient had been present on the MR table at the time of this event, a fatality or serious injury could have resulted. Removal of the stretcher likely required removal of the magnetic field, with consequent costs and downtime. (Courtesy E. Merkle.)

Direct Effects of the Static Magnetic Field

Unlike other organisms, humans lack the possibility of directly experiencing magnetic fields, at least at a conscious level.[1,2] However, *when a person moves within a magnetic field, and especially through a spatial magnetic field gradient, electrical currents are generated inside the body* due to electromagnetic induction (Faraday's law). These currents are caused by the change in magnetic flux through the conducting tissues of the body, and their effects are mostly noticeable in the head. At the same time, the magnetic field exerts mechanical forces (Lorentz forces) on the fluid inside the bony labyrinth, thus inducing a sensation of movement.[3]

The combination of these phenomena gives rise to a series of physiologic effects:
- Vertigo
- Nausea
- Metallic taste
- Reduction of hand-eye coordination
- Magnetic phosphenes (appearance of lights at the periphery of vision)

These effects are limited to the time during which the subject is exposed to the magnetic field, and generally pose no particular safety risk. *They are more severe when the temporal rate of change (dB/dt) of the magnetic field is higher because the induced currents are stronger.*

When moving in a nonuniform magnetic field, the temporal rate of change is proportional to the spatial gradient and to the speed at which the subject is moving in this field. Note that although this effect generally worsens with higher field strengths, that is not always the case, because it is also dependent on factors such as the type of magnet and type of shielding.

As seen in Fig. 19.2, the highest spatial gradient is in the vicinity of the entrance of the bore. Because of this, fast movements in this region—for example, while moving the patient table or while reaching inside the bore—have the strongest physiologic effects.

It should be mentioned that sensitivity to the direct effects of the static magnetic field is subject dependent and is usually not a cause of concern. *MR personnel should, however, be aware of these potential effects and act accordingly, limiting movement speed for themselves and for patients while in the scanner room, especially near the bore entrance.*

Indirect Effects of the Static Magnetic Field

The most important effect to take into account when considering MR safety is not directly related to the action of the B_0 magnetic field on the human body, but rather to the effects that the field has on surrounding or implanted objects. Specifically, objects that are ferromagnetic or metallic can be attracted to the bore or can be otherwise affected, which can

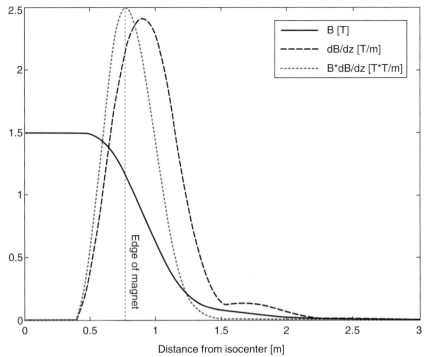

FIG. 19.3. Plot of B_0-field-related quantities for a 1.5-T commercial magnet as a function of the distance (z) from the isocenter. The solid line (*B*) represents the field strength, the dashed line (dB/dz) represents the rate of change of the field intensity in space (spatial gradient), and the dotted line (B*dB/dz) is the magnetic pull factor, a quantity proportional to the force exerted on a ferromagnetic object placed at that distance.

potentially result in damage to equipment, injury to patients and personnel, or even death.

The indirect effects of the static magnetic field include attraction and torque (on magnets or ferromagnetic materials) and magnetic forces secondary to electromagnetic induction (on conductive materials). The attraction forces are the most dangerous aspect of an MRI machine. These are the forces that can be responsible for objects flying toward the center of the magnet, seriously injuring patients and staff (see Fig. 19.2). *Attraction forces act on a class of materials that are called ferromagnetic. When ferromagnetic materials are immersed in a magnetic field, they exhibit a strong magnetization* (an internal magnetic field), which interacts with external magnetic fields. The degree of magnetization that a material experiences in response to the applied external field is called *susceptibility*. The larger this value, the stronger the attraction that will act on the object.

The magnitude of the attraction force acting on an object is proportional to the volume of the object, the intensity of the magnetic field B_0, and the spatial gradient of the external magnetic field.

As we can see from the plot in Fig. 19.3, the highest magnetic pull is generally experienced around the edge of the magnet. Similarly, the force decreases quite steeply with the distance from the magnet. It is therefore very important to bear in mind that *a small movement toward the scanner can result in a sudden increase in force.* For this reason, *all potentially ferromagnetic objects must never be brought inside the scanner room,* or appropriate and strict measures must be followed when this is inevitable (e.g., monitoring equipment should be bolted to the floor).

ANSWERS: STATIC MAGNETIC FIELD

1. **B. Temporary loss of hearing**
2. **C. At the edge of the magnet**

Magnetic Materials

Given the potential dangers of attraction forces on ferromagnetic objects, it is important to understand what types of materials are ferromagnetic. Iron is the best-known ferromagnetic material. Its degree of magnetism depends primarily on its crystalline structure but also on the chemical composition of the alloy. Some iron alloys, such as some forms of stainless steel, are nonferromagnetic, whereas pure iron or other steel alloys are strongly magnetic, thus experiencing great attraction to the scanner. Similarly, metallic nickel is ferromagnetic, but some alloys, such as nitinol (nickel-titanium alloy), are nonmagnetic and can be used in a static magnetic field without experiencing any significant force. Table 19.1 lists the characteristics of some common ferromagnetic and nonferromagnetic materials.

Depending on the geometry of the object, the induced magnetic field might not be parallel to the external field; instead it might follow the object's shape. In this case, an additional torque is applied to the object, which tends to try to align its main axis with the external magnetic field. The intensity of this torque is proportional to the B_0 field and can be problematic in the setting of indwelling implants because they can be displaced. It is important to note that, because of the proportionality described earlier, the magnetic attraction is zero at the isocenter of the external magnetic field (spatial gradient = 0), whereas the torque is maximum in the same location.

In addition to the forces that act on ferromagnetic materials immersed in a static magnetic field, other mechanical forces are generated on every conductive object that is moved while inside an external magnetic field. These are forces that oppose movement of the object, which will tend to stay still in its position or deviate from the desired trajectory. However, these forces will not be experienced unless one tries to move the object. They are the result of currents that are induced in conductive materials in a changing magnetic field (Faraday's law), which in turn generate a magnetic field opposing the change (Lenz's law). These currents, and therefore the resulting forces, are larger when the conductive object presents a large surface. Because they only counteract an existing movement, these forces do not usually present significant safety concerns but should be taken into account when moving equipment in the scanner room.

Table 19.1 COMMON MATERIALS AND THEIR SUSCEPTIBILITY VALUES

Material	Density (g/cm³)	Susceptibility
Gold	11.85	-34×10^{-6}
Copper	8.92	-9.63×10^{-6}
Water, 37°C	0.933	-9.05×10^{-6}
Aluminum	2.70	20.7×10^{-6}
Titanium	4.54	182×10^{-6}
Nitinol 50	6.45	245×10^{-6}
Stainless steel (nonmagnetic)	8.0	$3.52–6.7 \times 10^{-3}$
Nickel[a]	8.9	600
Stainless steel (magnetic)[a]	7.8	400–1100
Iron[a]	7.87	0.2×10^{6}

For ferromagnetic materials, the susceptibility is not constant and depends on the applied field; the maximum differential values are tabulated. The magnetism of stainless steel depends on the crystal configuration. The martensitic configuration is strongly magnetic, whereas the austenitic configuration is weakly magnetic.

[a]Strongly magnetic materials that present significant danger in an MRI environment.

Data from Schenck JF. The role of magnetic susceptibility in magnetic resonance imaging: MRI magnetic compatibility of the first and second kinds. *Med Phys.* 1996;23:815–850.

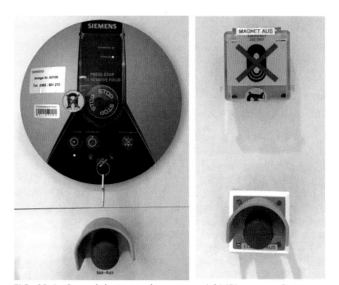

FIG. 19.4. Quench buttons of a commercial MRI scanner. Buttons are generally installed outside *(left)* and inside *(right)* the scanner room. The emergency electrical switch is visible below the button. This latter switch does not disable the magnetic field.

Preventing Accidents Due to Magnetic Attraction

The introduction of ferromagnetic objects inside the scanner room is the single most important aspect to control regarding MR safety. Fatal accidents have been reported due to the introduction of iron objects (e.g., oxygen tanks) into the scanner room, especially in emergency situations.

If possible, the space adjacent to the MR room should be clearly divided into different zones.[4] In any case, in the vicinity of the scanner, all objects that are ferromagnetic should be clearly identified, and *nonmagnetic versions of critical equipment should be ready for use and clearly labeled as such.*

Identification of potential ferromagnetic implants or foreign objects in the body of a patient before scanning is a requirement and is accomplished by way of a careful patient history. All identified implants should then be investigated further and in the deepest possible detail. In case of uncertainty, a ferromagnetic detector can be used. Weakly ferromagnetic implants can be tolerated when they are small and firmly attached to the body (e.g., orthopedic prostheses).

Quenching

A superconducting magnet can be quenched in case of emergency. During a quench, the liquid helium is forced to boil off quickly, causing the magnet to lose its superconductivity. As a result, *the current circulating in the* *superconducting wire would quickly be eliminated, and the magnetic field would decrease to zero.*

All superconducting MR scanners have a quench button that should be protected from being accidentally pressed and should ideally be placed both inside and outside the scanner room (Fig. 19.4).

Quenching is a measure that can and must be taken in case of entrapment, when removing the magnetic field is needed to rescue a person. However, it has some important drawbacks: first of all, *the removal of the magnetic field is not instantaneous.* It can take up to 1 minute for the magnetic field to reach a negligible value. It is therefore not safe to press the quench button and immediately enter the room with ferromagnetic material. A second drawback is that the quenching resistors are cooled by the liquid helium normally used for maintaining the superconductivity. The liquid helium rapidly expands into gas and needs to escape the room. A quench pipe is installed for this purpose, but if it is not properly maintained, then gaseous helium could fill the scanner room, potentially causing cold burns (due to its low temperature), overpressure inside the room, and risk of asphyxiation. Lastly, the helium needs to be replaced and the magnet ramped up before the scanner is operational again, causing considerable costs and economic losses.

In view of these problems, *a quench should only be treated as an emergency measure when no other possibilities are available.* Ideally, before initiating a quench, all personnel should be evacuated from the room.

1. What is the best way to deal with peripheral nerve stimulation during a clinical MRI scan?
   A. Avoid it by reducing the slew rate.
   B. Peripheral nerve stimulation cannot happen in a commercial scanner.
   C. Tell the patient not to cross the legs and keep the arms along the body.
   D. Inform the patient of the possibility of it happening, but that it is not harmful.

2. What is the safest way to prevent hearing damage due to gradient acoustic noise?
   A. Using earplugs and earmuffs
   B. Scanning at lower field strength
   C. Reducing the scan time
   D. Reducing the flip angle

ANSWERS: QUENCHING

1. **D.** Inform the patient of the possibility of it happening, but that it is not harmful.
2. **A.** Using earplugs and earmuffs

Gradient Fields

During image acquisition, to enable spatial encoding of the MR signal, time- and spatial-varying magnetic fields are activated by the MR sequence. These fields vary linearly in space; they have a value of zero in the isocenter and increase along each of the three spatial orthogonal directions inside the scanner—conventionally indicated as x, y, and z, where z is usually the direction of the main magnetic field, B_0. The strength (in megatesla per meter) and rate of change of these gradients are controlled by the sequence. Typical maximum strengths for clinical systems are 40 to 120 mT/m, and typical maximum switching rates are of the order of hundreds of hertz.

Because the gradients increase linearly, the maximum absolute value of the magnetic field can be found at the edge of the imaging field of view. Any direct effect of these fields is therefore stronger at this position.

Direct Effects

The gradient fields are time-varying magnetic fields. *When a time-varying magnetic field interacts with a conductive material, currents are induced in the material* due to Faraday's law in a manner proportional to the rate at which the gradient changes.

Because the human body is also conductive, currents are also induced within it. These currents can interfere with the physiologic signaling of neurons, causing depolarization of peripheral motor neurons (peripheral nerve stimulation). Occasionally, peripheral nerve stimulation results in a sensation of mild muscular twitching in the patient during the scan.

Higher gradient strengths and faster switching rates increase the magnitude of this effect. However, the possible gradient strengths and switching rates of commercial MRI scanners are purposefully limited by the manufacturer so that painful or dangerous stimulation cannot occur.[5]

Indirect Effects

The time-varying magnetic fields produced by the gradient coils are superimposed on the static main magnetic field. The interaction between these fields generates forces acting on the gradient coils, which consequently vibrate. *The result of this vibration is the characteristic loud noise associated with an MRI scan.*

Depending on the hardware characteristics of the scanner and on the particular MR sequence, sound pressure levels can reach 130 dB, which is conventionally considered to be the threshold for pain.[6,7] For comparison, this is in the range of noise from a pneumatic drill (Table 19.2 lists reference noise levels). One of the consequences of unprotected exposure to such noise levels is a threshold shift or elevation of the hearing threshold following cessation of the noise. Threshold shifts can last for minutes to hours after exposure (transient threshold shifts) or can be associated with permanent hearing loss (permanent threshold shifts).

To protect the subject and occasional personnel present in the room during acquisition, it is necessary to use appropriate hearing protection—namely, earplugs and earmuffs. Correct use of earplugs and earmuffs can provide a protection of up to 40 dB, thus bringing the MR noise to acceptable levels.

Another indirect effect of the gradient system is the *induction of currents and variable magnetic forces on conductive objects inside the scanner.* This is a major source of concern in the setting of active *implanted devices such as pacemakers, which can be damaged or lead to fatal malfunctions by these currents* (see "Active Devices" later in this chapter).

Table 19.2 EXAMPLE NOISES AND THEIR NOISE LEVELS

Noise	Level (dB)	Comments
Breathing	10	Limit of hearing
Whisper	20	
Quiet rural area, quiet bedroom	30	
Quiet library	40	
Living room	50	
Conversation at 1 m	60	
Vacuum cleaner	70	Beginning of irritating sound level
Busy road	80	
Motorcycle at 8 m	90	Hearing protection for prolonged exposure
Power lawn mower	100	
Car horn at 1 m	110	Threshold of discomfort
Chain saw	120	
Jet aircraft takeoff at 16 m	130	Threshold of pain
Shotgun	140	Risk of eardrum rupture

The decibel scale is logarithmic; an increase of 3 dB corresponds to a doubling of the sound pressure.

Radiofrequency Field

To generate an MR signal, the magnetizations of the nuclei within the patient need to be perturbed from their equilibrium state (i.e., alignment along the B_0 field) into an excited state. This is achieved by using a variable magnetic field (B_1 field) that is emitted by the transmit coil. This magnetic field varies in time at the Larmor frequency. The Larmor frequency is a function of the imaged nucleus (the hydrogen nucleus is standard in clinical MR applications) and increases linearly with the intensity of the B_0 field (Table 19.3). For practical field strengths, this frequency is similar in order of magnitude to radiowaves; therefore, this B_1 field is also called the radiofrequency (RF) field.

Although it is the magnetic field component that is actually useful for the excitation, an electric field (conventionally identified by the letter E) is always associated with it according to Maxwell's laws of electromagnetism. Because of the conductive nature of biologic tissues, *this electric field generates electrical currents inside the body that in turn cause heating.* This heating, both at a global and localized level, is the main safety concern associated with the RF field.

According to Ohm's law, the dissipated energy inside the tissue is proportional to the square of the induced electric field and is quantified by the SAR. SAR is a local quantity—defined for every point inside the body—expressed in watts per kilogram of tissue and is dependent on the tissue characteristics and local intensity of the electric RF field elevated to the power of 2. These quantities vary, depending on the spatial location and on time, and usually a time- and space-averaged value is calculated (e.g., whole-body or head SAR, averaged over a time window of 6 minutes).

Due to this averaging, the SAR becomes lower with longer repetition times because the RF pulses are executed less often and are of longer pulse durations, a parameter that can usually be controlled, at least broadly (e.g., by selecting low SAR, normal, or fast pulses in the sequence parameters). On the other hand, it increases with the square of the main magnetic field and with the square of the flip angle. To summarize this into a proportionality formula:

$$SAR \propto \left(B_0^2 \times \alpha^2\right) / (\tau \times TR)$$

where B_0 is the static field strength, α is the flip angle, τ is the pulse duration, and TR is the repetition time of the sequence. The actual proportionality constant is evaluated by mathematical models and is internally handled by the software of the

Table 19.3 LARMOR FREQUENCIES FOR HYDROGEN NUCLEI AND WAVELENGTHS IN AIR AND TISSUE

B_0 (T)	Larmor Frequency of ^{1}H (MHz)	Wavelength in Air (cm)	Wavelength in Tissue (cm)	Resonant Lengths in Air (cm)	Resonant Lengths in Tissue (cm)
0.2	8.5	3521	390	1760, 6280, ...	195, 585, ...
0.3	12.8	2347	260	1173, 3520, ...	130, 390, ...
1.0	42.6	704	78	352, 1056, ...	39, 117, ...
1.5	63.9	469	52	235, 704, ...	26, 78, ...
3.0	127.7	235	26	112, 352, ...	13, 39, ...
7.0	298	100	11	50, 150, ...	5.6, 16.7, ...
9.4	400	75	8	37, 112, ...	4.1, 12.4, ...

MRI system (considering the patient's weight and possibly height), which continuously monitors the SAR and restricts operation according to its mode of operation.

The human body has a natural capacity for heat dissipation, so constant exposure within certain SAR levels normally causes only limited increases in body temperature.[8] This is taken into account when defining the acceptable irradiation levels for the patient under different operating modes of the scanner.

The normal operating mode of the scanner is considered a mode in which no particular physiologic stress to the patient is expected. The increase in core temperature of the subject is limited to 0.5°C, corresponding to a whole-body SAR limit (averaged over a 6-minute window) of 2.0 W/kg.

The first-level controlled operating mode is a mode in which physiologic stress can be achieved. The increase in core temperature is limited to 1°C, corresponding to a whole-body SAR of 4.0 W/kg. This mode should never be used for patients with impaired thermal regulation, infants, or unconscious patients without appropriate monitoring.

The second-level controlled operating mode is a mode in which these limitations can be exceeded and is normally not accessible in conventional diagnostic scanners. Further SAR limits are summarized in Table 19.4.

These considerations about the physiologic temperature increase are valid under two assumptions, both (partially) under the control of the operator:

1. The subject's thermal regulation is not impaired by the subject's condition or by external factors—for example, the room temperature is cool, there is sufficient airflow, or the subject is not excessively covered.
2. There is no element that could focus the electric field distribution and make it deviate from the standardized models used (e.g., resonant electromagnetic induction, antenna effect).

The second assumption is associated with focal heating due to geometric conformations of conductive materials inside or outside the body. These materials can act as linear antennas locally focusing the intensity of the electric field or as resonant coils that couple with the magnetic field. In both cases, a local increase in temperature of a much higher magnitude than what was predicted by the models can be observed.[9] The most dangerous geometries are large loops or straight conductors of a length equal or close to the resonant lengths (see Table 19.3).

Table 19.4 SPECIFIC ENERGY ABSORPTION RATE (SAR) LIMITS FOR MRI[a]

Body Region	LIMIT (W/KG)		
	Normal Mode	First-Level Controlled	Second-Level Controlled[b]
Whole body	2	4	>4
Partial body			
Head	3.2	3.2	>3.2
Not head[c]	2–10	4–10	>(4–10)
Local SAR[d]			
Head, trunk	10	20	>20
Extremities	20	40	>40

Radiofrequency exposure must observe all SAR limits—for transmit coils with highly inhomogeneous field, local SAR over a small region might be reached before partial- or whole-body SAR limits, whereas for more homogeneous coils, partial- or whole-body limits might be reached first.

[a]As defined by the IEC 60601-2-33 norm.

[b]Second-level controlled cannot be enabled for routine diagnostics.

[c]Partial-body SAR scales linearly with the ratio between the patient mass exposed and total patient mass.

[d]Local SAR values are averaged over 10 g of tissue.

This effect can have three causes:

1. Incorrect positioning of the patient
2. Presence of external conductive material
3. Presence of conductive implants

The patient must therefore never be positioned so that the arms and hands form a closed loop or their legs are crossed. Touching the bore can also form a dangerous conductive loop. The patient must also not touch any external cable in the bore (e.g., monitoring cables; Fig. 19.5).

In case of suspected impaired thermal regulation or implants, it is important to keep the SAR at a minimum. According to the formula above, reducing the SAR can be achieved by the following:

- Switching to a lower-field system
- Reducing the flip angle
- Increasing the pulse duration
- Increasing the TR
- Changing the sequence type (e.g., from spin echo to gradient echo)

Correct positioning

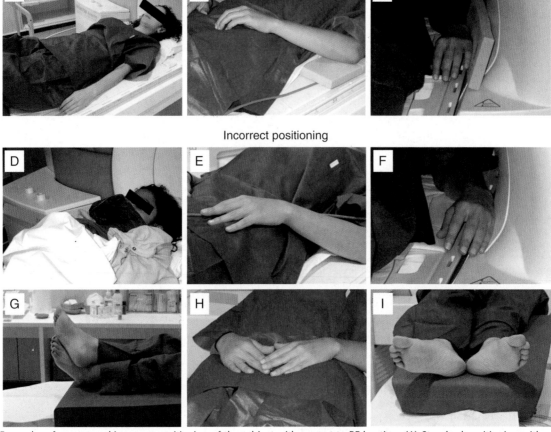

Incorrect positioning

FIG. 19.5. Examples of correct and incorrect positioning of the subject with respect to RF heating. (A) Standard positioning with unimpaired heat dissipation and arms alongside the body. (B–C) Demonstration of using padding to avoid contact with a monitoring cable or the bore. (D) Excessive covering of the subject that might lead to a global rise in temperature during scan. (E–F) Contact with conducting elements of the scanner or other equipment might result in contact burns. (G–I) Formation of conductive loops with the limbs with potential focal heating at contact points.

1. What is SAR?
   A. A measure of the intensity of the RF field
   B. A measure of the RF power converted into heat inside the body
   C. The rise in temperature experienced by the subject during a sequence
   D. The intensity of the acquired MR signal

2. How can SAR be reduced?
   A. Scanning at a lower field strength
   B. Increasing the RF pulse duration
   C. Reducing the flip angle
   D. All of the above

ANSWERS: SPECIFIC ENERGY ABSORPTION RATE

1. **B. A measure of the RF power converted into heat inside the body**
2. **D. All of the above**

FIG. 19.C2

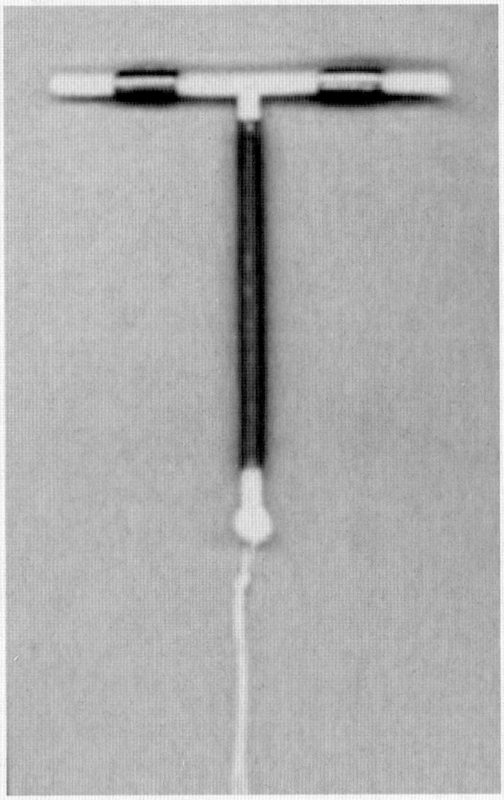

1. A patient with a copper intrauterine contraceptive device (IUD, no other information available) is scheduled for a chest MRI. Can the examination be performed?
   A. Yes, at any field strength
   B. Yes, but only at 1.5 T
   C. Yes, but only at 3T
   D. No
2. Should a specific scanning protocol be used?
   A. Only normal mode SAR should be used.
   B. Spin echo–type sequences should be avoided.
   C. The scanning protocol should last less than 30 minutes.
   D. No special adaptation is necessary.

FIG. 19.C2. ParaGard intrauterine contraceptive device.

Discussion

The IUD is made of copper and plastic, so magnetic pull is not an issue. The only concern in this case is focal heating due to the antenna effect. Geometrically, the IUD could exhibit focusing of the electric field because it is a thin elongated shape; however, these devices are small (≈30 mm in length), much shorter than the critical length of 13 cm at 3 T (see Table 19.3). This patient can therefore be scanned without particular adaptations of the protocol. However, verbal contact with the patient throughout the scan is advised.

It is worth noting that although not common in the United States, Canada, and Europe, stainless steel IUDs exist,[10] but their safety in an MR environment has not been assessed.

Implants and MRI

Patients with implants need to be treated with special care before and during MRI scanning because indwelling implants may carry additional risks. In general, every implant should be classified with respect to its category of risk—MR safe; MR conditional; MR unsafe (Fig. 19.6).

MR safe is an implant (or any object) that is safe in all MR environments and scanning conditions, independent of the magnetic field or RF power levels. In practice, only objects made of nonmagnetic and nonconductive materials fall into this category.

At the opposite end of the spectrum lies the MR unsafe classification. Objects in this category cannot be considered safe in any MR environment. Usually these are ferromagnetic objects that can cause a significant projectile or displacement hazard or active devices whose functionality can be compromised by exposure to the magnetic field.

The MR conditional category contains everything that can be safely scanned, provided that certain conditions are met. In principle, every device or implant manufacturer should provide an MR classification sheet and a list of required conditions for scanning. When scanning such a device, all these conditions must be met. These typically include the following:

1. *Allowed field strength(s).* It is important to note that safety at *a higher field strength (e.g., 3 T) does not imply that the device is also safe at a lower field strength.* This is because of the different resonant lengths for the antenna effect.
2. *Maximum spatial field gradient.* This is a measure of the rate at which the static magnetic field varies in space and is specified by the manufacturer.

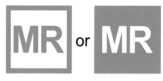

MR Safe

MR Conditional

MR Unsafe

FIG. 19.6. Symbols used in labels indicating the safety of objects and devices with respect to MR environments, as recommended by the American Society for Testing and Materials.

3. *Maximum RF field intensity* (in terms of $B_{1,rms}$ or SAR). Commercial MRI scanners give an estimation of the SAR and, in some cases, of $B_{1,rms}$ before the start of the acquisition. This aids in planning and adjusting the scan protocol. When the $B_{1,rms}$ value is available, it is advised that this parameter be used instead of SAR because it is independent of patient characteristics.

4. *Maximum gradient slew rate* (in Tesla per meter per second). This is also a characteristic of the scanner and is provided by the manufacturer.

5. *Scanning region restrictions. Some devices restrict scanning to specific body regions; for example, some MR conditional pacemakers do not allow scanning of the thorax.*

6. *Allowed transmit coils* (body coil or local transmit coils). It is important to remember that most of the coils used in MRI are only *receive* coils, whereas the excitation is performed by the *body coil* integrated into the scanner bore. Only some coils (typically the knee coil and some head coils) are transmit or receive coils.

7. *Other restrictions* (e.g., total scan time, indications to fix the device to avoid displacement).

CASE 19.2 ANSWERS

1. **A. Yes, at any field strength**
2. **D. No special adaptation is necessary.**

CASE 19.3

1. A patient with a Senza Spinal Cord Stimulation System (Nevro) implanted in the lumbar spine needs to undergo head MRI at 1.5 T. Can the MRI be performed?
   A. Yes, the MR can be performed regardless of the MR environment or conditions.
   B. Yes, but only if a transmit-receive head coil is used.
   C. Yes, but only if the body coil is used for transmission.
   D. No.

2. What protocol can be used?
   A. Normal operating mode must be used.
   B. No special protocol adaptations are needed.
   C. The scan time must be less than 15 minutes.
   D. Both A and C

Discussion

This stimulator is an active device; thus the appropriate guidelines must be followed. These guidelines can be found on the manufacturer's website (http://www.nevro.com/Physicians/MRI/Guidelines). The device is MR conditional at 1.5 and 3 T; however, the manufacturer specifies that only a transmit-receive RF head coil should be used. Often, head coils are receive only, and the body coil performs the excitation. If this is the case with the available MR scanner, then the scan cannot be performed.

If the system is equipped with a transmit-receive head coil, the correct procedure to scan the patient safely involves the following:

1. Confirm that the device and the leads are from the same manufacturer and that no other leads are present.
2. Turn off the device.
3. Confirm that the maximum slew rate of the gradient system is below 200 T/m per second (common value for commercial scanners).
4. Prepare a protocol with an effective scan time of up to 15 minutes.

The guidelines mention that the SAR should be lower than 3.2 W/kg. However, this is the SAR limit for the head at the normal operating mode and at the first-level controlled operating mode; therefore this constraint is already fulfilled by the scanner constraints.

Active Devices

The scanning of active devices—devices that are equipped with electronic or electromechanical components with an independent power source, such as pacemakers or infusion pumps—is in principle only possible when they are MR conditional and the conditions for the specific device (as indicated in the device's manual or brochure) are known and respected. When these indications are not followed, malfunction of the device, in addition to the known hazards of MRI, especially severe in the case of implanted electrodes,[11] can occur, with potentially fatal consequences.

Even when following the appropriate instructions, scanning patients with implants (especially active implants) carries an elevated risk for complications. For this reason, appropriate monitoring and emergency procedures should be implemented.[12] In particular, an MR-safe procedure for resuscitation and cardiac defibrillation should be defined. This usually involves taking the patient out of the scanner room or using MR-safe crash carts and oxygen tanks.

CASE 19.3 ANSWERS

1. **B. Yes, but only if a transmit-receive head coil is used.**
2. **C. The scan time must be less than 15 minutes.**

CASE 19.4

1. A patient with a 10-year-old mechanical aortic valve prosthesis is scheduled for MRI at 3 T. The heart valve manufacturer and model are unknown. Can the examination be performed?
   A. Yes
   B. Yes, but it must be performed at 1.5 T.
   C. Yes, but only if the chest region is excluded.
   D. Without additional information, it is not safe to scan at any field strength.

2. What protocol can be used?
   A. The normal operating mode must be used.
   B. No special protocol adaptations are needed.
   C. The scan time must be less than 15 minutes.
   D. Both A and C

Discussion

A heart valve replacement can be made of various metallic materials; thus it is conductive and potentially ferromagnetic and both attraction and heating issues must be considered. However, the valve has a small volume and is already subject to significant mechanical stress due to blood flow and cardiac movement. Regarding heating issues, the valve is also small with respect to the RF wavelength and it is placed inside a major vessel, where the blood is an excellent medium to remove excess heat. The patient can be safely scanned without any special protocol. This recommendation can also be confirmed by checking the related page on the MRI safety website (http://www.mrisafety.com/SafetyInfoFromList.asp?LSub=33).

Passive Implants

Obtaining MR safety information for particular implants may not always be possible or practical. Because a large number of passive implants can still be safely scanned in the absence of such information, especially those manufactured in the past 20 years, it is sometimes possible to make a safety decision based on a few assumptions about the implant itself. In this case, *the two most important concerns are magnetic attraction and RF heating.*

The material of the implant is of crucial importance when considering magnetic attraction. If the material is known to be nonferromagnetic, then significant attraction forces can be ruled out; however, *if the material is unknown, the following aspects should be considered:*

1. *Is the implant small (and possibly flexible)?*
2. *Is it firmly attached to the body (e.g., orthopedic implants, onset of fibrosis)?*
3. *Is it located in a body region where a small displacement or force can be tolerated (e.g., not in the brain)?*

In the case of an affirmative answer, it is reasonable to assume that the implant will not experience harmful forces. For example, cardiac valves need to withstand strong physiologic forces and are therefore firmly attached to the tissue: they generally pose no safety problems. On the other hand, *aneurysm clips might be ferromagnetic and could cause significant damage when immersed in a magnetic field, with one fatal accident reported.*[13]

For unknown vascular implants (outside the head), a minimum of 6 weeks after surgery is recommended to ensure fibrosis onset and firm attachment of the implant to the wall. Intracranially vascular fibrosis does not occur; therefore extra care must be taken to ensure that implants are MR safe.

Assessing safety with regard to potential RF heating requires consideration of several variables. Conductive implants have the potential to focus the electric field due to the antenna effect, depending on their positioning and geometry. The following configurations yield higher risk:

1. *Thin implants with a sharp tip (e.g., electrodes)* because the electric field is focused at the tip
2. *Implants with a length close to the resonant length* (note that this is dependent on the field strength; see Table 19.3)
3. *Implants parallel to the axis of the bore* because they are parallel to the electric field

One should also take into consideration the sensitivity of the adjacent tissue (e.g., deep brain stimulation electrodes have a high damage potential[11]) and the extent of local perfusion (because blood helps dissipate heat).

Finally, whenever an implant is present, it is important to monitor the patient closely and maintain voice contact throughout the scan. However, it should be understood that even with these safeguards in place, asymptomatic heat damage could still occur because pain receptors are not present in some deep tissues.

Additional information on implants and their behavior in MRI can be found at http://www.mrisafety.com.

Piercings

Decorative piercings are a popular form of body modification. Body piercing jewelry is usually made of biocompatible metals, which are typically conductive and, in some cases, can exhibit ferromagnetic behavior. Therefore the presence of such jewelry on the patient during an MRI scan can carry the risk of magnetic pull, vibration due to currents induced by the gradients, and RF heating.

For safety purposes, the removal of all jewelry is recommended before an MRI scan. However, this is sometimes not possible for practical reasons. In this scenario, similar considerations apply as for other passive implants. Depending on the location of the piercing, bandages or patches can be applied to reduce magnetic pull and vibrations. Contrary to implants, however, jewelry is usually superficially located and is therefore in close proximity to pain receptors. This allows for the patient to detect increased temperatures due to RF heating. It is therefore important to inform patients about this possible adverse event and to monitor them by keeping constant voice contact throughout the scan.

Tattoos and Permanent Makeup

Tattoos and permanent makeup consist of ink that is permanently applied under the skin. This ink can be composed of a variety of compounds and often contains metals. As a result, artifacts can be generated in the immediate vicinity of the tattooed site, which needs to be considered during image acquisition and interpretation.

The main MR safety concern for tattoos and permanent makeup is the potential for conductivity resulting in possible RF heating. RF burns in tattoos and permanent makeup are rare and usually mild (up to second-degree burns), and most spontaneously resolve. However, there have been many reported cases of serious incidents in the literature, including burns on eyelids due to permanent makeup.[14-17]

As with piercings, it is important to inform the subject of the possibility of heating at the site of the tattoo and to maintain verbal contact with her or him throughout the scan. Applying a cold compress on the tattoo might also serve as a preventive measure.

CASE 19.4 ANSWERS

1. **A. Yes**
2. **B. No special protocol adaptations are needed.**

TAKE-HOME POINTS

1. An MRI scanner uses three different types of magnetic fields to produce images—the static magnetic field, gradient fields, and RF field. Each of these has associated safety considerations that should be reviewed prior to scanning a patient.
2. The static magnetic field is always active, even when the scanner is not scanning or is turned off.
3. The main safety issue with the static magnetic field is its capability to exert an attractive force on ferromagnetic objects. This force is proportional to the volume of the object and increases rapidly while approaching the magnet. It can be strong enough to make small and large objects fly toward the magnet, which might lead to a fatal accident.
4. The gradient fields are responsible for the acoustic noise that can be heard during an MR acquisition. This noise can be strong enough to cause temporary or even permanent hearing damage. Therefore the patient (as well as anyone else in the scanner room during the examination) needs to be protected with earplugs or earmuffs.
5. The RF field is associated with heating. SAR is a measure of how much power the subject's body is absorbing as heat. It is based on mathematical models; that is, it is not an actual measure and is only valid as long as certain conditions are met.
6. For obese patients, infants, those with a high fever, and persons with impaired thermal regulation, SAR estimations might be incorrect, and restricting the SAR limits is advisable.
7. To avoid overheating, the patient must not be overly covered in clothes and blankets while lying in the scanner. To avoid burns, the patient should be positioned to avoid forming conductive loops—no crossing of legs, clasping of hands, or touching the magnet bore.
8. When scanning patients with implants, extra care must always be taken.
9. Active implants must always be correctly identified and scanned according to the guidelines of the manufacturer.
10. A decision to scan passive implants can be made based on some general considerations when exact information about the implant is not available. In particular, a passive implant can be generally considered safe if it is small, firmly attached to the body, and embedded in a tissue that can withstand some thermal and/or mechanical stress.
11. Tattoos and piercings that cannot be removed are at risk of RF heating, and the patient should be properly informed and monitored.

References

1. Baker RR. *Human Navigation and Magnetoreception*. Manchester, England: Manchester University Press; 1989.
2. López-Larrea C, ed. *Sensing in Nature*. New York: Springer; 2012.
3. Roberts DC, Marcelli V, Gillen JS, et al. MRI magnetic field stimulates rotational sensors of the brain. *Curr Biol*. 2011;21:1635–1640.
4. Expert Panel on MR Safety; Kanal E, Barkovich AJ, Bell C, et al. ACR guidance document on MR safe practices: 2013. *J Magn Reson Imaging*. 2013;37:501–530.
5. International Commission on Non-Ionizing Radiation Protection. Guidelines for limiting exposure to time-varying electric and magnetic fields (1 Hz to 100 kHz). *Health Phys*. 2010;99:818–836.
6. Billings BH, Gray DE, American Institute of Physics. *American Institute of Physics Handbook*. New York: McGraw-Hill; 1972.
7. Hattori Y, Fukatsu H, Ishigaki T. Measurement and evaluation of the acoustic noise of a 3 Tesla MR scanner. *Nagoya J Med Sci*. 2007;69:23–28.
8. Ahlbom A, Bergqvist U, Bernhardt JH, et al. Guidelines for limiting exposure to time-varying electric, magnetic, and electromagnetic fields (up to 300 GHz). *Health Phys*. 1998;74:494–521.
9. Dempsey MF, Condon B, Hadley DM. Investigation of the factors responsible for burns during MRI. *J Magn Reson Imaging*. 2001;13:627–631.
10. Bilian X. Chinese experience with intrauterine devices. *Contraception*. 2007;75:S31–S34.
11. Henderson JM, Tkach J, Phillips M, et al. Permanent neurological deficit related to magnetic resonance imaging in a patient with implanted deep brain stimulation electrodes for Parkinson's disease: case report. *Neurosurgery*. 2005;57:E1063.
12. Sommer T, Luechinger R, Barkhausen J, et al. Members of the Working Group on Cardiovascular Imaging, German Roentgen Society (DRG). German Roentgen Society statement on MR imaging of patients with cardiac pacemakers. *Rofo*. 2015;187:777–787.
13. Klucznik RP, Carrier DA, Pyka R, et al. Placement of a ferromagnetic intracerebral aneurysm clip in a magnetic field with a fatal outcome. *Radiology*. 1993;187:855–856.
14. Franiel T, Schmidt S, Klingebiel R. First-degree burns on MRI due to nonferrous tattoos. *AJR Am J Roentgenol*. 2006;187:W556–W556.
15. Tope WD, Shellock FG. Magnetic resonance imaging and permanent cosmetics (tattoos): survey of complications and adverse events. *J Magn Reson Imaging*. 2002;15:180–184.
16. Wagle WA, Smith M. Tattoo-induced skin burn during MR imaging. *AJR Am J Roentgenol*. 2000;174:1795–1795.
17. Vahlensieck M. Tattoo-related cutaneous inflammation (burn grade I) in a mid-field MR scanner. *Eur Radiol*. 2000;10:197.

Note: Page numbers followed by "b", "f", and "t" indicate boxes, figures, and tables, respectively.